Contents

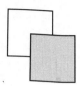

HOUSING AND PUBLIC POLICY
Citizenship, choice and control

edited by
Alex Marsh and **David Mullins**

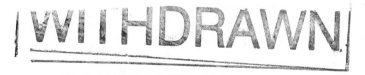

Avril Robarts LRC

OPEN Liverpool John Moores University
Bucki

Open University Press
Celtic Court
22 Ballmoor
Buckingham
MK18 1XW

email: enquiries@openup.co.uk
world wide web: http://www.openup.co.uk

and
325 Chestnut Street
Philadelphia, PA 19106, USA

First published 1998

A catalogue record of this book is available from the British Library

ISBN 0 335 19925 9 (pb)   0 335 19926 7 (hb)

Library of Congress Cataloging-in-Publication Data
Housing and public policy : citizenship, choice, and control / edited
  by Alex Marsh and David Mullins.
      p.   cm.
  Includes bibliographical references and index.
  ISBN 0-335-19926-7. – ISBN 0-335-19926-9 (pbk.)
  1. Housing policy – Great Britain – Citizen participation.
I. Marsh, Alex. II. Mullins, David. 1955–
HD7333.A3H6768 1998
363.5'0941–DC21   98-4871
                                                                        CIP

Typeset by Type Study, Scarborough
Printed in Great Britain by Biddles Ltd, Guildford and King's Lynn

The editors and contributors

Patricia Kennett, Lecturer in Comparative Policy Studies, School for Policy Studies, University of Bristol.

Peter Lee, Lecturer in Urban and Regional Studies, Centre for Urban and Regional Studies, the University of Birmingham.

Alex Marsh, Lecturer in Urban Studies, School for Policy Studies, University of Bristol.

David Mullins, Senior Lecturer in Housing Studies, Centre for Urban and Regional Studies, the University of Birmingham.

Alan Murie, Professor of Urban and Regional Studies, Centre for Urban and Regional Studies, the University of Birmingham.

Pat Niner, Senior Lecturer in Housing Studies, Centre for Urban and Regional Studies, the University of Birmingham.

Moyra Riseborough, Lecturer in Housing Studies, Centre for Urban and Regional Studies, the University of Birmingham.

Bruce Walker, Lecturer in Economics, Institute of Local Government Studies, the University of Birmingham.

Preface

The origins of this book lie in a conversation between one of the editors (Alex Marsh) and Alan Murie around Easter 1996. They reflected upon the fact that during the 1990s the housing research team at the Centre for Urban and Regional Studies (CURS) (in which we include Bruce Walker as 'an honorary CURS person') had undertaken a number of research projects on diverse aspects of contemporary housing policy for a range of statutory and voluntary-sector clients, but the output of those projects was largely confined to policy reports and official publications. This observation started the process of thinking about writing some more reflective and accessible pieces which drew upon this research and set it in the context of wider political and economic debates. Pursuing this line further led to the identification of three concepts – citizenship, choice and control – which recur in contemporary debates and to which the research undertaken at CURS clearly related, but which had not been developed to any significant extent in the housing studies literature.

This book aims to advance understanding of the impact of changing housing policy by presenting an analysis based on the three concepts (citizenship, choice and control) in combination. It explores the extensive changes in housing policy and rapid restructuring of housing provision that have occurred in Britain since 1979 from the perspective of citizenship, choice and control. Existing housing debates utilize these concepts, but this book emphasizes the benefit of combining them and seeks to provide an integrated analysis. It aims to examine critically topics in three broad areas. First, it is concerned with the ways in which policy change, legislative reform and changes in the broader economic environment have affected the experience of citizenship, choice and control among housing consumers. Second, it analyses changes in the locus of control and the extent of choice between housing providers brought about by housing policy in Britain since 1979. Third, it emphasizes the importance of recognizing changes in the balance of power – between producers of housing and between producers and consumers – that have resulted from shifting policy priorities.

The book has very much been a collaborative effort. Discussion and debate among members of the housing team has involved much sharing of ideas and generated some momentum behind the project. This was particularly valuable because in the early stages of the project an institutional move put some geographical distance between us.

Alex Marsh and David Mullins

Acknowledgements

Our first acknowledgement and most heartfelt thanks go to all the contributors. Any collection such as this would be nothing without contributions, but in this case the process of completing the manuscript was much more interactive and collaborative than is often the case. Through their cooperation and responsiveness to the gentlest of pressure (!) they made the job of editing the book almost a pleasure. We would particularly like to thank Alan Murie for his initial enthusiasm for the project, his input into the development of the idea, and his support throughout.

The editors and the contributors are, of course, grateful to all our research clients and to the many thousands of individuals who took part in the research reported in this book.

We would like to thank the Council of Mortgage Lenders for permission to use Table 1 from Freeman, A., Holmans, A. and Whitehead, C. (1996) *Is the UK different? International Comparisons of Tenure Patterns*, London, CML as Table 1.1 and the Scandinavian University Press for the use of Figure 1 from Murie, A. (1993) 'Privatisation and restructuring public involvement in housing provision in Britain', which appeared in *Scandinavian Housing and Planning Research*, 10: 145–57, as Figure 6.2.

Census data and associated products used throughout Chapter 3 are Crown copyright, reproduced with the kind permission of the controller of Her Majesty's Stationery Office. Local base and small area statistics are a subset of the 1991 census, Crown copyright (ESRC/JISC purchase). The samples of anonymized records (SARs) used in Chapter 3 were provided through the Census Microdata Unit of the University of Manchester with the support of ESRC/JISC/DENI.

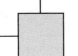

1

Processes of change in housing and public policy

Alex Marsh

Acceptable housing – or the lack of it – is a central feature of all our lives. How much housing costs in relation to household income and the quality and quantity of what we get for our money are issues which keep returning to centre-stage in policy debates. More fundamentally, how the state should intervene in the housing market to assist households who are unable to secure adequate accommodation for themselves is an issue facing governments across the globe. The way in which these issues have been approached varies between societies and within societies at different points in time.

This book seeks to examine the way in which public policy towards housing has developed in Britain and how policy has attempted to resolve the perennial problem of how to ensure that the British population is adequately housed. It focuses primarily upon the last two decades because this period has witnessed rapid policy innovation and the vigorous pursuit of distinctive solutions to old problems. In the course of the discussion we draw on the way in which other societies have addressed the same problems in order to understand better the particularities of the paths pursued in Britain.

Before examining housing and public policy in more detail, we need to clarify the forces influencing the housing system and the nature and origins of public policy. The remainder of this chapter therefore attempts three tasks. First, because current public policy is only one of the influences on the housing system, it locates policy in the context of the other factors influencing the way in which populations are housed. Second, it explores the notion of 'public policy'. It asks where the content of such policy originates and explores the nature of the institutions and processes that put it into effect. Finally, in order to provide some reference points for the subsequent discussion of housing and public policy, it introduces three themes – citizenship, choice and control – which it argues can be seen running through much of the policy debate and development that has occurred during the last two decades.

Sources of change in housing

The roots of change in the housing sphere lie in three broad areas. Demographic and social change directly influence the number of households that require shelter. Economic change determines the type and quantity of housing that is built, the nature of demand from housing consumers and how much they are able to pay for housing. Public policy influences the type, quantity and cost of housing. It is not only policies which are formulated under the label 'housing' that influence housing production and consumption in this way: wider welfare and economic policies also have a substantial impact upon what occurs in the housing sphere. Further, when we are considering the impact of policy upon housing it is essential to recognize the legacy of past policy (Malpass and Murie 1994: 129–32). The impact of present and future policy depends in significant ways on the outcomes of policies pursued in the past.

Demographic and social change

The demographic and social changes that have occurred in industrialized countries over recent decades have been dramatic and it is not unreasonable to expect change to continue. Increasing longevity has accounted for an increase in the number of adults to be housed, while declining fertility rates have reduced the average size of the nuclear family among many social groups within the population. Fundamental social changes include: the erosion of kinship ties; the stresses on, and possible disintegration of, the extended family household; the desire for independence on the part of young adults; the decision to marry being made later or not at all; and increased rates of marital breakdown. These trends have contributed to a decrease in average household size and, in particular, an increase in the number of single-person households. This increase is occurring at both ends of the life cycle. Older households, which tend to be small, are increasingly continuing to live independently rather than with relations or in institutions. Many young people are choosing to leave the parental home and establish separate households as single people or with other unrelated adults rather than on entry to marriage.

All these changes have considerable implications for housing need and demand. A concern with the shortage of housing relative to population played an important role in driving housing policy in the early post-war period (Holmans 1987), while contemporary debates are focusing on how housing and planning policy should cope with the rapid growth in the number of households over the coming decades (DoE 1996).

Economic change

A number of related processes of economic change have a direct bearing upon the housing sphere. These changes are operating at both the macroeconomic level – encompassing a fundamental change in the industrial structure of the British economy – and the microeconomic level in terms of the deregulation of markets. Public policy has played a central role in shaping some of these processes.

The period following the Second World War was marked in Britain and elsewhere by low levels of unemployment, high job security and rising household incomes. The stability and predictability of the economic environment favoured the growth of owner occupation in particular. However, the economic crisis of the 1970s and early 1980s was accompanied by a massive rise in unemployment and a dramatic decline in the level of economic activity in Britain. This decline was particularly sharp in manufacturing industry and was therefore felt particularly badly in regions such as northern England and the West Midlands, and in Scotland and Wales where local economies were founded on such industry.

During the 1980s the nature of the British economy was transformed: there was a major shift in employment from manufacturing to the service sector and some commentators heralded the arrival of a 'post-industrial' society. The changing profile of economic activity had a geographical impact as employment growth shifted towards the south east of England where many firms in financial and professional services are based. Local housing markets in this part of the country overheated badly as a result.

The macroeconomic policies pursued by governments during the 1980s and early 1990s were at least in part the cause of these changes in the economy. Policy during the period was by no means entirely consistent but there was a focus on the use of monetary policy – mainly the manipulation of interest rates – in order to achieve low inflation. High real interest rates are typically accompanied by high exchange rates which make exporting difficult and hence partly account for the decline in manufacturing. The period 1990–2 was particularly notable in this respect because interest rates were kept high in order to maintain the value of sterling within the European exchange rate mechanism. More important from a housing perspective is the fact that relying upon interest rates as the key instrument of economic management has a direct impact upon the housing sphere within the British institutional framework. Much housing finance for owner occupation is provided on a variable-rate basis and thus rises in interest rates for the purposes of economic management feed rapidly through to the housing sector and have a significant impact upon the cost of housing consumption.

At the microeconomic level the 1980s witnessed major changes in the way the British economy functioned. Government believed that in order for Britain to compete in the increasingly competitive and 'global' economy, markets needed to be more flexible. Most attention was directed towards the labour market and a programme of labour market deregulation was prescribed. This was intended to facilitate the creation of a more flexible, pliant and responsive workforce. The deregulation of the labour market opened up the possibility of more insecure employment. This change in the economic structure has led commentators to argue for a corresponding restructuring of housing provision (e.g. Maclennan 1994).

Further aspects of economic change that have a direct bearing upon housing are located within the housing sphere itself. Changes in the structure of the house-building industry and technological and organizational change in the processes of housing construction can impact upon the cost of newly-constructed housing. Similarly, changes in the structure of the housing finance industry and processes of financial innovation which create new financial instruments can change the accessibility of housing finance to potential home buyers and change the costs of housing finance to those who secure a loan. Many of these changes are driven by the competitive pressures generated in the increasingly internationalized macroeconomy.

Public policy

The third broad source of change in housing is public policy. As noted above, such policy may come under the label 'housing' policy or it may, by convention, be located within other policy areas such as social security.

Active government policy towards housing in Britain has its origins in nineteenth-century concerns with public health (Malpass and Murie 1994, ch. 2) and government has influenced the way in which housing markets operate since that time. Such influence is exerted through three forms of policy intervention: direct, regulatory, or fiscal. Direct intervention is most obvious in the case of the construction of property to let at subsidized rents by government or its agents. Regulatory intervention occurs when governments decide that 'unfettered' market forces lead to undesirable consequences and intervene to curb the way markets operate by, for example, regulating the level of rents that can be set or determining minimum acceptability standards for dwellings for human habitation. Fiscal intervention alters the way in which housing consumption or production is financed by providing tax expenditures and/or subsidies (see Hills 1991 for a detailed discussion). Because of public spending and government department conventions, fiscal interventions are perhaps the most difficult to locate clearly under the heading 'housing'. A prime example in Britain is the personal subsidies paid to low-income tenants through the housing benefit system: throughout the 1980s housing benefit was seen as the main component of government policy towards housing and yet the housing benefit system is the responsibility of the Department of Social Security.

Government involvement in the housing market attempts to influence the amount of property of particular types that is produced and/or consumed, the cost of accommodation, or its quality. Many types of intervention are directed primarily at one of these targets but also have implications for the other two. Some, such as building regulations or minimum standards, are intended principally to influence the quality of accommodation but also have direct effects upon the quantity and cost of accommodation available. Others, such as rent control, address the cost of accommodation but arguably affect both the amount of rented accommodation and its quality indirectly. All three forms of involvement – direct, regulatory and fiscal – are present in the current British housing system, but the emphasis on particular types of intervention has waxed and waned over time for a variety of reasons.

Tracing the contours of change in housing

These three broad influences upon the housing sphere (i.e. demographic and social change, economic change and public policy) do not act entirely independently of each other: they are – to a greater or lesser extent – interrelated. So, for example, economic change which impacts upon incomes and employment can affect the rate at which independent households are formed. If economic circumstances worsen, unemployment rises and incomes stagnate, then young people may postpone forming independent households either through choice or necessity. In contrast, public policy which attempts to increase the number of accessible, affordable dwellings available may lead to an increase in the rate of household formation because the costs of setting up an independent household are lower.

These examples suggest that the causal processes involved here do not run exclusively from external factors – economic, demographic and policy changes – to effects and outcomes in the housing sphere. Rather, housing and wider economic, social and political processes stand in a subtle, complex two-way relationship. The possibility of a relationship running from housing to demographic change can be debated (Bramley and Watkins 1995; Holmans 1995), but the tracing of these lines of influence and causal relationships is a project which has yet to be fully realized.

A key point in understanding change in housing is that in most industrialized countries the majority of housing is provided in the private sector and allocated through market mechanisms, either in the owner occupied or privately rented sector. Table 1.1 shows the tenure structure of 12 industrialized countries. The way in which some countries define tenures differs somewhat and thus the picture presented in the table is best taken as a broad impression of the differences. Nonetheless, the table indicates that only in The Netherlands does social rented housing come close to accounting for the accommodation of half of all households. Market provision is clearly of central importance in most countries.

Because market provision dominates, economic and wider social processes play a fundamental role in determining the way in which housing is produced and consumed. On the face of it this suggests that policy is not the predominant influence shaping change. Indeed authors such as Ball *et al.* (1988) have used comparative research to demonstrate that much of the pressure for change that occurs in systems of housing provision is driven by wider economic forces. This means that, while there is room to manoeuvre in terms of domestic policy agendas and there remains considerable variation in the structure and operation of the housing systems in different countries (as illustrated by Table 1.1), governments tend to face similar issues and have tended to follow a limited range of options, despite political differences.

It is important here to recognize that housing produced and consumed in the private sector is not immune from government influence. It is a mistake to consider the 'private sector' as somehow separate from, and outside the influence of, government. Through fiscal and regulatory intervention, government policy plays a key role in shaping the way in which markets function. That the private sector, in Britain at least, is treated as entirely separable and separate from the public sector is as much a rhetorical stance as reality. Further, overt and direct intervention in the market is clearly a policy, but, equally, consciously failing to act or intervene when one has the

Table 1.1   Proportion of households by tenure, in selected industrialized countries (%)

Country	Owner occupation	Social renting	Private renting	Other private	Total	Date of source
USA	64.2	2.0	33.8	–	100.0	1991
UK	67.6	22.6	9.8	–	100.0	1994–5
Sweden	55.0	22.0	23.0	–	100.0	1991
Spain	78.4	1.1	13.8	6.6	99.9	1989
The Netherlands	47.3	40.2	11.2	1.3	100.0	1993–4
Japan	59.8	7.0	26.4	5.1	98.3	1993
Ireland	76.8	13.9	7.7	1.6	100.0	1987
Germany	38.0	15.0	43.0	4.0	100.0	1987
France	54.4	14.5	25.1	6.0	100.0	1990
Finland	78.4	10.7	9.5	1.4	100.0	1992
Canada	62.7	5.6	31.7	–	100.0	1991
Australia	70.0	6.0	19.0	5.0	100.0	1994
Average	**62.7**	**13.6**	**20.9**	**2.6**	**99.9**	

Source: Freeman *et al.* 1996, Table 1.

capacity to do so is *also* a policy. During the early 1990s there were periods of turmoil in the British housing market during which commentators made strident demands for the government to intervene, but the government followed a policy of non-intervention.

Accepting that private markets play the key role in providing housing, it is nonetheless true that in many industrialized countries a substantial minority of households rely upon housing provided by organizations operating entirely outside the private sector. Further, non-market housing has often acted as a safety net for those unable to secure accommodation privately and thus much housing-related policy change has a disproportionate impact upon the most vulnerable in society. The fact that most direct intervention through housing policy is focused upon particular groups in society means that housing policy differs from other components of the post-war British welfare state, such as the health service or education, which aspired to cater for the needs of all. Because most people do not feel that they rely on the state for housing, housing policy is arguably on a different, perhaps less secure, footing than services such as health and education which in Britain are almost universally popular. This suggests that there is more likely to be debate and disagreement regarding the appropriate role and extent of housing policy.

The policy process and the state

Having located public policy as one of the key influences upon housing, this section examines the nature of public policy in more detail.

Study of the policy process has developed rapidly over the last two decades. During this period a number of competing interpretations of policy making and the policy process have emerged and fundamental questions regarding the aims of policy have been raised. In this section we briefly discuss some of the key issues that have been identified: a more detailed discussion can be found in Ham and Hill (1993) and Hill (1993) brings together many of the important contributions to the literature.

A simple account of the policy process would start by drawing a distinction between three broad stages of the process: the policy decision (or 'policy making'), policy implementation and policy outcomes. The decision stage of the process encompasses – as well as the policy decision itself – the formulation of policy and the evaluation of policy options before a decision is taken. Once a decision has been taken the implementation stage begins. During implementation the various provisions of the policy are implemented either by the policy-making body or by other individuals or organizations empowered to do so. Finally, after an appropriate period of time, the outcomes of the policy will become evident: they can be evaluated and, if appropriate, form the input into future policy.

This simple, linear account of the process requires close scrutiny. We start by focusing upon the idea of a policy decision and consider how we might go about identifying a policy.

How can policy be identified?

What is meant when one refers to 'a policy'? A situation in which a group of people sit down together and formally decide on a course of action might be considered a clear-cut case of a policy being made. Similarly, the passage of a piece of legislation through Parliament might be considered to indicate that a policy decision had been taken and a policy determined. Subsequent decisions or pieces of legislation would then be seen as representing changes in policy, however subtle. Yet, this decisional approach is a rather static and episodic view of policy making. When we attempt to situate a particular decision within its context we may discover that it is in fact one of a number of decisions or pieces of legislation which appear to be directed at a broader objective. If this is the case, then it may be better to conceive of each decision as simply a step in the working-out of a more fundamental *policy stance* (Friend *et al.* 1974). If particular decisions or legislative acts are better viewed as part of such a stance, then analysing them outside their context could be seriously misleading. However, determining whether a particular decision is consonant with an existing policy stance or represents a shift in stance may present considerable analytical difficulties. An extension of the notion of policy stance is the view that particular decision points should not be given undue prominence because policy is in fact in a continuous state of transformation in the light of evolving circumstances and fluctuating pressures upon policy makers. If such a view of policy is accepted then to talk of distinct points at which decisions or policy changes occur ceases to be meaningful.

A second difficulty raised by basing analysis upon decision-making episodes or overt policies is that these may not represent accurately the views of the policy-making body. There are a number of ways in which overt policy and the policy maker's views may part company. Once it is conceded that policy as expressed does not accurately reflect the true position of the policy maker it renders the analysis and interpretation of policy a considerably more subtle and demanding task.

The justification a policy maker offers for a particular policy may primarily be a rhetorical device designed to persuade the relevant audience of the appropriateness of the policy. Underlying the policy may be an entirely different agenda and the policy maker could hold the expectation that the policy will yield outcomes substantially different to those identified in the proffered justification. Determining whether the rhetoric attached to a particular policy disguises the intention is complicated by the fact that because of the nature of the policy process itself (discussed below) the outcomes of a policy may differ from those identified as being likely when the policy is first implemented. The key to identifying whether policy makers are using a rhetorical smokescreen to cover their true purposes is *intention*, which inevitably makes analysis more difficult because the evidence needed to bring such intentions into focus is likely to be less easily accessible.

A related argument, presented by Edelman (1971), suggests that some policies have a *symbolic* purpose and their objective is to demonstrate that action is being taken, rather than that the issue or problem is being addressed seriously. Symbolic policies may either be demonstrably inappropriate or ineffective from the start or a potentially effective policy may be rendered little more than symbolic by being starved of sufficient resources. Bramley (1993: 132) notes that symbolic policy 'seems rather commonplace, but perhaps this depends how stringently one defines it'. Ham and Hill (1993: 15) observe that 'This suggests . . . that students of the policy process should be wary of taking policy-makers too seriously. Policies may be intended to improve social conditions, but that should be part of the object of enquiry rather than an assumption of research'. The key to identifying symbolic policies is again to identify the intention behind them.

The idea that policy may not represent the true views of the policy makers receives further support by drawing on theories of power (see Ham and Hill 1993, ch. 4) and in particular the concept of 'non-decision making' which has its origins in the work of Bachrach and Baratz (1962). Taking a decisional approach to the analysis of policy assumes that all issues of importance are brought out into the open, discussed and decided upon. The notion of non-decision making suggests that this is a superficial reading of the policy process. Three mechanisms through which non-decision making may work have been suggested (Clegg 1989: 77–8). First, powerful actors may fail to acknowledge the demands or views expressed by the relatively powerless. Such views may simply be ignored entirely or be ruled inadmissible because, for example, they are not presented in an 'officially' recognized and accepted form. A second means by which non-decision making may occur is through the 'rule of anticipated reaction' identified by Friedrich (1937): if person B anticipates that relatively powerful person A will oppose a view or opinion that person B wishes to express then person B may decide not to raise the issue. The third way in which non-decision making may occur is through the 'mobilization of bias': this moves the discussion a stage further by suggesting that powerful actors may exert such control over the operation of the political system – including the values, beliefs and opinions of less powerful actors – that certain issues not congenial to the powerful are never raised nor demands ever made.

If powerful actors are able to ensure that certain issues are kept off the agenda then one is presented with a situation in which power is being exercised but where the principal evidence for this is that nothing happens. Clearly the identification of a non-decision-making process presents formidable analytical problems, although some studies (see Newton 1975) seem to offer support for the idea (see Clegg 1989 for an extended discussion).

These concerns all signal the need for a sensitive interpretation of policy formulation and policy decisions. The discussion so far has accepted the assumption that once a course of action has been decided upon then the implementation of that course of action is unproblematic. This simple view of policy and implementation also demands further scrutiny.

Implementing policy

Since Pressman and Wildavsky (1973) highlighted implementation as an important element in understanding the policy process a large literature on implementation issues has developed. There has also been detailed work within housing studies which explicitly draws on an implementation perspective (Malpass and Means 1993).

A distinction can be drawn between top-down and bottom-up models of implementation. The top-down model starts from a clear separation between the policy-making and implementation stages of the policy process and views policy making as an activity undertaken by those 'at the top'. Policy is then handed down for those 'lower down' to implement. Those who adopt such a model of the policy process are frequently concerned with diagnosing why particular policies fail to deliver the outcomes promised and under what conditions policy can be successfully implemented. A range of preconditions for success have been identified through reflection upon policies that have not been successfully implemented. According to Ham and Hill (1993: 101) the most important are that:

- the policy to be implemented should be as clear and unambiguous as possible;
- the implementation structure is as simple as possible, keeping links in the chain to a minimum;
- outside interference should be prevented;
- policy makers must have control over the implementing actors.

Pressman and Wildavsky (1973) document the way in which complex implementation structures involving several organizations or departments of government can lead to a serious 'implementation deficit'. Unless each organization involved executes its part in implementing the policy with complete success the individually small failures will result in a large deficit overall.

The bottom-up model of implementation offers a fundamentally different understanding of the policy process. Authors writing from this perspective deny that a clear distinction can always, if ever, be made between the policy-making and implementation stages of the process, even in situations where different organizations appear to have responsibility for the different stages. In contrast, the bottom-up model sees most policies as the product of negotiation and compromise which may continue throughout the policy process. Barrett and Hill (1984: 222) argue that many policies represent compromises at a number of levels: they are compromises between conflicting values; they often involve compromise with key interests within the implementation structure; and they often involve compromise with key interests upon which implementation will have an impact. Barrett and Hill go on to observe that when policies are framed it is often without attention being given to the way in which underlying forces, particularly economic forces, will undermine them.

There are a number of reasons why policy makers may wish to leave key decisions to what might otherwise be characterized as the implementation stage. Some of these reasons are a recognition of the complexity of the process of delivering policy so, for example, it may be thought that decisions are better made by implementors because they will have all the facts available to them or because they are better equipped than anyone else as a result of specific training or competence (Ham and Hill 1993: 107). Alternatively, Ham and Hill suggest it might be felt that it is politically inexpedient to try to resolve conflicts at the policy-making stage (p. 108). Fimister and Hill (1993) examine central government's approach to social security, housing and community care during the 1980s. They demonstrate that key decisions about how policies were to work in practice were avoided at the legislative stage and those organizations charged with implementing the policies had to attempt to resolve fundamental contradictions. Allowing such ambiguity to persist into implementation may serve the purposes of policy makers, particularly if a policy is primarily symbolic.

There are thus reasons why policy makers might wish to leave key decisions to those implementing a policy, but it is also the case that some divergence between policy-makers' intentions and policy outcomes will occur because individuals implementing the policy have some measure of discretion. Implementors may use their discretion disruptively (Lipsky 1980) but they may, working within the framework laid down by policy makers, arrive at interpretations and actions entirely at odds with the original intentions of policy makers simply because no policy can be so closely specified that implementors need do no more than follow the rules in all circumstances. If implementation relies upon organizations who are independent of the policy-making body then the scope for policy outcomes which diverge from the policy objectives increases.

This is particularly germane in the case of housing policy because central government in Britain has never adopted a strategy of direct involvement in the housing market. It has relied upon a range of local-level organizations – principally local authorities but more recently also housing associations – to implement policies formulated centrally. Where the centrally formulated policies take the form of guidelines or regulations which give a degree of discretion to local organizations we would expect to observe that the outcomes of a particular policy would vary between localities as local organizations decide for themselves on how best to put central government's wishes into practice. The scope for variation between areas is enhanced by the fact that local authorities are mostly party-political controlled organizations who have local priorities and may well be under the control of political parties in opposition nationally. At least part of the story of the policy towards housing since 1980 is the playing out of this tension.

Although both top-down and bottom-up models have their advocates, it can be argued that neither provides an adequate description of the policy process on its own. Even those who have been centrally involved in the debate have conceded that the distinction is not always useful, but that the key point to come out of the debate regarding the need to take account of the 'downstream' elements in policy processes is valid (Hill 1997). There have been attempts at synthesis (Sabatier 1986) which seek to bridge the gap between the two models and which may be taken further in future. Also, empirical evidence suggests that the models may be appropriate to understanding the policy process at different times, in different places or at different levels of government.

Organizational change in the policy process

The organizations involved in the policy process in an area such as housing are by no means fixed over time. One key feature of the policy process is what has been termed 'meta-policy' (Dror 1986) which is directed towards restructuring the way in which policy processes function to deliver particular outcomes, rather than at a particular set of outcomes. Such meta-policy is thus principally about changing the means by which policy is delivered rather than the ends of policy itself (Ham and Hill 1993: 106). This may entail changing the nature and extent of the involvement of existing organizations in the policy process or encouraging the participation of other organizations. Yet, changing the structures through which policy is delivered will not only change the means but may also result in some modification of policy outcomes. This is particularly true where meta-policy change results in a new set of independent organizations becoming involved in the policy process and the objectives of such organizations are not fully congruent with those of existing organizations.

Between 1980 and its defeat at the 1997 general election the Conservative government exercised its power to alter 'the rules of the game' in this way extensively. In particular it presided over (see, for example, Gray 1994):

- A reduction in the reliance upon local authorities for provision of services.
- An explosion in the number of quangos run by government appointees.

- Extensive privatization of utilities and other services.
- Restructuring of the National Health Service with the abolition of district health authorities and the transfer of power both upwards to regional health authorities and downwards to GPs and hospital trusts.
- The creation of executive agencies such as the Benefits Agency and the Highways Agency within central government departments.
- A complete restructuring of the way in which the subnational arm of government is administered through the creation of government offices for the regions.

The incoming Labour government placed many of these changes under review: at least some of the 'rules of the game' are likely to alter once again. The important point for our discussion is that all these changes make the analysis of the policy process more complex but, perhaps more fundamentally, they make identification of what should be counted as within the ambit of 'public policy' more difficult.

What determines policy content?

Having examined the way in which the policy process operates it is necessary to briefly consider what influences the nature and content of policy itself. One reading of public policy formation and change might see policy as the product of clashing political ideologies. Such a reading would focus upon the debate in various policy-making fora and on policy as the outcome of such debate: little attempt would be made to locate the political debate within its wider social context. However, a range of approaches to understanding policy in liberal democracies go beyond a focus on political ideology and attempt to understand the influences which lie behind particular policy positions. The most frequently discussed perspectives include pluralism, neo-pluralism, elitism and Marxism (see Dunleavy and O'Leary 1987; Ham and Hill 1993; Gray 1994 for detailed accounts).

These approaches adopt very different starting points. Pluralism, for example, sees policy making as a competition between social groups to get their views onto the agenda, with no single group having a monopoly of influence. The focus is thus on the agency of particular groups. This sort of approach has been criticized by Marxist-inspired writers who seek to take account of the way in which agency is structured by broader influences. It is important to recognize that we are studying policy making in capitalist societies and the overriding need to assure capital accumulation places demands on the nature of policy. Ginsburg (1992: 14), for example, argues in the context of an analysis of welfare states that analysis needs to consider the relative contributions of both agency and structure because if there is an exclusive focus on agency 'the undertowing effect of the deep structures of economic development or ideological power is inevitably missing'.

Although these approaches start from different positions it can be argued that, as each is critically appraised and modified, they have converged. Neo-pluralists conceive of the policy process as an unequally weighted affair, with many groups in society wishing to influence public policy but only a few in a position to make a real impact (Gray 1994: 98). Neo-pluralists see some groups as enjoying a close relationship with public policy makers – often because they control resources, such as expertise, that the government needs – while other groups find themselves outside the usual networks of consultation which inform policy making and hence have a much harder time getting their views heard and consequently have a more marginal effect upon policy.

Marxist approaches, on the other hand, have broken with strong economic determinism and allowed that the state has some autonomy and that capital is differentiated and so may place conflicting demands upon policy. As Ham and Hill (1993: 38) observe, if you allow that the state is not heavily constrained by capital and that capital is differentiated into a number of groups that have to compete to see their interests furthered by policy, then the Marxist approach starts to lose its distinctiveness and to come close to a neo-pluralist perspective.

Approaches which might be loosely termed neo-pluralist are therefore particularly central to current thinking. This modified concept of the policy process has been captured more formally in the concept of the *policy community* (Rhodes 1988). Within each policy area there is a policy community which encompasses the key participants in the policy process from both inside and outside government. The policy community for other policy areas will have a different composition and thus the overall process of public policy making is relatively fragmented. Members of a policy community – the 'insiders' – have privileged access to the policy process, while those who find themselves outside the community find it considerably more difficult to influence policy. This difficulty in influencing policy will increase the more central a policy is to the concerns of a particular policy community (Gray 1994: 100).

Analysing housing policy

In order to guide the examination of public policy towards housing, presented in the chapters that follow, this section identifies three themes which have recurred throughout the post-war period and which have particular salience in the debates of the 1980s and 1990s. The first theme is *citizenship*, which addresses the issue of what individuals are entitled to by virtue of being citizens of a particular society. What it means to be a citizen at the end of the twentieth century is one of the most wide ranging and fundamental debates that has been occurring among both political and academic commentators over the last decade. The second theme, which has been prominent in policy debate and development, is the issue of *choice*. As we approach the millennium as part of an increasingly consumption-oriented society many would see, or would like us to see, the defining characteristic of individual agency as the ability to exercise choice. Yet, the idea of choice encompasses more than simply consumerism. The importance of *control* – where the locus of control over a particular resource or activity lies – has already been alluded to in our discussion of central-local relations. However, there are a number of different aspects of policy change which can be illuminated through an examination of the issue of control and thus this forms the third theme used to guide the discussion.

Citizenship

The notion of citizenship stretches back to the ancient Greeks, but was first articulated in respect of developments in industrial societies in the late nineteenth century. It has subsequently re-emerged in policy and academic debates in Britain on two occasions: during the period immediately following the Second World War and over the last decade. The first two periods of concern with citizenship were associated with the implementation of public policies which increased the scope of welfare provision in industrial societies. The current interest in citizenship also accompanies changes in the scope of welfare, although these changes now take the form of the retreat of the state and reductions in provision.

What, then, is meant by 'citizenship'? The original Greek formulation was principally concerned with political rights and participatory democracy: which members of society – which citizens – were allowed to participate in debates about the government of their city-state? Certain groups in society, notably women and slaves, were excluded from the forum where policy was made because they were not considered full citizens. This conception of citizenship can be linked to Hirschman's (1970) idea that one mechanism for registering views is through 'voice'. That is, individuals and groups of citizens can voice their dissatisfaction by taking political action through democratic processes.

More recent debates concerning citizenship have explored the concept in more depth. Hill (1994: 9) observes that '... citizenship is both status, derived from membership of a collectivity..., and a system of rights and obligations that incorporates justice, equality and community'. Thus, one is a citizen of a particular collectivity, which is now typically viewed as the nation state. A key concern is therefore who should be considered a citizen of a particular society, and as such have particular entitlements, and who should not. In the contemporary context of extensive mobility on the one hand and fiscal constraint on the other, this means that the issue of migration between states – and which residents are to be considered citizens – is of fundamental concern (see Garcia 1996). The second element of Hill's definition of citizenship as a system of rights and obligations goes to the heart of much of the academic debate in the post-war period. The particular features she identifies – justice, equality and community – have been at issue since the advent of the modern welfare state and Marshall's (1950) seminal contribution.

Marshall attempted to account for the development of citizenship rights since the eighteenth century. He identified three components to citizenship rights: civil, political and social. Civil rights are those necessary for individual freedom. These encompass liberty of the person, freedom of speech, thought and faith, the right to own property and to conclude valid contracts, and the right to justice (Marshall 1963: 74). Political rights are the rights to participate in an exercise of political power, as a member of a body invested with political authority or as an elector of such a body (p. 74). The social element of citizenship meant 'the whole range from the right to a modicum of economic welfare and security to the right to share to the full in the social heritage and to live the life of a civilized being according to the standards prevailing in the society. The institutions most closely connected with it are the educational system and the social services' (p. 74). Marshall provided an account of the development of citizenship rights by arguing that the development of civil rights was associated with the eighteenth century, the development of political rights with the nineteenth century and the development of social rights with the current century. The development and elaboration of citizenship rights over time is portrayed as a result of broader social and economic forces such as industrialization, the decline of the peasantry, the rise of working-class movements, economic prosperity, and the stability of the international economic order (Barbalet 1988). In Marshall's account there is the clear suggestion that the establishment of civil and especially political rights facilitated the later development of social rights. Other factors such as warfare (Giddens 1982; Turner 1986) and the rise of egalitarian ideologies (Turner 1986) have been suggested as playing an important role in the expansion of citizenship rights, but their role has been questioned (Barbalet 1988).

Hill (1994) emphasizes the priority given to the social rights of citizens within the Marshallian approach since it is these rights which ensure the prerequisites needed for citizens to fulfil their role as autonomous individuals. The assumption is that welfare services are an essential part of building citizenship and the entitlements of citizens underpinned the welfare reforms of the 1940s through to the 1960s. Much of the literature on citizenship has taken the role of the welfare state in ensuring social rights as its focus. Perhaps the most sophisticated analysis of welfare states in this vein is Esping-Andersen's (1990) work on the extent to which particular industrialized societies are 'de-commodified': to what extent, because of the welfare state's guarantee of social rights, has citizens' access to resources been disconnected from reliance upon selling the commodity 'labour power' in the labour market?

Hill (1994: 9–10) goes on to identify two further distinctions central to an understanding of citizenship in the Marshallian tradition. First, a distinction can be drawn between the formal and substantive rights possessed by citizens. Thus although citizens may formally possess rights they may lack the means, be they financial, educational or whatever, to exercise those rights. Second, a distinction between procedural rights and actual outcomes: procedure may be open and fair but this is a separate issue from whether individuals are entitled to a particular outcome.

Marshall's account of the growth of citizenship has proved extremely influential and the citizenship debate of the 1980s and 1990s has to some extent been conducted as a dialogue with Marshall (e.g. Bulmer and Rees 1996). A number of aspects of Marshall's account have been subject to searching criticism (see, for example, Barbalet 1988; Turner and Hamilton 1994a, 1994b; Bulmer and Rees 1996). Here we note three of the most relevant.

First, Marshall's account may be a valid description of the development of rights in England, but there is a considerable body of evidence documenting the way in which developments in other countries took a very different path (see, for example, Brubaker 1992; Kennett 1995; Garcia 1996). Marshall's periodization cannot therefore easily be generalized.

Second, the discussions of citizenship by Marshall and many other writers have a tendency to be blind to the differential citizenship of groups within the population, particularly women and those from minority ethnic groups (see Lister 1993). A related issue which citizenship debates often fail to address is the citizenship status of groups such as children and those who are mentally impaired. Citizenship rights, such as the right to an adequate income, have often been formulated with the interests of men needing to earn a 'family wage' in mind. The need of both single and married women for access to an adequate independent income, the unevenness of caring responsibilities within the home and the relative 'time poverty' of working women in particular are not issues that have featured prominently in discussions of citizenship. The invisibility of these divisions has significant implications for the ability of citizenship as a concept to address debates concerning access to housing. Access to housing is one aspect of the housing system which is intimately linked to some of the very divisions which citizenship has often tended to neglect. A focus upon housing issues coupled with a sensitivity towards the possibility of differential citizenship provides an opportunity for work within housing studies which can make a valuable contribution to advancing broader citizenship debates.

Third, Marshall has been criticized for failing to emphasize the social struggle that underpins the definition and redefinition of citizenship rights (see, for example, Giddens 1982; Turner 1986). Marshall notes that citizenship rights – particularly the development of social rights – principally benefit the working classes and therefore that differences between social classes are eroded. But he does not explore in detail the possibility that the expansion of rights will be resisted by those in other social classes.

More recent authors draw attention to the role played by the struggle of the working class and the reaction to this struggle. Hirschman (1991) argued that it is entirely expected that any change in social rights that favours the working class will be met by a sustained reaction from other groups in society – any change in the rights attached to citizenship is likely to be countered by a 'rhetoric of reaction'. He identifies three key 'reactionary' arguments: the perversity thesis, the futility thesis, and the jeopardy thesis (p. 7). The perversity thesis is that any action to improve some feature of the political, social or economic order is likely to exacerbate the condition that it is trying to remedy. According to the futility thesis any attempt to transform society will fail because there is no way it can make any difference, while the jeopardy thesis views the cost of some proposed change or reform as too high because it would endanger some previous highly-valued accomplishment.

Barbalet (1988) argues further that focusing on struggle alone is not sufficient. Social struggle will only achieve its aim once the object of struggle is accepted within a particular society as legitimate. It is therefore necessary to examine the contexts in which struggle occurs: why do some struggles succeed, with the demands made for increased rights accepted, and why do others fail to secure the changes in rights desired? It may be that claims to rights only succeed when supported by a coalition of social classes which provides the necessary support for change (Esping-Andersen 1990). It is only if the ruling classes see it as in their interests to grant extensions of rights that such rights are likely to achieve acceptance; the alternative may be repression of the demands of the relatively powerless (Barbalet 1988: 36).

We can refine our understanding of the legitimacy of citizenship rights by distinguishing between moral and legal rights. A person could claim to possess moral rights – including the right to be considered a citizen – by virtue of their residence within a society, without such a right being enshrined in law. It is this disjunction which forms the basis for the struggle to gain legal recognition for particular rights. When discussing the rights of citizens we need to distinguish between rights claimed as moral rights (perhaps as part of policy debate) and those which are recognized as legal rights. In terms of thinking about changes in the rights attached to citizenship status we can hypothesize that a right – such as the right to affordable and secure accommodation – has to be widely recognized as a legitimate moral right within a particular society before it is likely to become law. Whether moral rights are, in themselves, inviolate or the product of the political and social philosophy of a particular social group at a particular point in time is a separate question. Freeden (1991), for example, adopts the position that moral rights are conventional and are therefore open to redefinition or downgrading in importance relative to other rights.

As we have witnessed over the last fifteen years in the British context, any perspective on rights that sees increasing citizenship rights as an inevitable accompaniment to broader social and economic progress is an inadequate tool for analysing policy development. Legal rights can be removed as well as augmented. As Rees (1995: 316) observes: 'The truth is that given an adequate Parliamentary majority, rights may be enacted, added to, abridged or abrogated with relative ease in the United Kingdom. It makes little difference whether they are classed as civil, political or social'. Thus the question of how rights can be removed by policy makers without sustained opposition is of vital importance in analysing contemporary developments. Does the removal of a legal right indicate that it has ceased to be viewed as a legitimate moral right or can some constellation of economic and social factors allow governments to remove a legitimate moral right with impunity?

Marshall (1950) does not examine the interaction between the three different types of citizenship right at length, but notes the way in which civil and social rights can conflict and gives some pointers towards explaining why social rights are therefore vulnerable. Social rights, in terms of guaranteed welfare provision funded through taxation, tend to be given emphasis in times of economic boom. In times of economic recession and fiscal constraint, civil rights – associated with market provision and freedom – are emphasized and they have the potential to undermine established social rights. Civil rights give each person 'the power to engage as an independent unit in the economic struggle' and because of this they make 'it possible to deny [a person] social protection on the ground that [he/she] is equipped with the means to protect [him- or herself]' (Marshall 1950: 33–4). As Barbalet (1988: 21) comments, '[recent] developments in advanced capitalist societies have given these notions a new voice'.

Much of the discourse on citizenship in recent years has been concerned with the content of citizenship rights and obligations, and is thus very much in the realms of political philosophy. Recent debates have shifted the focus onto the obligations of citizens rather than their rights. The conservative right have championed the idea of the active citizen with the focus being on the contribution that the citizen can make to their society. The concept of the 'active citizen' has been picked up by the centre-left and given a slightly different gloss. The most recent development is the emergence of communitarian thinking as an underpinning for policy (e.g. Etzioni 1993; Demaine 1996; Driver and Martell 1997). It is not necessary here to engage directly with these positions, but it is useful to note that when the terms 'citizenship' and 'citizen' are used in contemporary political discourse they may be referring to very different concepts: if we wish to engage in, or analyse, such debates it is vital to do so with the knowledge that the basic concepts require examination.

In order to employ the concept of citizenship analytically we need to distinguish between citizenship as a theoretical concept and a particular definition of citizenship as a political philosophy. It is not, however, always possible to disentangle these two uses of the term citizenship. In his recent work Turner (1993: 3) argues that a general theory of citizenship should move away from viewing citizenship as rights and obligations and towards viewing it as a set of practices. The idea of 'practices' offers the possibility of a more dynamic account of citizenship rights which change historically. Turner argues that such a theory would be concerned with four issues:

1 The *content of citizenship*: the exact nature of the social rights and obligations of citizens.
2 The *type of such obligations and rights*: whether citizenship is active or passive.
3 The *social forces* which produce such practices.
4 The *social arrangements* whereby such benefits are distributed to different sectors of society.

On the basis of the framework proposed by Turner we can argue that a general theory of citizenship would start from the assumption that in all societies citizens have rights by virtue of their status as citizens, but that the precise composition of those rights are a product of negotiation and struggle between social groups. As particular rights become accepted as legitimate they may become incorporated into the legal rights of citizenship. But as the social and economic context changes and policy debates continue legitimate moral rights and/or legal rights may be redefined. This redefinition may lead to either the expansion or contraction of the rights attached to citizenship status. At a less fundamental level, rights may remain unchanged but the way in which particular legal rights are ensured or the entitlements they establish are distributed may change.

Such a general theory is thus primarily an analytical tool which does not in itself seek to argue that the expansion of legal rights for a particular group represents an unambiguous 'social advance', although it would certainly view such a change as indicating that the interests of one or more groups in society have been advanced relative to the interests of others. Equally the removal of legal rights would be considered as an alteration to the rights attached to citizenship and this change would be disadvantageous to particular groups, but it would not be viewed as an unambiguous backward step. To argue that changes in rights represent either social advance or retreat would require an explicit engagement with political philosophy or ideology.

Choice

Embodied in the Marshallian notion of citizenship is the idea of autonomy, the ability to choose. In the context of housing, the ability to exercise choice as an attribute of citizenship has received increasing emphasis. However, choice has featured in policy discussion beyond debates couched in terms of citizenship. The rise of thinking influenced by behavioural models drawn from economics has led to choice being conceived principally in consumerist terms. Individuals are viewed as consumers who make rational decisions regarding their consumption of public goods and services. If they do not like what they get from a particular supplier then they can exercise what Hirschman (1970) termed the 'exit' option: they can simply take their business elsewhere. If many consumers decide to exit from a particular supplier then it sends a signal to the supplier that their good or service is not meeting with consumers' approval. This acts as a spur to remedy the problem: failure to act may lead to terminal decline as they are competed out of business.

The government's promotion of the extensive use of performance indicators in many areas of the public sector is partly aimed at giving consumers the information necessary for them to make choices over whether their current supplier is providing an acceptable service. The creation of the *Citizen's Charter* and its offspring in the early 1990s was also based on a consumerist view of public service users who need to be informed about acceptable service standards and the right to redress in individual cases where service falls short (see Oliver and Heater 1994). Although they focus on users as consumers, both charters and performance indicators can also be seen as oriented towards the exercise of 'voice' by dissatisfied users: the demands of individual consumers for better services will lead to service improvement, thus obviating the need to exit.

Choice is not restricted to consumers, however, and with the rise of the notion that local authorities should act as enablers rather than direct providers we can see that choice plays a role in the provision of services also. Whereas in the 1970s local authorities became large bureaucratic organizations responsible for both the planning and provision of services within a locality, the enabling authority as conceived by the 'new right' is a strategic authority which decides on the nature and level of services required and then contracts with independent organizations to provide the services. At the contracting stage the local authority is offered a choice of alternative suppliers. Choice thus became intimately associated with competitive processes as the Conservative governments of the late 1980s and early 1990s created quasi-market mechanisms in welfare services. The appropriateness of the quasi-market approach to service provision has been explored at length by a number of authors (see Le Grand and Bartlett 1993) and is being reviewed by the Labour government.

A number of concerns have been raised about equating choice with consumerism and market mechanisms. The issue of effective demand is of fundamental importance: it is only those with adequate resources that are in a position to choose, and such people are not necessarily those in need. In quasi-market situations such as education the government ties resources to individuals' choices, and there is concern that quasi-markets are replicating the undesirable aspects of market mechanisms by delivering good quality services to some but denying access to adequate services to others. Further it has been argued that in many public sector services there are no alternative suppliers available and thus consumers are unable to exercise the exit option – which is fundamentally important if systems based on consumer choice are to deliver service improvements – even if they wanted to. A similar concern is that simple economic models of consumer choice cannot be applied in particular contexts, not because market mechanisms are by definition inappropriate, but because a range of preconditions for choice are not present (see, for example, Walker and Marsh 1998). Finally, when thinking about the provision of welfare services it can be argued that the government has impoverished the notion of local government by focusing on issues of choice in service provision and by viewing citizens primarily as consumers (Burns *et al.* 1994).

Choice can, however, be seen in terms other than those of market exchange and alternative views of choice have dominated political debate during particular periods. First, it is important to distinguish between choice at the point of exchange and choice in use. The focus of choice in housing (quasi-)market participation is choice of landlord or tenure: it is about choice at particular points in the housing consumption cycle. But when we distinguish between a dwelling as a physical structure or asset and a dwelling as a home then there are a whole range of choices not associated with relocation/tenure choice that are de-emphasized by conceiving of choice in market terms. As was explored in the 'choice in welfare' debate of the 1970s, with carefully designed systems it is possible to give those who rely on managed welfare systems choice over the way in which they experience particular services. Viewing market systems as synonymous with choice and administered systems as inevitably about lack of choice is therefore inappropriate.

A second alternative conception of choice which dominated earlier debates on welfare was the idea of choice through the ballot box. With the focus directed towards the choices of individual consumers through the exit option, choice in welfare through democratic participation, as a manifestation of voice, has been relatively neglected.

Control

As with choice, at one level the idea of control is implicit in the notion of citizenship: citizens are in a position of independence and therefore have control over their resources. However, the idea of control can be explored from a number of further angles which can provide an insight into changes in public policy. There are several ways in which the issue of control can be thought of as central to the analysis of policy. Most, if not all, policy changes shift the balance of power – and therefore the locus of control – in a particular situation in favour of one or other of the parties involved, regardless of whether this is the intention of policy or recognized in policy debate.

The most well-established concern is the effect of legislative change on central-local relations noted earlier in this chapter. Central government retains the ultimate power to determine at which level primary responsibility for policy formulation and implementation lies, and over time meta-policy change has changed the location of responsibility. Such change is often explicit as government legislates to relocate functions. But, equally importantly, through reform of financial frameworks, for example, the shifting balance of power is not so immediately apparent. More recent concerns of particular relevance in the housing context are issues of partnership and the introduction of new stakeholders in service provision (Reid 1995). At the local level partnership approaches and 'enabling' are now widespread in the delivery of a range of services which have conventionally been located in the public sector. It is important not to accept the rhetoric of partnership uncritically and to retain a concern with issues of control. Although in principle strategies can be formulated jointly by partners, this ignores the reality of social interaction: it is typically the relatively powerful players in a particular situation who shape the agenda. Thus issues of control remain pertinent to partnership approaches.

New stakeholders have become involved in the provision of welfare services in Britain, the principal group being private financiers. This brings with it issues of control: who shapes activities and directions? Here again the influences may be subtle and control may not necessarily be exercised overtly. Analogously with Friedrich's (1937) rule of anticipated reaction, those social housing providers seeking private finance may act on a mis-apprehension of what private funders expect, thereby voluntarily relinquish-ing some control over the nature of their own activities. In the housing context, the issue of the control exercised by funders can be extended to the case of individuals seeking funding for house purchase. Here there are issues of access to ownership, but equally there is the fact that the use of the home is not entirely within the hands of the owner-occupier, particularly while there is an outstanding mortgage attached to the property.

Moving the analysis to a broader level it is necessary to recognize that control over the fate of a particular asset or activity is not entirely in the hands of the owner. Within the housing context there is, for example, the impact of the local environment upon the standards of housing consumption and asset values. Even though owners have control over their own asset, if their enjoyment of this asset and its value are contingent on, for example, neighbourhood effects, then in a real sense owners are largely powerless to control one important aspect of their enjoyment of their asset. At a still broader level, as we noted at the start of this chapter, the control over the fate of a household's housing consumption is contingent on broader macro-economic and labour market conditions that individual households cannot influence. So, for example, the negative equity experienced by many home-owners in the early 1990s removed some of the control that they had over their housing consumption by making it difficult for them to adjust con-sumption to the level they might desire. Similarly, labour market change and the transfer of risk-bearing onto individual households (see Forrest and Kennett 1996) means that in a real sense the degree of control – and more importantly the degree of security – that owners have over their housing consumption has been reduced significantly in recent years.

A final area of control relates to the balance of power between producer and consumer, in terms not only of the rights of each party but also in terms of the context in which producer-consumer interactions take place. The rights of the two parties are determined by legislation and case law and, in the case of housing, we have seen important legislative changes recently. Some changes have switched control over a particular interaction in favour of producers, while others have increased the relative power of consumers. The context in which producer-consumer interactions take place is not something which is encompassed by the economic view of two equal parties freely entering into a voluntary contract. Yet the context – for example whether there is excess demand for private rented accommodation in a particular locality – will fundamentally affect the terms on which a particu-lar interaction will occur.

Citizenship, choice and control in the analysis of policy

We can bring these themes to bear upon an analysis of public policy in at least three ways. First, we can examine the rhetoric which is used to advance particular policies and to ensure that they are accepted. In the chapters that follow it will become clear that several of the policies that have been introduced since 1980 have been characterized by politicians in terms of one or more of our three themes. Second, although political debate may not be cast explicitly in terms of these themes, it may be the case that particular policies have implications which can be analysed in these terms. Particularly where the rhetoric surrounding a policy represents something of a smoke-screen, a focus upon the themes will allow the illumination of the intention behind policy. Finally, the outcomes of policy can be examined in the light of one or more of the three themes. Such an examination can seek to determine whether policy outcomes represent a realization of the objectives behind the policy or are more of an unintended or unanticipated result. Results other than those anticipated may be a product of an implementation deficit or an inevitable part of the constantly changing policy process, depending on which policy-process model is subscribed to. Alternatively, unintended or unanticipated results may be primarily a product of an interaction between the policy and other social and economic changes occurring at the same time.

Structure of the book

Each of the following chapters draws on one or more of our three themes to reflect on a particular aspect of policy.

The contingent nature of citizenship is best demonstrated through longitudinal and comparative study. In Chapter 2 Patricia Kennett explores the concept of citizenship as it has evolved in three advanced industrialized countries: Britain, Australia and Germany. The chapter highlights the different approaches to citizenship the three countries have taken and it seeks to demonstrate the way in which the discourse of citizenship has both inclusionary and exclusionary potential. It illustrates the way in which some groups in society, particularly women and members of minority ethnic groups, have a very different experience of citizenship than others.

Contemporary debates about citizenship and choice are increasingly being linked to the issue of social exclusion and the possibility that particular groups in society, especially those living in social housing, may find themselves socially excluded, which is typically interpreted in terms of a denial of the social rights of citizenship. In Chapter 3 Peter Lee examines the housing disadvantage experienced by those living in different tenures and in different areas. He counsels caution in relying on tenure as the indicator for targeting resources towards combating social exclusion.

Each of the next three chapters examines a particular sector of the housing market. Alan Murie considers the changing policy debates and experience of owner occupation in Chapter 4, while Moyra Riseborough and I focus on the changing nature of the private rented sector and the experience of private tenants in Chapter 5. In both cases the focus is on issues of choice, but in debates around owner occupation in particular the issue of choice has become intimately connected with notions of citizenship. The sector which has experienced perhaps the most rapid policy change and innovation in the last two decades is social housing. In Chapter 6 David Mullins considers how the 'rules of the game' in this sector have been changing as social housing provision has been restructured. Through an extended case study of Large Scale Voluntary Transfers (LSVTs) he explores the utility of a number of frameworks available to understand these changes and considers the implications of the changes for issues of choice and control.

The extensive policy change in the social housing sector has a number of dimensions and the next group of chapters focuses in more detail on some of the most important and varied dimensions of change. In Chapter 7 Bruce Walker takes a broad historical perspective to examine the way in which systems of housing finance and subsidy have been used as a mechanism to control the development and management of local authority housing. He highlights the way in which economic thinking about choice has played an important role in changing policy directions. Claims regarding the social rights of citizenship are central to understanding issues of access to social housing, which is the topic examined by David Mullins and Pat Niner in Chapter 8. They focus on developments in policy towards homelessness and the use of common housing registers, because these topics not only highlight changing conceptions of citizenship but are centrally concerned with issues of both choice and control. In Chapter 9 Pat Niner considers the 1990s phenomenon of charterism through an examination of the local authority performance indicator regime and a little-known charter which operates in the park homes sector. While charters are intended to empower the resident as an individual citizen and consumer, the chapter concludes that for a variety of reasons the capacity of charters to do so is limited and that the most evident feature of charterism has been the possibilities it offers for increased central control. Chapter 10 moves away from tenants as individual citizens and considers the implications of tenant involvement, as a collective activity, for enhancing user control and choice. Moyra Riseborough examines the rise of tenant involvement and then scrutinizes various representations of tenant involvement in the light of evidence gathered from research with tenants of sheltered housing schemes. The evidence points to the conclusion that increased tenant involvement should not be assumed to be an unambiguously good thing and, furthermore, that tenant involvement as it is currently practised may in fact reinforce inequalities within the tenant population.

In the final chapter David Mullins reviews the issues raised by the substantive chapters and focuses upon the nature and extent of the gap between the rhetoric and reality of housing policy. He highlights some of the interconnections between the three themes, as they are manifest in housing policy, and concludes by reflecting upon the role of policy in determining change in housing.

References

Bachrach, P. and Baratz, M.S. (1962) Two faces of power. *American Political Science Review*, 56: 947–52.

Ball, M., Harloe, M. and Martens, M. (1988) *Housing and Social Change in Europe and the USA*. London: Routledge.

Barbalet, J.M. (1988) *Citizenship*. Buckingham: Open University Press.

Barrett, S. and Hill, M. (1984) Policy, bargaining and structure in implementation theory: towards an integrated perspective. *Policy and Politics*, 12: 219–40.

Bramley, G. (1993) The enabling role for local housing authorities: a preliminary evaluation, in P. Malpass and R. Means (eds) *Implementing Housing Policy.* Buckingham: Open University Press.

Bramley, G. and Watkins, C. (1995) *Circular Projections: Household Growth, Housing Development and the Household Projections.* London: CPRE.

Brubaker, R. (1992) *Citizenship and Nationhood in France and Germany.* Cambridge, MA: Harvard University Press.

Bulmer, M. and Rees, A.M. (eds) (1996) *Citizenship Today: The Contemporary Relevance of T.H. Marshall.* London: UCL Press.

Burns, D., Hambleton, R. and Hoggett, P. (1994) *The Politics of Decentralisation: Revitalising Local Democracy.* Basingstoke: Macmillan.

Clegg, S. (1989) *Frameworks of Power.* London: Sage.

Demaine, J. (1996) Beyond communitarianism: citizenship, politics and education, in J. Demaine and H. Entwistle (eds) *Beyond Communitarianism: Citizenship, Politics and Education.* London: Routledge.

DoE (1996) *Household Growth: Where Shall we Live?* Cm. 3471. London: Stationery Office.

Driver, S. and Martell, L. (1997) New Labour's communitarianisms. *Critical Social Policy,* 17: 27–45.

Dror, Y. (1986) *Policymaking under Adversity.* New Brunswick, NJ: Transaction Publications.

Dunleavy, P. and O'Leary, B. (1987) *Theories of the State: The Politics of Liberal Democracy.* Basingstoke: Macmillan.

Edelman, M. (1971) *Politics as Symbolic Action.* Chicago: Markham.

Esping-Andersen, G. (1990) *The Three Worlds of Welfare Capitalism.* Cambridge: Polity Press.

Etzioni, A. (1993) *The Spirit of Community.* New York: Simon & Schuster.

Fimister, G. and Hill, M. (1993) Delegating implementation problems: social security, housing and community care in Britain, in M. Hill (ed.) *New Agendas in the Study of the Policy Process.* Hemel Hempstead: Harvester Wheatsheaf.

Forrest, R. and Kennett, T. (1996) Home ownership, social exclusion and the post-Fordist city. Conference paper, ENHR conference on 'Housing and European Integration', Helsingor, Denmark, 27–31 August.

Freeden, M. (1991) *Rights.* Buckingham: Open University Press.

Freeman, A., Holmans, A. and Whitehead, C. (1996) *Is the UK different? International Comparisons of Tenure Patterns.* London: Council of Mortgage Lenders.

Friedrich, C. (1937) *Constitutional Government and Democracy.* New York: Gipp.

Friend, J.K., Power, J.M., and Yewlett, C.J.L. (1974) *Public Planning: The Intercorporate Dimension.* London: Tavistock.

Garcia, S. (ed.) (1996) Special issue on citizenship and the city. *International Journal of Urban and Regional Research,* January.

Giddens, A. (1982) Class division, class conflict and citizenship rights, in A. Giddens (ed.) *Profiles and Critiques in Social Theory.* London: Macmillan.

Ginsburg, N. (1992) *Divisions of Welfare.* London: Sage.

Gray, C. (1994) *Government Beyond the Centre: Sub-National Politics in Britain.* Basingstoke: Macmillan.

Ham, C. and Hill, M. (1993) *The Policy Making Process in the Modern Capitalist State,* 2nd edn. Hemel Hempstead: Harvester Wheatsheaf.

Hill, D. (1994) *Citizens and Cities: Urban Policy in the 1990s*. Hemel Hempstead: Harvester Wheatsheaf.

Hill, M. (ed.) (1993) *The Policy Process: A Reader*. Hemel Hempstead: Harvester Wheatsheaf.

Hill, M. (1997) Implementation theory: yesterday's issue? *Policy and Politics*, 25: 375–85.

Hills, J. (1991) *Unravelling Housing Finance*. Oxford: Clarendon Press.

Hirschman, A.O. (1970) *Exit, Voice and Loyalty*. Cambridge, MA: Harvard University Press.

Hirschman, A.O. (1991) *The Rhetoric of Reaction: Perversity, Futility, Jeopardy*. Cambridge, MA: Belknap Press.

Holmans, A. (1987) *Housing Policy in Britain: A History*. London: Croom Helm.

Holmans, A. (1995) *Housing Demand and Need in England, 1991 to 2011*. York: Joseph Rowntree Foundation.

Kennett, P. (1995) Citizenship and social exclusion in Britain and Germany. *Research in Community Sociology*, 5: 225–48.

Le Grand, J. and Bartlett, W. (eds) (1993) *Quasi-Markets and Social Policy*. Basingstoke: Macmillan.

Lipsky, M. (1980) *Street-Level Bureaucracy*. New York: Russell Sage.

Lister, R. (1993) Tracing the contours of women's citizenship. *Policy and Politics*, 21: 3–16.

Maclennan, D. (1994) *A Competitive UK Economy: The Challenges for Housing Policy*. York: Joseph Rowntree Foundation.

Malpass, P. and Means, R. (eds) (1993) *Implementing Housing Policy*. Buckingham: Open University Press.

Malpass, P. and Murie, A. (1994) *Housing Policy and Practice*, 4th edn. Basingstoke: Macmillan.

Marshall, T.H. (1950) *Citizenship and Social Class*. Cambridge: Cambridge University Press.

Marshall, T.H. (1963) *Sociology at the Crossroads and Other Essays*. London: Heinemann.

Newton, K. (1975) Community politics and decision making: the American experience and its lessons, in K. Newton (ed.) *Essays on the Study of Urban Politics*. London: Croom Helm.

Oliver, D. and Heater, D. (1994) *The Foundations of Citizenship*. London: Harvester Wheatsheaf.

Pressman, J. and Wildavsky, A. (1973) *Implementation*. Berkeley, CA: University of California Press.

Rees, A.M. (1995) The promise of social citizenship. *Policy and Politics*, 23: 313–25.

Reid, B. (1995) Interorganisational networks and the delivery of local housing services. *Housing Studies*, 10: 133–50.

Rhodes, R. (1988) *Beyond Westminster and Whitehall*. London: Unwin Hyman.

Sabatier, P. (1986) Top-down and bottom-up approaches to implementation research: a critical analysis and suggested synthesis. *Journal of Public Policy*, 6: 21–48.

Turner, B.S. (1986) *Citizenship and Capitalism: The Debate Over Reformism*. London: Allen & Unwin.

Turner, B.S. (1993) Contemporary problems in the theory of citizenship, in B.S. Turner (ed.) *Citizenship and Social Theory*. London: Sage.

Turner, B.S. and Hamilton, P. (eds) (1994a) *Citizenship: Critical Concepts*, vol. I. London: Routledge.

Turner, B.S. and Hamilton, P. (eds) (1994b) *Citizenship: Critical Concepts*, vol. II. London: Routledge.

Walker, B. and Marsh, A. (1998) Pricing public housing services in the UK: mirroring the market? *Housing Studies*, 13: 549–66.

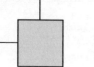

2

Differentiated citizenship and housing experience

Patricia Kennett

Introduction

This chapter utilizes a cross-national citizenship framework to understand processes that impact upon people's housing choices and opportunities. It draws on post-war developments in Britain, Germany and Australia to demonstrate that the boundaries of citizenship are socially constructed and vary over time and between nations. The post-war mode of integration in each of these countries was supported, in varying degrees, by an institutional framework built upon the incomplete citizenship of women and minority ethnic groups. Deconstructing the concept of citizenship highlights the differential way in which it has been bestowed and shows that it is as vital to look at those who are excluded as those who are included. Boundaries are constructed according to various exclusionary and inclusionary criteria, which relate not only to social class, but also to gender and racial divisions which, in turn, impact on people's housing experiences.

This chapter will begin by evaluating the contribution and limitations of Marshall's (1950) thesis to understanding differentiated citizenship. Housing issues in each of the countries will then be considered and embedded within a broad set of themes such as the context of welfare and the social relations of gender and ethnicity. The chapter will then emphasize the temporal and spatial specificity of the relationship between citizenship and housing, and the multidimensional nature of inclusion and exclusion.

Understanding citizenship

There is no overarching model of citizenship. It is subject to various political interpretations and social forces which change over time and from country to country. According to Marshall's (1950) influential thesis the notion of citizenship refers to the relationship between the individual and the state. His central theme was that the rights of citizenship involve national constitutional rights such as *civil* and *political* rights, as well as embracing *social* rights, each of which is closely associated with social and political institutions. The hallmark of advanced industrial democracies is the eventual institutionalization of all three levels and, in particular, social citizenship.

For Marshall, the citizenship rights that accrue to members of a political community integrate previously unintegrated segments of the population and serve to mitigate some of the inequalities of class, thus altering the pattern of social inequality. Marshall discusses 'class fusion' which he refers to as the 'general enrichment of the concrete substance of civilised life, a general reduction of risk and insecurity, and equalisation between the more or less fortunate at all levels' (Marshall 1950: 56). This leads '. . . towards a fuller measure of equality, an enrichment of the stuff of which the status is made and an increase in the number of those on whom the status is bestowed' (p. 29).

Marshall has been criticized for the evolutionary and Anglocentric nature of his thesis (Giddens 1982; Mann 1987), as well as its emphasis on class. Recent theoretical developments have enabled a more subtle and nuanced interpretation of citizenship. Anti-racist and feminist critiques, and theories of transition have contributed to an understanding of the contingent and differential nature of citizenship and its relationship with housing. For Smith (1989b: 148) it is the contingent nature of the citizenship framework which makes it a:

> comprehensive vehicle through which to explore systematic discrepancies between the obligations required of, and the rights extended to members of a nation-state. Enduring variations in the availability of these rights, or in the opportunities to exercise them effectively, can thus be conceptualised as forces shaping or structuring society.

Citizenship configurations and housing systems are not only the outcome of class struggle but, according to Williams (1994), also involve the interplay of the relations of other forms of social power such as racism and patriarchy, and are equally significant in the reproduction of 'race'- and gender-related inequalities. Whilst welfare states reflect the cultural, economic and political specificities of individual nation states they are also, to varying degrees, a product of the 'interrelation between capitalism, patriarchy and imperialism' (Williams 1994: 61). Marshall (1950) recognizes the contradiction between the rise of capitalism and citizenship development but he does not recognize citizenship rights as a process of constant struggle and negotiation. The progression from civil to political and social rights is not the smooth, inevitable process Marshall suggests, but has always been dependent on political struggles between social movements, groups and classes. Retrogression and the erosion of the rights of particular groups are an ever-present possibility.

Welfare, housing and citizenship

The concept of citizenship is encapsulated within the institutions and ideology of the welfare state. Britain, Germany and Australia represent variants of post-war social policy, each with its own particular 'web of welfare' and housing provision. These countries, particularly Germany with the merging of two fundamentally different systems, provide case studies for demonstrating the contingent and contested nature of citizenship.

Esping-Andersen (1990) investigates the degree to which social rights permit people to exist independently of the labour market by eroding the commodity status of labour in capitalist society. He also considers dimensions of stratification within welfare states which he saw as structuring the content of social citizenship. He classifies Britain and Australia as liberal regimes in which decommodification potential is low. Selectivism and residualism characterize the welfare states of the liberal regime, limiting the 'realm of social rights' and providing a 'blend of a relative equality among state-welfare recipients, market-differentiated welfare among the majorities, and a class-political dualism between the two' (p. 27). Castles and Mitchell (1992) have developed Esping-Andersen's thesis and have suggested that Australia belongs to a 'fourth world of welfare capitalism' in which the emphasis, particularly from the political left, has been on achieving equality in pre-tax, pre-transfer income rather than through welfare rights. This strategy has served to justify the flat-rate, means-tested benefits which characterize the Australian welfare system. Germany, in contrast, is classified as a conservative regime which reflects a strongly corporatist tradition and offers moderate decommodification potential. The dominant feature of this regime is the preservation of status differentials, and consequently the institutionalization of rights attached to class and status.

In each of these regime types the formulation of social rights was carried out not only against the backdrop of different historical legacies but also in the context of different ideologies, and therefore offers an opportunity to examine the contingency, flexibility and fragility of the social contract between the state and the individual.

Following the Second World War the ethos of egalitarianism prevailed in all three countries and trends were towards decreasing social inequality and the gradual inclusion of previously excluded or marginal populations. This was an era in which 'the concept of citizenship was given an invigorated meaning' (Tomlinson 1996: 4). The British context was that of an ideological commitment to social planning and to the welfare state. The post-war welfare consensus emphasized an explicit commitment to state intervention through universal access to direct public provision of welfare benefits. It accepted an extended role for the state in economic and social policy and implicitly guaranteed social rights of citizenship for the whole population. In reality the welfare citizenship of women, black people and the poor was not secured. As Ginsberg (1992a: 141) comments: '... the whole notion of welfare citizenship at the heart of the post-war consensus was ideological in the sense that it carried nationalist overtones and implied the exclusion of certain people from the benefits of citizenship'. Nevertheless, the post-war expansion in welfare enormously extended the range of state support for the individual.

At the core of the consensus in post-war Britain was the promotion of the ideal of universal citizenship, and the provision of mass housing can be seen as a particularly important component of this project. Though never fully socialized, according to Smith, 'housing [as shelter] was regarded by successive governments as one of the more prominent social benefits of British citizenship' (Smith 1989a: 175). In Britain between 1945 and 1952 over 80 per cent of all new dwellings were built by local authorities (Malpass and Murie 1987). The public sector stock in the period 1945–56 almost doubled as a proportion of the total stock. According to Harloe (1981) however, the universalistic basis of the provision of social housing for the working class was always in doubt. As Malpass and Murie (1987: 74) point out, access to the good quality council housing built during this period 'reflected the political and economic power of organised skilled labour – the better off working class, as distinct from the poor'. Thus in Britain it was the better off sections of the working class that were accommodated in social housing. At the same time, increasing affluence, a stable social contract and unionization also enabled members of the labour aristocracy to fuel the expansion of home-owning suburbia.

In Germany the end of the Second World War saw a devastated nation from which two very different German states were to emerge. They shared a common history but their economic, political and social systems were built on opposing ideological principles resulting in quite different formulations of citizenship rights. Like Britain, many German cities had experienced massive damage and destruction during the war (Power 1993) and housing policy was a central element of reconstruction. The East German system developed its interpretation of socialist philosophy incorporating the right to work, gender equality, guaranteed access to housing, and social benefits in old age and sickness through a centrally planned apparatus. Housing formed part of the national strategy and was incorporated into five-year economic plans set down by the Socialist Unity Party (SED) of Germany. It was acknowledged as a basic need; to be built, allocated and maintained by the state for all citizens. In 1949 the majority of dwellings were privately owned, though under state control. There was no market for either buying or renting and families seeking accommodation were allocated by the local housing department to both state housing and private rented housing (Dienemann 1993). During the 1950s and 1960s the emphasis was on the redevelopment of war-damaged inner cities, but as supply failed to meet demand the trend turned towards developing large satellite towns on the periphery of existing urban areas. Between 1960 and 1985 some 125 large developments of over 2500 units were built utilizing industrialized building methods (Power 1993).

In West Germany, the policy context that was to emerge reflected a variety of influences, in particular that of the United States through Marshall Aid (to support reconstruction after the Second World War), the legacy of national socialism and the 'spectre' of communism. This in turn impacted upon the development of the political system which was based on decentralization, with extensive functions devolved to regional and local governments. The ideological context of West Germany was enshrined within the basic law in the philosophy of the social market economy, which promoted the notion of the socially conscious state (*Sozialstaat*), whilst also encouraging an active role for the market, the family and voluntary welfare institutions. The concept of the social market economy, according to Ginsberg (1992a: 19), represented 'a liberal capitalist reaction to fascist and Stalinist conceptions of an authoritarian state, both of which were distrustful and destructive of the institutions of civil society'.

Underlying the notion of the socially conscious state was the principle of subsidiarity which, shaped by Catholic doctrine, combined and supported traditional notions of the 'family' and 'motherhood' and emphasized that the state would only intervene when the family's capacity to service its members was exhausted (Esping-Andersen 1990). From the 1950s a plurality of welfare associations re-emerged and there was an explicit commitment to the private world of marriage and family, all of which had been virtually abolished during the Nazi era. Langan and Ostner, building on Esping-Andersen's classification, refer to the German welfare state as a gendered status maintenance model 'supporting the male "normal worker" and the female "normal wife"' (Langan and Ostner 1991: 138). Thus the content of social rights within this regime were likely to uphold and reproduce various existing social divisions, including those between men and women.

The construction of housing was seen as a way of reinvigorating private industry, of accommodating the millions of refugees and displaced persons following the devastation of the war and as a means of reasserting the home as a private realm and thus strengthening the family unit. Consistent with the dominant economic philosophy of a social market economy in West

Germany the Christian Democrats encouraged a market system based on the promotion of home ownership and private tenancy. Given that incomes for the majority of the population were relatively low until the late 1960s and that there were alternative housing options, it is perhaps not surprising that home ownership actually declined during this period and even today only represents some 40 per cent of households. It was in this context that under the economic, social and political pressures of reconstruction, the 1950s became most notable as the high point of state intervention in housing policy (Jaedicke and Wollmann 1990). Housing production during the 1950s constituted almost 600,000 housing units a year, with never less than 50 per cent of the units being social housing. The main providers of social rented housing were limited-dividend housing companies, in keeping with the principles of a social market economy. Since the 1950s social housing subsidies have been available not only to social landlords, but also to commercial and private landlords. With grants tied to notions of controlled profit and cost rent, and to a period of 'social commitment' requiring landlords to chose tenants from those meeting income eligibility, the West German system of subsidy enabled a variety of tenure arrangements to develop. Up until the 1970s the belief was that housing needs had been met.

The merging of the two fundamentally different German systems in October 1990 offered the opportunity for innovation and fusion in the social system, a vision incorporated in to the Social Charter of the German Democratic Republic (GDR) (1990) in the early stages of the unification process. Yet, rather than innovation and fusion, Winkler (1994) has referred to social union in Germany as based on assimilation and standardization. The former GDR's social system, evolving through a centrally-planned economy, was rapidly displaced by the established system of social security based on the principles of the social-market economy, and incorporating features of the conservative regime of welfare. Thus, as implied in the Unification Treaty, West German welfare-state programmes were simply extended to the five new federal states. Whilst these developments were driven, to some extent, by the belief in the social and economic superiority of the West German system, and its ability to deal with the problems of transition, in reality the '. . . shortcomings, deficiencies, and injustices inherent in the West German social system have been exported to the East German setting' (Winkler 1994: 226). Winkler has characterized the former GDR as a society with a 'relatively low but rather equalised standard of living' (Winkler 1990: 111). More recently the impact of social union has indicated a different scenario: unprecedented hardship and social dislocation have emerged for many people in the East as an all-German social security system has developed incorporating an alternative mode of integration to that in the former East, and reasserting the conjugal family unit.

In Australia the strong emphasis on citizenship and equality translated into equality to participate in the labour market and receive a living wage, at least for the organized, white, male population. State intervention was concerned with wage regulation in and social protection through the labour market, resulting in the distinctive pattern of social policy outcomes labelled the 'wage earners' welfare state' (Castles 1988). The growth of mass mortgaged home ownership, occurring much earlier than in Britain, took place in the context of economic boom, rapid population growth, rising real wages and low levels of unemployment. It formed a vital part in reinforcing the nationalist slogan promoting 'the Australian way of life', as 'standards of living for ordinary people were almost constantly improving and many immigrants achieved their hopes in material assimilation to suburbia's desires' (Castles *et al.* 1992: 12). Ideologically home ownership fitted well with the notion of 'industrial citizenship' (right to strike, form trade unions, etc.) encapsulated within the 'wage earners' welfare state' which promoted individualism and limited direct state provision. According to Jayasuriya (1991: 32), industrial citizenship emphasized 'the industrial activity of men, rather than advocating political citizenship for men and women alike'. The maintenance of this system involved three main pillars which Castles (1988) has referred to as a policy strategy of 'domestic defence'.

The first was a system of compulsory conciliation and arbitration of industrial disputes with the aim of 'simultaneously achieving a social policy minimum (a 'fair' wage sufficient to support a breadwinner and a family) and of adjusting wage levels to take account of fluctuations caused by dependence on a highly unstable primary commodity market' (Castles 1993: 8). The second was a series of tariff and import controls which were used to protect domestic manufacturing from overseas competition, and the third involved the regulation of migration to control labour supply and exclude low-wage labour, minimize unemployment and protect wage levels negotiated through arbitration.

Jones (1996: 10) refers to the uniqueness of the Australian approach to social welfare as, more accurately 'a planned attempt to create a white society based on high wages in an economy sheltered from overseas competition'. This policy of 'domestic defence' was the inclusionary policy mechanism through which the government and an organized working class could attempt to ensure and maintain the social rights of the employed citizen (white and male) and which justified the principles of residualism and selectivism in the development of social policy which sought 'to encourage even the moderately affluent to provide for their own welfare in retirement and during troubled times in their lives' (Jones 1996: 10). Home ownership was constructed as the 'Australian Dream', and was maintained through the sale of state housing (which constituted 10 per cent of the stock during the 1950s) and then through tax concessions, low interest rates, State and Commonwealth government sponsorship for home ownership and the construction of houses for sale. Home ownership grew from 53 per cent of households to 70 per cent between 1947 and 1961 (Troy 1991) and has remained roughly the same ever since, with state housing playing a residual role, representing only 5 per cent of the total stock. State housing increasingly meets the needs of only the neediest, with most tenants now being single parents and one-person – mostly elderly – households and on social welfare benefits. This trend is likely to be perpetuated as targeting for specialized groups and more stringent means tests are introduced, and the numbers of needy, particularly amongst the homeless, single-parent and Aboriginal households, increases.

Patriarchal citizenship

In all three countries, amongst the democratic pledges, egalitarian values and universal principles, dimensions of inequality were created based around patriarchy and racism which severely affected people's housing options. Issues relating to class, race, gender, household type and sexuality have been major considerations in how a 'home' has been defined and who has been able to gain access. Though women have made substantial gains in relation to both civil and political rights an investigation of their social rights and status as citizens reveals, according to Pateman (1989: 35), 'the patriarchal character of ostensibly universal categories'. Women are incorporated as members of the family, a private sphere that is essential to, but separate and opposite from, the public sphere of civil society and the state, which are historically male constructs. The white male worker represents 'the individual', 'the citizen' in the public sphere, and is legitimated in the private sphere as the 'breadwinner'. A range of policies construct women as wives, mothers and carers in the private (domestic) sphere, regulating their social role and reinforcing their dependency. The form and specific historical source of patriarchy shifts over time and place and according to Pateman has evolved from the 'father' to the 'husband', with the state and the economy particularly significant as the site of patriarchy during the post-war years. This in turn is influenced by the social relations established between the state and the individual which vary across national boundaries and over time. To understand the position of women one must analyse the significance of the assumptions about gender and how these assumptions have influenced the discourse and legitimation for different patterns of participation, choice and citizenship. The case of a reunified Germany is particularly useful for exposing these processes and for highlighting their impact on women.

In West Germany for example, the rebuilding of a capitalist democracy after the Second World War included the political reconstruction of the family and legislation which served to protect and preserve 'patriarchal authority; women's economic dependence on men; the ideological elevation of motherhood; pronatal sentiments; and a normative conception of the "family" as an ahistorical social unit transcending class division' (Möller 1989: 139).

Notions of women's citizenship were subsumed within the family ideal, and were exemplified in the policies promoting marriage and the maintenance of the 'traditional family' during the 1950s. As mentioned earlier the direction of policies during this period was strongly influenced by Catholic doctrine, by events of the previous era and developments in the East. The legitimation for the subordination of women was the emphasis on 'the role of the family as the bulwark against communism and other forms of totalitarianism ... marriage and family were constructed such that "privacy" meant freedom from immediate state intervention' (Ostner 1993: 98) in contrast to the Nazi era in which, according to Ostner, '... the female, and to a lesser extent, the male body, became a state controlled terrain, a public space' (p. 99). Up until the 1977 Marriage and Family Rights Act, which encouraged notions of partnership and joint responsibility between husband and wife, the policy agenda towards women, according to Chamberlayne (1994: 185), was one of 'legal subordination' to their husband.

In contrast the GDR was founded in 1949 as a socialist state within the territory of the Soviet occupation zone. This dramatic transformation saw a reversal of Nazi policies and the living and working conditions of women in the GDR as the state sought to reintegrate women into the public sphere and to facilitate both career advancement and motherhood simultaneously. By the 1980s some 92 per cent of working-age women in the GDR were either in training or employed outside the home. The fall of the Sozialistiche Deutsche Arbeitpartei (SED) (Socialist Unity Party) government of the GDR in 1989 brought GDR citizens an extension of civil rights in relation to the right of speech, assembly, association and freedom of movement. But unification with the Federal Republic of Germany (FRG) in October 1990 saw the erosion of a number of social and economic rights, including guarantees of employment and affordable housing, free medical care and education, paid parental leave and day care. As Rosenberg (1991: 133) indicates, despite the fact that: '... only three per cent of the women in the five new Eastern states described housewife as their ideal job and 65 per cent stated that "they would work even if they didn't need the income" the West German social agenda and economic infrastructure are returning them to the private sphere whether they wish it or not'. The impact of these developments has been characterized as a massive attack on the rights of women, as the conservative welfare regime of a social market economy is imposed on the former socialist welfare state.

For East Germany the rapid transition to a market economy has seen dramatic changes in the social and labour market structure. The new *Länder* (regional states) have experienced steep increases in unemployment, which by January 1992 had reached 16.5 per cent, with an even greater number of East Germans either working a reduced working week (2 million) or participating in state subsidized job creation schemes (400,000), training programmes (450,000) or early retirement schemes (500,000). Over 60 per cent of registered job seekers were women; the unemployment rate among women had reached almost 22 per cent. Blue-collar workers represented 68 per cent of the unemployed (OECD 1992). The impact of the transition has been accompanied by the reduction of subsidies for services such as housing and health care, the reduction of facilities enabling women's participation in the labour market, and the virtual elimination of a system based on the social protection of women as independent individuals.

In post-war Britain, the importance of women's role as wives and mothers in ensuring the continuation of the British race was enshrined within the Beveridgian settlement in which women were treated as dependants of the male breadwinner. Policy supported and was directed towards the patriarchal family, particularly in areas such as housing and social security entitlements. The 'married women's option' exemplified this role assignment, with married women able to pay less social security contributions and therefore receive less benefits. Although this option was dismantled in the 1970s following the passage of equal opportunities legislation, little systematic state aid has ensued to assist women's integration into the labour market. Similar ideals were incorporated into the German constitution with the principle of universal social security for those active in the labour market, while for non-economically active women the assumption was that benefits would be derived from the male partner's contribution.

The two-tier system of welfare evident in Britain and Germany, divided between social insurance and social assistance, is not evident in Australia where, generally, only the latter is available. Because of this, the Australian system, though shaped by assumptions about the traditional sexual division of labour, has not been quite as deeply gendered (Orloff 1995). The unitary system and flat rate means-tested benefits for those outside the labour market 'does not offer different benefits to the clients of work-related versus family related programmes' (Orloff 1995: 46) thus exposing the unemployed as well as single parents to stigmatized, residual benefits. In other words, benefits programmes do not reward former wage-earners any more than those who have principally been carers. Nevertheless, the assumptions and influence of the male breadwinner model in all three countries has influenced the different terms on which women compete in the labour and housing markets and has shaped the terms on which the boundaries of women's citizenship have been drawn. For those women wishing, or forced, to establish independent households the patriarchal assumptions pervading housing systems, labour markets and social security systems during the immediate post-war period put them at a severe disadvantage.

In Britain and Australia for example, women would have been unlikely to have equal access to the capital through which the suburban home ownership ideal could be achieved. In Australia, because of the limited availability of social rented housing, women would have been reliant on the cheaper end of the private rental sector, which until recently received rent assistance well below the level equivalent to the benefits received by homeowners. In 1993 the Australian Department of Housing and Regional Development stated that there were '582,400 low-income households in "financial housing stress" [spending over 30 per cent of income on housing – the Australian average is 13.1 per cent], representing 6–7 per cent of all income units' (Jones 1996: 186). The report also indicated that over half of these were living in private rented accommodation. The report did not break down the findings by gender but it is a clear indication that many people in this sector are likely to be experiencing significant housing difficulties.

In Britain social rented housing remained an option. However, in the 1970s a British government report was to state that fatherless families were seriously disadvantaged in the housing market when compared to two-parent families and went on to state that 'much of the evidence received on the subject of local authority housing was concerned with discrimination in the allocation of tenancies, either against one-parent families in general, or against unmarried mothers' (Finer 1974: 381).

The introduction of the Housing (Homeless Persons) Act 1977 repre-sented a fundamental shift in policy and practice and made Britain the only one of the three countries to officially define homelessness and establish housing as a legal right. Whilst it was an opportunity to improve the status of women and their housing opportunities by overcoming the discriminatory allocation policies of local authorities, it also went some way to acknowl-edging homelessness as a housing problem rather than a welfare problem. The Act placed an obligation on local authorities to provide accommodation for those who were considered homeless and in priority need. This category included those with or expecting children as well as those considered vul-nerable because of old age, mental illness and handicap or physical dis-ability. Influenced by growing public pressure and an increasing awareness of homelessness as an issue this extension of citizenship rights can also be understood as an attempt to reconfirm the rhetoric of home and family and the citizenship of women based on their role as mothers.

However, the commitment to provide permanent accommodation to those considered eligible within the parameters of the legislation (a commit-ment which has since been eroded) also signalled the changing character of council housing which was to evolve from a tenure for middle income groups to a residualized tenure of last resort (Forrest and Murie 1983; Sommerville 1994).

Racial and ethnic identity, nationhood and citizenship

The most overt discussions of citizenship have been in relation to race and immigration. Issues relating to the citizenship of ethnic and racial minorities involve all levels of citizenship: civic, political and social. In addition, the relationship between citizenship, ethnicity and immigration has been central in defining identity and nationhood in all the countries. Castles *et al.* (1992) point to two distinct but interlocking processes in relation to dispossessed Australian Aboriginal people whose destruction and exclusion has been sought through physical and cultural genocide, and labour recruitment, settlement and incorporation of migrant populations. In post-war Australia, for example, the particular configuration of citizenship excluded the indigenous peoples (Aborigines and Torres Strait Islanders) whose presence preceded colonial settlement and who were never considered a useful source of labour and therefore never incorporated as industrial citizens. In fact, many of the legislative mechanisms explicitly excluded Aboriginal people from accessing social rights such as social security and award wages so that when they did work their conditions were often close to slavery. According to Bryson (1992) it was not until the mid 1960s that the trade union movement intervened to end their exploitation. Even though little concern was shown for immigrants, particularly those of non-British origin, they were at least able to participate in the labour market. This opened up the possibility of access to cheaper, suburban homes encircling all major Australian cities by the 1960s.

One of the first acts of the New Commonwealth Parliament in 1901 was to establish the White Australia policy through the Immigration Restriction Act which was to remain in force as the basis for immigration policy until the 1960s. According to Pearson (1995: 2):

> The vision of Australian nationhood set out in 1901 ... was, of course, racist and strongly committed to the notion of a perpetual British society in the South Pacific. The exclusion from citizenship of Aboriginal peoples showed that the vision of nationhood conceived of no place for the country's original inhabitants because they were of a different and inferior race.

By 1947 only 9 per cent of the Australian population was overseas-born and only 1 per cent (including Aborigines) was of non-European origin. After this period, though Britain remained the largest single source of immigrants, it was unable to meet population growth targets and the emphasis shifted to non-British, 'white' European immigrants. Maintenance of the White Australia policy involved emphasizing assimilation and cultural homogeneity. For Aborigines assimilation policies were, according to Castles *et al.* (1992: 21) 'a cloak for concealing the desperate socio-economic situation of many blacks, both urban and rural' and an attempt to destroy Aboriginal identity. Housing policy in the post-Second World War period was seen as an important tool with which to achieve Aboriginal assimilation. A 1957 Queensland Native Affairs Annual Report argues that: 'Housing has always held a very high priority in State Government policy aimed at the ultimate assimilation of the Aboriginal people into the white community. Equally with education, housing provides the medium of uplift without which assimilation could never materialize' (Heppel 1979: 1).

Aboriginal housing policy has largely been misdirected and unsuccessful in meeting Aboriginal needs. The much criticized segregation and 'protection' strategies of the 1930s, which had involved placing Aborigines on reserves under the Aboriginal Protection Authorities, was replaced in 1968 by policies emphasizing the construction of 'transitional housing' for those Aboriginal people living on reserves. It was envisaged that those living in transitional housing would be tutored and prepared for eventual residence in suburban-type housing along with the non-Aboriginal population, when it was felt they were ready. Whilst the failure of this policy can be attributed to lack of funds, poor quality housing and its paternalistic approach, it was also the case that throughout the 1950s and 1960s the numbers of Aboriginal people living on reserves, at whom the policy was directed, had dwindled. Significant numbers of Aboriginal people had already independently migrated away from the reserves and into mainly rented, poor quality housing in the towns and cities (Sanders 1993: 216). It was not until the Whitlam Government and the establishment of the second Commonwealth Aboriginal housing programme in 1972 that a more sustained and innovative approach to Aboriginal housing was adopted.

The referendum that occurred in 1967 was, according to Tomlinson (1996: 4) 'the first public recognition of Aboriginal citizenship in their own country' and was followed by a reassertion of Aboriginal identity and political action. There was greater involvement in Aboriginal affairs policy at a national rather than state level and self-determination and self-management became important policy goals. During the 1970s the Department of Aboriginal Affairs and the Commonwealth Aboriginal Land Rights Act (Northern Territory) were established and a range of Commonwealth Aboriginal housing programmes were initiated covering a range of different forms of housing provision. Public rental housing was provided specifically for Aborigines, Aboriginal community housing associations were established to provide and manage community-owned dwellings, hostel accommodation was provided throughout the country and low-interest loans were made available for home ownership.

This period of political and policy activity represented limited and stuttering progress but an important impetus towards Aboriginal citizenship was established. However, it is clear that the 'workers' welfare state' which established a living wage and various government schemes to assist home purchase has been unsuccessful in meeting the housing needs of the Aboriginal population. The unemployment rate of Aboriginal and Torres Strait Islander people is 38 per cent, almost five times the national rate, and approximately thirty per cent of Aboriginal and Torres Strait Islander people were considered to be homeless or living in sub-standard accommodation in 1996 (Healey 1997). Approximately 39 per cent were public authority tenants, 31 per cent live in private/community rental dwellings (Sanders 1993) and the rate of home ownership for Aborigines is about one third that of the population generally (Bryson 1992: 96).

The issue of 'appropriateness' and the recognition of cultural specificity has emerged as the policy discourse has moved from one of assimilation to multiculturalism and cultural pluralism. The Australian population is now one of the most ethnically diverse in the world. There is a growing awareness and sensitivity to the idea that housing provision needs to reflect and incorporate the cultural and psychological needs of the various ethnic communities and Aboriginal people as well as meet their economic and social needs. Funds have been channelled through ethnic organizations for education, welfare and cultural programmes and, for Aboriginal people, it is community-based provision which has the potential to be an important source of housing. Aborigines have chosen to distance themselves from the notion of multiculturalism and instead to find new meaning in the concept of citizenship through their particular claims as an indigenous people with legitimate rights to self-determination and the restitution of land.

In West Germany a strategy of labour importation was adopted in the 1950s. Rapid economic growth after the Second World War, and the reduction in the convenient labour source from East Germany following the construction of the Berlin wall in 1961 had led to the decision to recruit 'foreigners' as the most convenient and cheapest solution to labour shortage. The original guestworker concept of rotation was based on the perception that the migration of men and women was temporary and could be restricted according to labour-market needs. Wilpert (1983) argues that as this system could not be applied to workers from EC (European Community) countries, it encouraged high recruitment of Turkish and Yugoslav labour during the late 1960s and early 1970s. By 1981, Turks constituted 30.9 per cent of the economically active foreign population in West Germany. In 1981 over 50 per cent of the foreign population under 16 were Turkish. Women migrants formed a substantial part of the immigrant labour force and were subject to oppression in relation to their class, gender, and because they were migrants.

In West Germany the idea of ethnic homogeneity is built into the notion of citizenship itself (Baubock 1991). Brubaker (1989) has described German citizenry as a 'community of descent' (p. 369) which has had fundamental implications for the extent to which Germany's post-war immigrants have been incorporated as citizens. German citizenship law is based solely on the principle of *jus sanguinus* which reinforces the notion of descent and is constructed biologically. Brubaker refers to the German conception of nationhood as 'particularist, organic, differentialist and Volk-centred' (p. 386), emphasizing cultural, linguistic and racial community. No significance is given to birth in the territory and there is no mechanism for second or third generation immigrants to automatically become citizens. Citizenship is available only through naturalization, a purely discretionary decision of the state. According to Lash (1994) less than 10 per cent of German-born ethnic minorities have either citizen or resident status. *Jus sanguinus* applies to the extent that ethnic Germans (though usually not German-speaking immigrants who may have spent centuries outside Germany) have immediate citizenship, housing and welfare rights. According to Wilpert, the criteria for admission provides the basis for inequality within contemporary German society and 'supplies the logic and legitimacy for racist ideologies and institutional discrimination towards the collective of foreign workers and their descendants, who are not recognised as having accumulated similar rights [to ethnic Germans] within German society' (Wilpert 1991: 57).

The fall of communism in Europe and the destruction of the Berlin wall resulted in massive population flows into Germany which placed increasing pressure on a housing market already under strain. During the last six months of 1989 over 300,000 people crossed to the FR Germany. The total number of arrivals, including non-German immigrants brought the total immigration figures for 1981–91 to 1 million per year (Le Dem 1991). Former East Germans and ethnic Germans (*Aussiedler*) are entitled to compete for the diminishing number of homes in the West. However, the 1.8 million Turks, invited to Germany as guestworkers because of their value to the economy during the post-war 'economic miracle' and who may have been resident in Germany for up to three generations have no such automatic access to housing. Asylum seekers are redistributed to long-term hostel accommodation in any of Germany's 16 federal states, organized according to a strict quota system.

In Britain the post-war years saw policies to promote the notion of a tolerant and accommodating 'mother country' maintaining the image of a Commonwealth led and nurtured by Britain. The 1948 Nationality Act formally gave all members of the Commonwealth the full set of rights and privileges associated with British citizenship. This placed them on the same social, political and economic footing as Britons born in the UK. By 1958 about 125,000 West Indians and 55,000 Indians and Pakistanis had arrived as UK citizens under the 1948 Nationality Act. Although Commonwealth immigrants possessed the equivalent legal rights, Jacobs (1985) describes a system of informal racism operating throughout the welfare state, prohibiting access to welfare rights for black people which, in turn served to reduce the black British to the status of second-class citizens. Since then a series of restrictive and selective immigration and nationality acts has meant that black immigration with a view to settlement has virtually come to an end (Gordon and Klug 1985).

The circumstances of black men and women from the new Commonwealth (for example, the West Indies, India) indicate the flexibility of the 'universal' discourse of the post-war era. Indispensable for economic growth during the 1950s, they found themselves concentrated in inner-city areas in poor housing (Jones 1970; Cater and Jones 1979), in the lowest stratum of the labour market and forced to take jobs in Britain below their level of qualifications (Castles and Kosack 1973: 110). According to Sarre *et al.* (1989: 7) the 'newcomers were not able to exercise any locational choice, but were instead forced to act as a replacement population, settling in areas where they would not be in direct competition for jobs and housing with the indigenous population'. Public housing authorities made no special provision for housing single immigrant workers and exposed families to discriminatory eligibility criteria in relation to, for example, residential qualification (Rex and Moore 1967; Henderson and Karn 1987). As Smith (1989b: 52) records, only 6 per cent of the overseas-born black population had been accommodated in the local authority sector by the mid-1960s, in contrast to 20 per cent of Irish migrants, and one third of the English-born population.

The housing characteristics and conditions of the black minorities in Britain have certainly changed over the last three decades. There has been a significant tenure shift, with an increase in the number of ethnic minority households entering council housing (especially among the Afro-Caribbean population), and a growth in the proportion of owner-occupiers (especially among Asian communities). There has been some movement of households away from the inner city but as Smith (1989b: 173) comments 'Black owner occupiers – who are disproportionately clustered within the most depressed segment of the housing market – find it increasingly difficult to move to take advantage of the more buoyant sectors of the economy or to realise the capital stored in their homes'. Bangladeshi homeowners, for example, are over-represented in low quality, older, lower value dwellings, have disproportionately high levels of mortgage arrears and are over-represented among those homeowners not in arrears but having difficulties meeting housing costs (ONS 1997a).

Ginsberg (1992b) differentiates between *structural racism* (policy and administrative processes, particularly government immigration and housing policies, and the structure and functioning of the labour market); *institutional racism*, which manifests in 'the policy and administrative processes in local authority housing departments, building societies and estate agents' (Ginsberg 1992b: 109); and *subjective racism*, expressed by individuals as overt racial prejudice. All of these processes combine to create and perpetuate inequality in access to and allocation of housing for black people (see also Dhillon-Kashyap 1994). A number of reports (CRE 1984; Phillips 1986, 1987) have highlighted what Sarre *et al.* (1989: 186) refer to as 'unfair practice by local authority housing departments'. Historically denied access to local authority waiting lists, ethnic minorities and, in particular, women sole parents, are now likely to have access to the worst council housing in the least desirable locations.

The number of Afro-Caribbean households renting from the local authority increased from 2 per cent in 1961 to over 40 per cent throughout most of the late 1970s and 1980s (OPCS 1965; Brown 1984). This increase has tended to be interpreted as the outcome of changes in eligibility criteria and residence requirements and in terms of the class position and bad housing conditions experienced by Afro-Caribbean households. Peach and Byron (1993) argue that class position might explain the tenure pattern of Afro-Caribbean male heads of household, but the tenure patterns of female heads of household is the product of a much more complex interplay of class, gender, racism and family structure. Peach and Byron explain that the substantial over-representation of Caribbean households on council estates is not so much because of class structure but because of gender. Not only are female-headed Afro-Caribbean households concentrated in council housing, but they are also disproportionately located in the least desirable sections – hard-to-let properties on the worst estates. These findings support the earlier work of Mamma (1989) and Rao (1990) who found that black women – who are twice as likely as white women to suffer long periods of home-lessness (Dhillon-Kashyap 1994) – when accepted by a local authority as in 'priority' need, were most likely to be offered bed and breakfast accommo-dation and had to wait longer to be rehoused. Both studies revealed the relative powerlessness of black women to exercise choice in that they were given no opportunity to refuse the first offer of accommodation. According to Peach and Byron (1994) approximately 70 per cent of Afro-Caribbean households occupy flats and maisonettes, compared with 40 per cent of white tenants. They are also more likely to be on higher floors or in base-ments than their white counterparts. This clearly has implications for opportunities to purchase under the Right to Buy policies. Indian and Pakistani households are much less likely to live in council housing but when they do they tend to be in a slightly better position to buy than Afro-Caribbean tenants in that they have usually been allocated houses rather than flats or maisonettes.

Restructuring and redrawing the boundaries of citizenship

As economic conditions deteriorated from around the mid-1970s, the post-war consensus, to which most advanced western countries had subscribed in their own unique ways, began to crumble. According to Pierson (1991: 145), it was the end of uninterrupted post-war economic growth that weakened confidence as 'governments throughout the developed west were simul-taneously failing to achieve the four major economic policy objectives – growth, low inflation, full employment and balance of trade – on which the post-war order had been based'.

The institutional arrangements of the post-war period which had sup-ported specific configurations of citizenship were increasingly perceived as barriers and impediments to the deploying of new methods of production and consumption, while labour contracts and social legislation inhibited effective competition both within nation-states and in the increasingly important international markets. By the mid-1970s Australia, Britain and Germany had all abandoned Keynesianism and adopted a reconstructed political agenda. The political rhetoric of this period encompassed deregulation, privatization, the efficiency of the 'free market' and rolling back the frontiers of the state. The emergence of this alternative policy discourse has been accompanied by changes in the way citizenship is being constructed. According to Twine (1994: 42) the social rights of citizenship have been replaced by the 'civil rights of contract'. As the content of citizenship has changed so has the discursive context. The concern has moved from social rights to obligation and contract, epitomized in the *Citizen's Charter* in Britain. The 'consumer' and the 'active citizen' fit the ideological context of the market, which emphasizes individual responsibility and action.

Restructuring and rationalization have tended to reinforce social divisions with a shift towards greater inequality and an acceptance of much higher levels of unemployment, poverty and homelessness. Policies of the post-war era were aimed at preserving jobs, providing housing for the majority of the population, and maintaining the existing social structure. More recently there has been a recognition of a fragmented and individualized society in which the certainties of the past have given way to insecurity, risk (Albertson 1988; Beck 1992) and growing inequality since the 1980s. Of the three countries under discussion a recent study by Hills indicated that Britain had experienced the greatest rise in inequality followed by Australia, with a slightly less substantial rise in West Germany (Hills 1995: 66–7). In all three countries there has been a growth in long-term unemployment and a greater reliance on more basic forms of social assistance, particularly amongst young people and ethnic minority groups (Healey 1997).

Retrenchment and reorientation have been universal phenomena, but the precise form between countries has varied significantly. A given mode of integration and citizenship configuration will be influenced by the institutional arrangements of previous regimes and will also be a response to pressure from interest groups. In Britain, following the victory of the Thatcher government in 1979, government strategy, according to Krieger (1991: 53) involved 'a co-ordinated assault, with electoral appeals, policy agendas, and discourse united to reconstitute common sense, redefine the nation, and shatter traditional Labourist-collectivist solidarities'. The structural and institutional reforms regarding trade unions, the welfare state and supply-side economics and individualism have been more far-reaching than in either Australia or Germany.

In Australia, Keating introduced 'Working Nation' (1994) which proposed a different role for social policy and indicated the dismantling of the protective measures which had ensured high levels of employment and maintained the 'wage earners' welfare state'. According to Jones, strategies of economic rationalism (Pusey 1991) incorporating privatization and de-regulation, were embraced 'regardless of their effects on employment and wages. Government accepted the case for free trade and extensive structural change in the economy' (Jones 1996: 29).

The strength of the trade union movement in Australia and the insti-tutionalized system of state reconciliation and arbitration meant that the eventual outcome, according to Castles (1993: 9), was a 'hybrid and uneasy combination of economic rationalist solutions for freeing up markets and corporatist negotiation to buy-off trade union dissent'.

In Germany the Christian-liberal rhetoric of deregulation and a 'new realism' has dominated politics. However, the very strength of the insti-tutional arrangements through which the state sought to distance itself from the political domain has prevented any substantial dismantling of the forms established during the post-war period, as the voluntary sector, the church and the trade unions have become strong, influential and entrenched interest groups. Craft and industrial workers have maintained their numerical pos-ition in the labour force and remain a dominant class force. However some change in the balance of power between capital and labour has occurred and negotiations focusing on the introduction of a new flexibility in the organiz-ation of the labour market have become the focus of class struggle. Never-theless, elements of the neo-liberal strategy have penetrated the framework of cooperative federalism, as the rights of trade unions have been eroded, the non-profit housing sector has been deregulated, and notions of status differ-entials, rather than citizenship, have been strengthened in relation to social rights.

Housing and urban policy have been at the forefront of strategies aimed at marketization and liberalization in both Britain and Germany, while in Australia the emphasis on home ownership indicates continuity rather than change. As deregulation and privatization have become policy instruments in both Britain and Germany access to affordable housing has become increasingly difficult. In both countries the availability of social rented housing has diminished as a result of transfer to home ownership in Britain and the private rented sector in Germany. In Britain this has been ac-companied by the gradual reduction in the construction of local authority dwellings and an actual decline in the availability of council housing to rent for the first time since 1919 (Malpass and Murie 1987). By the beginning of the 1980s one third of all British households were still in the public sector, a situation that was to change following the introduction of the 1980 Housing Act and subsequent legislation. Since 1980 the number of local authority dwellings has fallen (by 2.2 million) through sales to sitting tenants and other transfers. More recently sales have been bolstered by Large Scale Voluntary Transfers, as dwellings are transferred from local authorities, usually to housing associations (ONS 1997b), who are envisaged as the future providers of social housing with local authorities confined to the role of strategic enablers.

A number of developments have occurred in the old *Bundeslander* (West German regional states) which have given rise to concern about the shortage of low-cost housing, referred to as the *Wohnungsnot* in Germany. A decline in the construction of new homes, lack of investment, policies of renovation which increased the living space for some while decreasing the amount of overall rental space, rising rents and the decline in the number of rent-controlled dwellings have all contributed to a worsening housing situation in Germany. Figures for 1994 suggest the need for 2.5 million units, including 1 million in the former GDR. An annual rate of construction of 500,000 homes is considered necessary to meet current needs (Comite Europeen de Coordination de l'Habitat Social 1994).

In the former GDR, old forms of social benefits have been dismantled (such as low cost housing and child care) while new types of social benefits (such as housing allowances) have been introduced to cushion the impact of 'enforced deindustrialization' and increased rents. Prior to unification large housing subsidies meant that rents in the GDR covered only one third of all housing costs and represented only 3–5 per cent of average income. In 1989 the housing programme, combined with management and maintenance costs, required an annual subsidy of 14 million marks, representing 10 per cent of national income (Knowles 1989). In October 1990 all state-provided and socially owned housing became the responsibility of limited dividend housing companies and housing cooperatives, subject to federal German law. Two years later rents had risen fourfold to approximately 12 per cent of income as subsidies were removed and attempts were made to cover management and maintenance costs in full (Power 1993). Despite a commitment to modernization and new construction a large percentage of the housing stock is now dilapidated and lacking in basic amenities, particularly in the 47 per cent of the stock built prior to 1919. Nearly a quarter of all dwellings have no internal toilet and 18 per cent have no bath or shower (*Der Spiegel* 1991). Deterioration and dilapidation permeates the housing stock and municipalities, experiencing financial crisis, are consequently keen to privatize it. The large social housing sector is therefore being transformed through privatization policies into home ownership, private renting and claims for restitution on older stock.

There are estimated to be around 1.8 million people either homeless or inadequately housed in the unified Germany. In the West, although the constitution incorporates a commitment to a decent home for all, the main emphasis has been on police law (*Polizgesetz*) or social welfare law (*Bundessozialhilfgezetz*), the former usually applied to single people, the latter to families. In the Länder of the former West Germany an estimated 50,000 women were homeless in 1992 (Geiger 1992), with more women than ever sleeping rough. Although increasing participation in the labour market has increased employment and housing opportunities for some, for others economic and housing insecurity have become commonplace (Bondi 1991). As gentrification diminishes the supply of affordable rented housing and hostel provision continues to cater predominantly to the traditional image of the homeless single male, so the options and choices for women have diminished. Housing problems in the East are estimated to be worse than in the West as stock is transferred to the private sector and subsidies are removed. It appears that 'whether Halle or Erfurt, Leipzig or Schwerin – for the first time in 40 years many communities in the East have discovered homelessness' (*Der Spiegel* 1992: 80). In the early 1990s in the new Länder (regional states of the former East, now in unified Germany) around 200,000 people were estimated to be homeless.

Germany faces major challenges and the drawing of the boundaries of citizenship is likely to be hotly contested. Population inflows, the legacy of major housing problems in the former GDR, the shrinking of the social rented sector as stock is transferred to the market and the rising rents in the deregulated private rented sector have contributed to a situation in which it is much more difficult for many people, particularly those on low incomes, to fulfil their housing needs.

Governments in Australia and Britain have consistently shown a commitment to promoting home ownership as 'the badge of citizenship' and have had considerable success. Home-ownership rates in Britain jumped from 55 per cent at the end of 1979 to 68 per cent in 1992. The prospects in Britain and Australia in the 1990s for many mortgage borrowers have been somewhat different than in the past. The expansion of owner occupation in Britain, supported over the past couple of decades by the sale of stock from the public sector (accounting for 46 per cent of home ownership growth between 1981 and 1991 (Forrest and Murie 1994) has included a greater proportion of those on lower and less secure incomes, vulnerable to changing economic circumstances and more sensitive to the impact of volatile interest rates. Lower- and middle-income households have found it more difficult to meet their rising housing costs. Negative equity, mortgage arrears and repossessions have become more commonplace in both countries. In Australia the erosion of the strategy of 'domestic defence' and the 'wage earners' welfare state', ensuring full (white male) employment and a 'fair wage' has undermined the institutional basis on which mass-mortgaged home ownership was developed. Increasingly, single people in Britain and Australia have experienced constrained choice in housing systems which are oriented towards 'family' households, and have faced difficulties in societies where the idealized tenure – owner occupation – increasingly requires two incomes to enter and sustain it (Smith 1990: 68). The German housing market has operated in a very different environment to that in Britain and Australia. Fixed-rate loans, lower levels of gearing and substantial deposits are the norm in Germany, with first-time buyers usually in their late 30s and early 40s (Muellbauer 1992). The relatively low rate of return in housing has not created the same opportunities for speculation and the accumulation of wealth as it has in Australia and Britain.

Conclusion

This chapter has considered the nature of the state and the social relations of welfare in a historical and cross-national perspective in order to show that citizenship has been shaped by ideology, historical legacy and social struggle relating to issues of class, race, ethnicity and gender. The boundaries of citizenship interact not only with class struggle, but with other forms of social power such as racism and patriarchy. The significance and constitution of these social relations changes over time and place and such relations are institutionalized through the nation state and its articulation with the inclusionary/exclusionary boundaries of citizenship.

Ideals of nationhood encompass notions such as unity, commonality and equality but these occur within a context in which the policies and discursive practices attached to the provision of social rights are exclusionary and/or differentiated along the lines of class, race and gender. Thus citizenship for some can be partial and discriminatory. As Bovenkerk *et al.* (1990: 487) have argued: '... the degree of exclusion and the mechanisms by which exclusion is effected may not differ a great deal from one country to another, but the discourse does. This reflects separate national traditions and sensitivities and this needs to be clearly grasped conceptually and analytically'.

The Keynesian era of welfare capitalism was experienced in different ways in Britain, Germany and Australia, as a result of the differences in the balance of class forces and cultural and political traditions and expectations. The principle of universalism and the rhetoric surrounding the notion of citizenship was, in all three countries, more an ideal than a reality. For many women and black people access to full citizenship was an illusion. The boundaries of citizenship were drawn in such a way as to deny opportunity to exercise the social rights of citizenship and instead offer only institutionalized second-class status in relation to the labour market and welfare services, or complete exclusion.

More recently, restructuring processes, the reorientation of the welfare state and a redefining of citizen/state relations have resulted in a worsening of living standards for a substantial minority of people, particularly for minority groups and single parents. There has been an increased prevalence of dispossessed and impoverished populations to be found in many urban areas. The pattern of social integration and citizenship seems to be one in which more people will be at risk of poverty and constrained in the pursuit of full participation in the norms of society. Yet differentiated citizenship could be inclusionary and empowering. As the meaning of citizenship becomes more complex and the role of the nation state is diluted by the increasing number of supranational organizations in a new global order, there is potential for people to find new meanings and interpretations to the concept of citizenship, and alternative sites of struggle through which to emphasize the complementarity rather than the contradictions between difference and equality in the construction of social rights.

References

Albertson, N. (1988) Postmodernism, post-Fordism and critical social theory. *Environment and Planning D: Society and Space*, 6: 339–65.
Baubock, R. (1991) Migration and citizenship. *New Community*, 18: 27–48.
Beck, U. (1992) *Risk Society: Towards a New Modernity*. London: Sage.
Bondi, L. (1991) Women, gender relations and the inner city, in M. Keith and A. Rogers (eds) *Hollow Promises? Rhetoric and Reality in the Inner City*. London: Mansell.
Bovenkerk, F., Miles, R. and Verbunt, G. (1990) Racism, migration and the state in Western Europe: a case for comparative analysis. *International Sociology*, 5: 475–90.
Brown, C. (1984) *Black and White Britain*. Aldershot: Gower.
Brubaker, W.R. (1989) Immigration, citizenship and the nation-state in France and Germany: a comparative historical analysis. *International Sociology*, 5: 379–407.
Bryson, L. (1992) *Welfare and the State*. London: Macmillan.
Castles, F. (1993) *Families of Nations: Patterns of Public Policy in Western Democracies*. Dartmouth: Aldershot.
Castles, F. and Mitchell, D. (1992) Three worlds of welfare capitalism or four? *Governances*, 5: 1–26.
Castles, F.G. (1988) *Australian Public Policy and Economic Vulnerability*. Sydney: Allen and Unwin.
Castles, S., and Kosack, G. (1973) *Immigrant Workers and Class Structure in Western Europe*. London: Harper & Row.
Castles, S., Kalantzis, M., Cope, B. and Morrissey, M. (1992) *Mistaken Identity: Multiculturalism and the Demise of Nationalism in Australia*. Sydney: Pluto Press.
Cater, J. and Jones, T. (1979) Ethnic residential space: the case of Asians in Bradford. *Tidjschrift voor Economische en Sociale Geographie*, 70: 86–97.
Chamberlayne, P. (1994) Women and social policy, in J. Clasen and R. Freeman (eds) *Social Policy in Germany*. London: Harvester Wheatsheaf.
Comite Europeen de Coordination de l'Habitat Social (1994) *Germany*. News bulletin no. 1, Paris: l'Observatoire Europeen du Logement Social.
CRE (Committee for Racial Equality) (1984) *Race and Council Housing in Hackney: Report of a Formal Investigation*. London: CRE Publications.
Der Spiegel (1991) 41: 158–60.
Der Spiegel (1992) 6: 80.
Dhillon-Kashyap, P. (1994) Black women and housing, in R. Gilroy and R. Woods (eds) *Housing Women*. London: Routledge.

Dienemann, O. (1993) Housing Problems in the former German Democratic Republic and the 'New German states', in G. Hallett (ed.) *The New Housing Shortage: Housing Affordability in Europe and the USA*. London: Routledge.

Esping-Andersen, G. (1990) *The Three Worlds of Welfare Capitalism*. Cambridge: Polity Press.

Finer, M. (1974) *Report of the Committee on One-parent Families*. Cmnd. 5629. London: HMSO

Forrest, R. and Murie, A. (1983) Residualisation and council housing: aspects of the changing social relations of housing tenure. *Journal of Social Policy*, 12: 453–68.

Forrest, R. and Murie, A. (1994) Home ownership in recession. *Housing Studies*, 8: 227–40.

Geiger, M. (1992) Understanding the relationship between welfare and extreme poverty: the example of homeless single women. *Fraunforschung*, Institut Frau und Gesellschaft 10 Jahrgang, Heft 1 & 2: 6–18.

Giddens, A. (1982) Class division, class conflict and citizenship rights, in A. Giddens (ed.) *Profiles and Critiques in Social Theory*. London: Macmillan.

Ginsberg, N. (1992a) *Divisions of Welfare: A Critical Introduction to Comparative Social Policy*. London: Sage.

Ginsberg, N. (1992b) Racism and housing: concepts and reality, in P. Braham, A. Rattsani and R. Skellington (eds) *Racism and Anti-Racism: Inequalities, Opportunities and Policies*. London: Sage/Open University.

Gordon, P. and Klug, F. (1985) *Immigration: A Brief Guide*. London: Runneymede Trust.

Harloe, M. (1981) The recommodification of housing, in M. Harloe and E. Lebas (eds) *City, Class and Capital*. London: Edward Arnold.

Healey, K. (ed.) (1997) *Poverty in Australia*. Balmain, NSW, Australia: The Spinney Press.

Henderson, J. and Karn, V. (1987) *Race, Class and State Housing: Inequality and the Allocation of Public Housing in Britain*. Aldershot: Gower.

Heppel, M. (ed.) (1979) *A Black Reality: Aboriginal Camps and Housing in Remote Australia*. Canberra: Australian Institute of Aboriginal Studies.

Hills, J. (1995) *Joseph Rowntree Foundation Inquiry into Income and Wealth*. York: Joseph Rowntree Foundation.

Jacobs, S. (1985) Race, empire and the welfare state: council housing and racism. *Critical Social Policy*, 13: 6–40.

Jaedicke, W. and Wollmann, H. (1990) Federal Republic of Germany, in W. van Vliet (ed.) *International Handbook of Housing Policies and Practices*. London: Greenwood Press.

Jayasuriya, L. (1991) Citizenship, democratic pluralism and ethnic minorities in Australia, in R. Nile (ed.) *Immigration and the politics of ethnicity and race in Australia and Britain*. London: Sir Robert Menzies Centre for Australian Studies, University of London.

Jones, M. (1996) *The Australian Welfare State*. St Leanards, NSW, Australia: Allen & Unwin.

Jones, P. (1970) Some aspects of the changing distribution of the coloured population in Birmingham 1961–6. *Transactions of the Institute of British Geographers*, 50: 199.

Keating, P. (1994) *Working Nation: The White Paper on Employment and Growth.* Canberra: AGPS.

Knowles, A. (1989) The other side of the wall. *Housing Review*, 38, July–August: 106–8.

Krieger, J. (1991) Class, consumption and collectivism: perspectives on the Labour Party and electoral competition in Britain, in F. Fox Piven (ed.) *Labour Parties in Post-Industrial Societies.* Cambridge: Polity Press.

Langan, M. and Ostner, I. (1991) Gender and welfare: towards a comparative framework, in G. Room (ed.) *Towards a European welfare state.* Bristol: SAUS Publications.

Lash, S. (1994) The Making of an underclass: neo-liberalism versus corporatism, in P. Brown and R. Crompton (eds) *Economic Restructuring and Social Exclusion.* London: UCL Press.

Le Dem, J. (1991) The costs of German reunification. *Contemporary European Affairs*, 4(2/3): 88–100.

Lund, B. (1996) *Housing Problems and Housing Policy.* London: Longman.

Malpass, P. and Murie, A. (1987) *Housing Policy and Practice*, 2nd edn. Basingstoke: Macmillan.

Mamma, A. (1989) *The Hidden Struggle.* London: London Race and Housing Research.

Mann, M. (1987) Ruling-class strategies and citizenship. *Sociology*, 21: 339–54.

Marshall, T.H. (1950) *Citizenship and Social Class.* Cambridge: Cambridge University Press.

Möller, R. (1989) Reconstructing the family in reconstruction Germany. *Feminist Studies*, 15: 137–69.

Muellbauer, J. (1992) Anglo-German differences in housing market dynamics: the role of institutions and macroeconomic policy. *European Economic Review*, 36: 539–548.

OECD (Organisation for Economic Cooperation and Development) (1992) Labour market reforms in Central and Eastern Europe and the rise of unemployment. *Employment Outlook*. Paris: OECD.

ONS (Office for National Statistics) (1997a) *Ethnic Minorities.* London: Stationery Office.

ONS (Office for National Statistics) (1997b) *Social Trends*, vol. 27. London: Stationery Office.

OPCS (1965) *Census 1961, England and Wales.* London: Commonwealth Immigrants in the Conurbations.

Orloff, A. (1995) Gender in the liberal welfare states: Australia, the United Kingdom and the United States. Conference paper, ISA Research Committee 19 conference 'Comparative Research on Welfare State Reforms', University of Pavia, Italy, 14–17 September.

Ostner, I. (1993) Slow motion: women, work and the family in Germany, in J. Lewis (ed.) *Women and Social Policies in Europe: Work, Family and the State.* Aldershot: Edward Elgar.

Pateman, C. (1989) *The Disorder of Women.* Cambridge: Polity Press.

Peach, C. and Byron, M. (1993) Caribbean tenants in council housing: race, class and gender. *New Community*, 19: 407–23.

Peach, C. and Byron, M. (1994) Council house sales, residualisation and Afro-Caribbean tenants. *Journal of Social Policy*, 23: 363–83.

Pearson, N. (1995) An optimist's vision, in N. Pearson and W. Sanders *Indigenous Peoples and Reshaping Australian Institutions: Two Perspectives*. Discussion paper no. 102. Canberra: Centre for Aboriginal Economic Policy Research, ANU.

Pearson, N. and Sanders, W. (1995) *Indigenous Peoples and Reshaping Australian Institutions: Two Perspectives*. Discussion paper no. 102. Canberra: Centre for Aboriginal Economic Policy Research, ANU.

Phillips, D.A. (1986) The institutionalisation of racism in housing: towards an explanation, in S. Smith and J. Mercer (eds) *New Perspectives in Race and Housing*. Glasgow: University of Glasgow.

Phillips, D.A. (1987) *What Price Equality? A Report on the Allocation of GLC Housing in Tower Hamlets*. GLC Housing Research and Policy Report No. 9: London: GLC.

Pierson, C. (1991) *Beyond the Welfare State? The New Political Economy of Welfare*. Oxford: Polity Press.

Power, A. (1993) *Hovels to High Rise. State Housing in Europe since 1850*. London: Routledge.

Pusey, M. (1991) *Economic Rationalism in Canberra: A Nation-building State Changes its Mind*. Cambridge: Cambridge University Press.

Rao, N. (1990) *Black Women in Public Housing*. London: London Race and Housing Research Unit, Black Women in Housing Group.

Rex, J. and Moore, R. (1967) *Race, Community and Conflict*. Oxford: Oxford University Press.

Rosenberg, D. J. (1991) Shock therapy: GDR women in transition from a socialist welfare state to a social market economy. *Signs: Journal of Women in Culture and Society*, 17: 129–52.

Sanders, W. (1993) Aboriginal Housing, in C. Paris (ed.) *Housing Australia*. South Melbourne: Macmillan.

Sarre, P., Phillips, D. and Skellington, R. (1989) *Ethnic Minority Housing: Explanations and Policies*. Aldershot: Avebury.

Smith, S. J. (1989a) Society, space and citizenship: a human geography for the 'new times'? *Transactions of the Institute of British Geographers*, 14: 144–56.

Smith, S. J. (1989b) *The Politics of 'Race' and Residence*. Cambridge: Polity Press.

Smith, S. J. (1990) Income, housing, wealth and gender inequality. *Urban Studies*, 27: 67–88.

Social Charter of the GDR (1990) *Resolution of the Volkskammer of the German Democratic Republic*, 7 March, Berlin.

Sommerville, P. (1994) Homelessness policy in Britain. *Policy and Politics*, 22: 163–78.

Tomlinson, J. (1996) Citizenship and sovereignty. *Australian Journal of Social Issues*, 31: 2–18.

Troy, P. (1991) *The Benefits of Owner Occupation*, working paper no. 29. Canberra: Urban Research Programme, ANU.

Twine, F. (1994) *Citizenship and Social Rights*. London: Sage.

Williams, F. (1994) Social relations, welfare and the post-Fordism debate, in B. Loader and R. Burrows (eds) *Towards a Post-Fordist Welfare State?* London: Routledge.

Wilpert, C. (1983) From guestworkers to immigrants: migrant workers and their families in the FRG. *New Community*, 11: 137–42.

Wilpert, C. (1991) Migration and ethnicity in a non-immigrant country: foreigners in a united Germany. *New Community*, 18: 49–62.

Winkler, G. (ed.) (1990) *Sozialreport '90: Daten und Fakten zur sozialen Lage in der DDR*. Berlin: Die Wirtschaft.

Winkler, G. (1994) Social policies at a crossroads, in M.D. Hancock and H.A. Welsh (eds) *German Unification: Processes and Outcomes*. Boulder, CO: Westview Press.

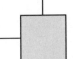

3

Housing policy, citizenship and social exclusion

Peter Lee

Introduction

In Britain there is a renewed concern about social inequality and multiple deprivation. New and wider divisions in contemporary British society are seen as having serious social, economic and political consequences (Hills 1995). In a period of economic change some sections of the community have not shared in rising incomes and wealth, and the economic, demographic, social and welfare restructuring which has occurred since the mid-1970s has left a wider gap between those on the highest incomes and those on the lowest (HMSO 1993). These trends have been repeated in other nation states both within and outside the European Union (Esping-Andersen 1990), and are alternatively explained by changes in the mode of regulation of capital, the drive towards flexible labour markets (Kennett 1994) and the fragmentation of welfare states in line with the globalization of capital (Jordan 1997).

Increasing polarization and inequality has rekindled interest in the spatial pattern of deprivation. Social and economic changes at the national and global level are increasingly being translated into spatial differences, with more visible boundaries being created within cities and regions. In the United States, some have viewed these divisions as posing a threat to the stability of society and the emergence of an underclass (Wilson 1987; Murray 1990). In Europe, the emergence of the term 'social exclusion' mirrors this, especially where the focus is upon excluded groups and communities (Room 1995a), and there is a concern that certain sections of society are being cut off from the mainstream. This emphasis echoes a concern that fragmentation of the welfare state and increasing inequalities are having negative spatial outcomes.

More important, however, is the emphasis and policy proposals that result from this analysis. The use of spatial urban policies to combat social exclusion is increasingly seen as the most effective strategy. For example, in England the Single Regeneration Budget (SRB) put a greater emphasis on local priorities and local involvement, and on tackling the needs of the most deprived areas. The statement by the minister for regions, Richard Caborn, illustrates how parts of the city are equated with social exclusion: 'The SRB is one of our most useful tools for tackling social exclusion – pockets of need which may not be targeted in main programmes' (DoE 1997: 1). Similarly, the new British Labour government announced a special task force to combat the worst aspects of social exclusion and in the process emphasized particular estates and parts of cities to be targeted (Mandelson 1997). The measurement of deprivation and its relationship to policy is also becoming increasingly salient in other areas of government. For example, the allocation of resources to local authorities under the Housing Investment Programme (HIP) changed again from a wholly discretionary system to one where 50 per cent is based on housing deprivation (DoE 1997b).

Emerging in the face of increasing polarization and inequality, therefore, are policy prescriptions to combat poverty and social exclusion that have an explicitly spatial focus. The role that housing policy can play in combating social exclusion, where the focus is on particular parts of the city, will be increasingly emphasized. What is contested, however, is how changing definitions of poverty and social exclusion link to notions of citizenship and how this is best represented by social policy (Levitas 1996; Jordan 1997) and the best way in which deprivation or social exclusion can be measured spatially (Lee et al. 1995). Moreover, the way in which housing is perceived as contributing to social exclusion – particularly the way tenure is used in the research process – will significantly influence this agenda as well as influencing the design of effective policies and our understanding of how social exclusion persists over time.

This chapter attempts to address some of these issues by locating housing in the debate on deprivation and poverty. Within this debate there needs to be a separation between housing deprivation per se and the processes of disadvantage that result from the consumption and distribution of housing (Murie 1983). After considering housing deprivation, the chapter, therefore, turns attention to how housing connects to European debates on social exclusion and how social exclusion reflects attempts at refocusing the concept of social citizenship within the framework set out by T.H. Marshall (Marshall and Bottomore 1992). What emerges is the way in which spatial aspects of social exclusion connect to housing conditions and consumption. Housing has not featured as prominently as it might warrant in debates about poverty, but concern with the relational elements of space and exclusion should see housing located more centrally in these debates.

Relative housing 'deprivation' and housing poverty

Historically, because of the links between housing and community health, measures of adverse physical housing conditions have been used to compare the empirical associations between housing, deprivation and poverty. In Britain adverse physical conditions normally refer to one of four measures:

1 Housing that is unfit for human habitation or below tolerable standards (BTS).
2 Housing in disrepair.
3 Housing that lacks basic amenities such as a bath/shower or toilet.
4 Overcrowded housing.

The worst of these aspects of housing deprivation had been radically transformed by the mid-1970s and the number of households exposed to poor housing conditions showed a major decline in Britain. The problems faced by those with least choice and bargaining power in the housing market are, therefore, very different today than in the past. Changing definitions of housing deprivation and its relative nature are reflected in changes in the way housing deprivation is measured. The 1951 census did not include a question on housing tenure and the only question relating to housing deprivation referred to the presence of an internal hot or cold running tap. For the first time, the 1991 census of population asked respondents whether their home had central heating. As almost 100 per cent of dwellings in the UK have access to hot and cold running water the question was not repeated in 1991. Meanwhile, as Table 3.1 shows, the last three population censuses have shown a consistent and dramatic decline in the proportion of households experiencing all the main recorded housing deprivations.

Table 3.1 Percentage of households experiencing housing deprivation, Great Britain 1971–91

Housing deprivation	1971	1981	1990
Lacking WC (toilet)	1	–	–
Lacking bath or shower	9	2	1
Lacking central heating	65	41	22
Overcrowding[1]	9	5	3

[1] Below bedroom standard: number of rooms divided by number of people standardizing for age and mix of children's sex.

Source: HMSO (1992: 149, 241.)

However, these traditional 'housing deprivations' have not been elim-
inated. For example, although overcrowding is low by historical standards,
0.5 million people continue to live at a density of more than 1.5 persons per
room (OPCS 1991a). Regional variations mean that overcrowding is most
strongly associated with inner city and metropolitan areas such as Inner
London, the North West of England, Birmingham and the larger Scottish
cities. For example, nine of the ten local authorities with the severest problems of overcrowding (households with more than one person per room) are
London Boroughs (OPCS 1991b). In addition Glasgow, Manchester, Black-
burn and Birmingham all have significant problems: for certain wards in
these cities the rate of overcrowding was between eight and fourteen times
the average of less than 2 per cent for Great Britain as a whole (OPCS 1991b).

Regional variations also persist with housing conditions. In 1991 some 1.4
million dwellings in England (7.1 per cent of the stock) were regarded as
unfit due to structural inadequacies leading to damp, condensation or
subsidence. In Northern Ireland where 7.5 per cent (41,000) of the stock
was unfit, the proportion was similar to England. In Wales, problems of unfit
housing are more prevalent with almost one in seven homes unfit (151,000).
Figures for Scotland appear to be lower (4.7 per cent) because of differences
in the measurement of housing fitness (Leather and Morrison 1997).

Reasons given for the unfitness of housing differ according to evidence
from the separate house conditions surveys for England, Scotland, Wales
and Northern Ireland. Dampness, for example is less of a problem in
England than in the other countries cited. Just over 22 per cent of unfit
housing in England was due to problems of dampness, whereas in the other
countries the figures were 49 per cent, 38 per cent and 51 per cent respectively (Leather and Morrison 1997). Geographically the highest rates of unfit
private sector dwellings are in local authorities in South Wales, rural areas of
Cornwall and a corridor running north from High Peak through central
Lancashire to the North of England. The Highlands and Islands of Scotland
also register large proportions of unfit private sector dwellings as measured
by BTS (Leather and Morrison 1997).

However, using housing deprivation alone as a guide to generalized disadvantage or poverty can be erroneous. Demographic factors such as
changes in household size and household type as well as income poverty
need to be taken into account. An issue of concern, therefore, is the role
that life cycle and demography plays in housing and deprivation and how
far different indicators of housing and generalized poverty coincide. In
terms of demography the numbers suffering multiple housing deprivation[1]
between 1971 and 1991 declined for all household types. Thus, whilst
more than one in five households with children suffered multiple housing

---

[1] Households experiencing more than one of the following housing deprivation indicators:
overcrowded housing, shared access to dwelling space, and shared amenities.

Table 3.2 Percentage of households with multiple housing deprivation, Great Britain, 1971–91

Type of household	1971	1981	1991
Pensioner couple	2.0	0.5	0.1
Single pensioner	6.3	1.9	0.5
Couple with children	23.3	8.6	0.9
Couple with no children	11.3	4.4	1.0
Single with children	19.5	3.6	1.2
Single person	16.7	6.8	3.0

Source: Dale et al. 1996, Tables 4.3, 4.4 and 9.5.

deprivation in 1971 this had declined to less than one in a hundred by 1991 (see Table 3.2).

Demographic change has led to smaller household sizes which has reduced problems of overcrowding and thereby led to a reduction in housing deprivation. The proportion of households of different types suffering multiple deprivation has decreased so significantly that it is single-person households (below pensionable age) that are now at greatest risk. Partly this is attributable to a rise in student numbers indicated by the proportion of economically active young people in work dropping from 92 per cent to 73 per cent over the period 1973–92 (HMSO 1995), but also represented amongst this group are a growing percentage of households living in private rented accommodation, many on low incomes due to a decline in value of benefits, student grants and 'entry-level' wages (HMSO 1995).

Table 3.3 Household type by income and housing deprivation, Great Britain, 1979–91

% whose family type is:	Bottom 10% of income distribution (after housing costs)		Households in multiple housing deprivation	
	1979 (%)	1991 (%)	1981 (%)	1991 (%)
Pensioner couple	20	6	3	2
Single pensioner	11	5	7	6
Couple with children	41	49	46	27
Couple with no children	9	11	18	20
Single with children	9	11	8	10
Single person	10	18	18	35
Total	100	100	100	100

Source: Dale et al. 1996, Tables 4.4 and 9.5; DSS 1993, Table D1 (AHC).

When income poverty and its relationship to housing deprivation is taken into account then the picture becomes more complex. Table 3.3 shows what proportion of the lowest income decile are represented by a range of different household types and what proportion of households in multiple housing deprivation are of each type. For example, families (couples with children) represent a growing proportion of the *income poor* – 49 per cent of all households in the lowest decile in 1991 were families with children compared to 41 per cent in 1979. Yet, such households are increasingly less likely to figure amongst those suffering the worst aspects of *housing deprivation* as they represent 27 per cent of all households suffering multiple housing deprivation in 1991 compared to almost half of such households in 1981. Meanwhile, (due to lower wages for entry-level occupations) single person households have taken up an increasing proportion of households in the lowest 10 per cent of household incomes and at the same time they have tended to occupy the worst dwelling types. Between 1981 and 1991 their representation among households suffering multiple housing deprivation rose from 18 per cent to 35 per cent.

Due to the interaction between benefits, employment and housing policy, housing tenure has increasingly served as a framework for understanding the relationship between housing and deprivation and housing and income poverty. The residualization of council housing has meant that the debate concerning the relationship between income poverty and housing has focused upon the relationship between tenure and poverty. However, while the residualization of council housing has served as a focus for the relationship between poverty and housing since 1979 (and the sale of council housing), the process was well under way before then. For example, in 1967 almost half (45 per cent) of households in receipt of means-tested social assistance benefits (supplementary benefit) were council tenants. By 1971 this figure had risen to 52 per cent and by 1979 it had exceeded 60 per cent. During this period the proportion of the housing stock which was council housing had risen only very slightly – from 29 per cent in 1967 to 32 per cent in 1979 (Murie 1983: 187–8).

The process of residualization and income polarization has continued after 1979. Demographic changes such as smaller household sizes and a growth in one-parent families coupled with a polarization in the income structure have resulted in a concentration of the poorest sections of the community in council housing. Between 1980 and 1991 the percentage of households with incomes in the bottom decile of British household incomes living in council housing increased from 17 to 30 per cent (HMSO 1983; 1992). These trends are explained by the increasing proportion of council tenants dependent upon state benefits and the decline in the value of state pensions and benefits which have not kept pace with inflation or earnings growth.

In discussing the residualization of council housing, however, it is important to recognize two related features of housing deprivation that shape the debate: housing deprivation, when analysed by tenure, is more of a relative problem in the private rented sector and more of an absolute problem in the owner-occupied sector; and regional trends in residualization mean that what is happening to the council housing tenure across the country is not always going to be apparent in what is happening to different cities or neighbourhoods. Therefore, despite the residualization of council housing and the funnelling of the poorest households into the social rented sector, it is the private rented sector that continues to represent the worst aspects of housing deprivation. For example, more than one in ten households in the private (furnished) rented sector share amenities and more than half of unfurnished rented households have no central heating. Meanwhile, levels of housing deprivation (no central heating and shared amenities) amongst households renting from a local authority are considerably lower at 24.4 per cent and less than 1 per cent respectively (see Table 3.4).

Regional variations in housing deprivation by tenure depart significantly from national trends. For example, while for Great Britain as a whole the proportion of council tenants with no central heating was less than a quarter (OPCS 1991b), only 13 per cent of council tenants in the London Borough of Tower Hamlets had no central heating compared to more than half (53 per cent) of such households in Liverpool. Furthermore, the role that different tenures play in housing different ethnic groups combined with the inter-action between employment and material deprivation, provides significant data on regional variations of deprivation by tenure. Table 3.5 presents evidence from four major urban areas which demonstrates this relationship forcefully. In Birmingham, Bradford and Liverpool the majority of the non-white population suffering each of the types of deprivation shown are not living in council housing. For example, less than 8 per cent of Bradford's

Table 3.4   Tenure by housing deprivation, Great Britain, 1991

	No central heating (%)	Shared amenities (%)	Overcrowding (>1 person per room) (%)
Owned outright	18.4	0.1	0.6
Buying	11.2	<0.1	0.2
Private rented furnished	33.5	10.5	5.0
Private rented unfurnished	50.0	1.4	2.1
Rented with job	21.3	0.8	2.3
Housing association	19.1	1.4	3.0
Local authority	24.4	0.5	4.0
Scottish homes	27.5	0.1	5.0
Great Britain	18.4	0.6	2.3

Source: OPCS 1991b.

Table 3.5 Percentage of all non-white households (by measures of deprivation) living in council housing

	% of each category living in council housing			
Non-white headed households with:	Tower Hamlets	Birmingham	Liverpool	Bradford
No earner in household	83.9	35.8	23.0	7.8
No car	79.8	33.7	30.3	9.5
Long-term illness in household	84.7	22.0	18.2	8.7
Head of household unemployed	82.1	29.9	27.8	9.6

Source: Lee and Murie 1997.

non-white headed households with no earner live in council housing, whereas almost 84 per cent of such households in Tower Hamlets live in council housing.

When comparing white headed households to households headed by a member of a minority ethnic group the differences in the tenure characteristics within cities are more clearly highlighted. Whereas Table 3.5 showed that in Bradford less than 10 per cent of the non-white population without a car live in council housing, for the white population in the same city 35.2 per cent of households without a car live in the sector (see Table 3.6).

These data indicate that the polarization between tenures for different

Table 3.6 Percentage of all white households (by measures of deprivation) living in council housing

	% of each category living in council housing			
White headed households with:	Tower Hamlets	Liverpool	Birmingham	Bradford
No earner in household	70.0	41.4	41.2	30.6
No car	66.4	45.7	42.3	35.2
Long-term illness in household	71.0	39.3	36.8	28.1
Head of household unemployed	67.1	47.4	43.1	38.4

Source: Lee and Murie 1997.

income and economic groups is more striking in the white population than in the non-white population. These findings are important because policies designed around limited perspectives on housing tenure and its interaction with life-cycle, deprivation and incomes can exclude parts of the housing sector where particular social groups face problems which are equally severe. Tables 3.5 and 3.6 illustrated this with regard to the social and economic deprivation experienced by different ethnic groups. Policies which seek to target social assistance through a focus on council estates, for example, are likely to be more effective in achieving this in relation to the white population than the non-white population. The announcement of a special task force to combat the worst aspects of social exclusion by the British government emphasizes the role that tenure plays in understanding poverty and social exclusion as there is a specific focus on council housing estates in the recent government policy proposals (Mandelson 1997). Such policies are not sufficiently attuned to the different housing market experience of the non-white population in different cities or neighbourhoods.

Housing and social exclusion

Accounting for these policy responses emphasizes the way in which social analysis of housing has been pushed in the direction of viewing the relationship between housing and deprivation or poverty in tenurial terms alone. The dramatic changes to council housing over the past 20 years and the fact that much policy in Britain – on topics such as housing finance – is tenure-specific, have perhaps inevitably strait-jacketed discussion and led the debate along tenurial lines. Yet this can be misleading. The evidence reviewed here suggests that there is greater differentiation in terms of deprivation between tenures than in the past. To provide an adequate analysis of the changes that have occurred it is necessary to develop alternative perspectives.

The process of residualization of council housing has played a large role in the way that housing is related to debates on poverty and social exclusion and mirrors the wider poverty debate in Britain. The evolution of this debate has traditionally followed an empiricist or inductive approach to analysis of social division and social rights. Poverty debates have emphasized the 'standard of living' concept developed by Townsend (1979) and Mack and Lansley (1985) which tends to focus upon expenditure and consumption but ignores choice or the processes that determine housing consumption. Graham Room contrasts this 'Anglo-Saxon' approach with the theoretical debates that have taken place on the continent (Room 1995a). These debates revolve around notions of inclusion, the rights and obligations of citizens and surface in the term 'social exclusion'. Meanwhile, Jordan (1997) identifies two established methods of social policy analysis which have shaped the poverty and social exclusion debate and offer different perspectives on the role of the welfare state: economic individualism has lead Anglo-Saxons to study the welfare state as a response to 'socially undesirable consequences of market interactions' (Jordan 1997: 86), whereas compulsory collectivism offers a perspective of the welfare state as an organizing principle for societies. It is the principle of 'compulsory collectivism', as part of a French tradition of social analysis, that 'society is seen by intellectual and political elites as a ... number of collectivities, bound together by sets of mutual rights and obligations ... rooted in some broader moral order' (Room 1995a: 6).

Thus while poverty refers to the outcome of a process (measured by the distribution of resources and incomes), the term social exclusion refers to the mechanisms and relations of the process and the interaction between different elements that lead to exclusion. These elements are measured by inadequate social participation, lack of social integration and lack of power (Room 1995b). A starting point for linking housing and social exclusion is to connect housing to the four aspects of social exclusion identified by Room (1995a); these are: the *concentration* of exclusion on population groups or areas; the *persistence* of exclusion over time; the *compound* nature of disadvantage which creates exclusion; and the *resistance* to existing or traditional policy solutions. These themes and how they relate to housing are now considered in turn.

The concentration of exclusion

The concept of social exclusion is especially relevant to housing because of the explicit spatial references. Illustrative is that some accounts of social exclusion suggest it has emerged in the context of transition within communities through the twin processes of immigration and spatial polarization. As Castillo (1994: 625) notes 'the city provides a visible spatial embodiment of the cleavages of a dual society'.

Concentration of exclusion and the relevance of housing location in the social exclusion debate is especially relevant in the British context because of the volume of council house sales. Research has shown that during the 1980s much of the better stock in the high demand areas was sold off (Kerr 1988). Inevitably this has meant that in many areas the only households becoming new tenants of council housing were those who were classified as homeless or drawn disproportionately from those outside the labour market (Forrest and Murie 1988; Prescott-Clarke *et al.* 1988, 1994). This pattern is being repeated in the non-profit, voluntary, housing association sector as it has grown. Its tenants and new tenants have a similar profile to council tenants and recently concern has been expressed about creating 'ghetto' estates (Page 1993). Low-demand housing areas tend to be poorly served by other services and poorer households are less likely to have the resources to seek better services elsewhere. Consequently those living in these areas are less able to avail themselves of opportunities which could increase their incomes and bargaining power and enable them to move on. Without strategic policy initiatives to alter this cycle of disadvantage, housing-market position and residential location begin to determine a person's wider life chances.

The debate about inner-city housing or peripheral estates is a debate about the quality and quantity of health, education and leisure services, the proximity to employment and training services, and the adequacy of transport facilities to access these resources as much as it is a debate about housing itself. Even where housing deprivation *per se* is not so evident, for example in dwellings which are modern and well equipped, the neighbourhoods in which they are located may offer poor local resources for residents. This is the case for new estates built on land that has required a change of use such as inner-city brown-field sites (Page 1993). In such cases environmental deprivation may be high especially where the land was previously contaminated. Households may be cut off from the mainstream due to a combination of poor infrastructure on brown-field developments and a reluctance of capital to invest, given the opportunity of attractive green-field or edge-city sites being released by local authorities.

As certain areas and parts of the market become more strongly associated with poor people and represent poor social environments those with choice in the housing system are less likely to move to such areas. As a result the social and income mix in these areas is further eroded. The common features of these households – relating to incomes and expenditure patterns and lack of access to information networks, and other resources which could change household circumstances in the short term – exacerbates problems for residents and affects the reputation of areas. The stigma and reputation of areas further affects residents in seeking jobs and in a variety of other contexts. Households living in areas with limited resources are likely to be disproportionately dependent on local facilities – shops, schools, health services, transport services, jobs and training, yet these areas tend to be deprived in terms of the key local services which can be accessed.

The persistence of exclusion

The role that time plays in the relationship between poverty and housing deprivation is often overlooked. This means that analysis often fails to identify the persistence of social exclusion. As noted earlier, the profile of household types suffering housing deprivation has changed significantly in recent years so that young single-person households now represent the majority household type suffering multiple housing deprivation and account for 35 per cent of all such households (see Table 3). In Marshall's benign view of social rights, the provision of services represented an incremental process driving towards long-term reduction of inequalities (Marshall and Bottomore 1992: 34). In this model Marshall recognized that inequalities would persist as 'the target is perpetually moving forward, and the state may never be able to quite get within reach of it' (p. 35). Marshall used as an example the case of housing where two households of similar needs are treated differentially and likened this to an element of *chance* in the system which in turn leads to inequality. In this view of social rights inequalities persist as a 'fair balance needs to be made between collective and individual elements in social rights' (p. 35) but equity is enshrined as an incremental process. Demographic trends such as the increase in smaller households and the delay of child-rearing put additional pressure on housing markets so that an element of chance creeps into the provision of decent housing.

However, what is important, and often overlooked in defining social exclusion (especially in relation to housing), is *how long* housing deprivation endures and whether there exist mechanisms for the incremental improvement of housing services within Marshall's benign model of the welfare state, the length of time poverty is endured within a particular tenure and whether persistent housing deprivation or poverty has an effect upon escaping poverty or escaping to tenures of 'choice'.

Altering the time frame makes a considerable impact on our understanding of social exclusion and how it relates to housing. This has an important bearing upon the relationship between social (housing) rights and inclusion. There is considerable evidence, as Walker has shown, that the choice of accounting period for studying poverty has 'non-trivial' consequences on the numbers found to be in poverty. A *reduction* of the accounting period from 12 months to one month, for example, *increases* the official poverty rate in the United States by almost a quarter (Walker 1995: 105). Looking at lifetime earnings rather than relying on cross-sectional analysis of earnings dampens the polarization effect of earnings and income structures. Therefore, extension of the accounting period similarly reduces the numbers found to be in poverty, but brings us closer to identifying those who are potentially socially excluded. This perspective can be extended to the analysis of housing tenure and its interaction with other policy areas. As an example, students suffering housing deprivation are not considered to be socially excluded as they are likely to have opportunities to move on to better accommodation. In considering the role of housing in disadvantage it is therefore important to weigh up both the length of time poverty is endured as well as prospects for moving on to different tenures or housing arrangements of choice.

The compound nature of exclusion

Because social exclusion requires a shift in focus from distributional issues to relational issues, examination of the interaction between housing and other policy areas can throw up the compound nature of exclusion. The interaction, for example, between benefits, incomes and housing finance has implications for the ability of households to take up employment or move beyond the poverty trap; the effects of unhealthy or unsuitable housing have compounding effects for life chances through debilitating effects on health. Housing's role in this process can be summarized in three ways: breaking out of housing circumstances not of choice because of the effects of housing policy (e.g. housing finance and the poverty trap); breaking into the housing market and out of homelessness; and the direct effects of housing consumption on health.

Breaking out: housing and the poverty trap

Changes in the arrangements for housing finance and subsidy in Britain over the past two decades have involved a shift from capital to individual subsidies in the council and housing association sectors and the consequent emergence of higher rents and high rates of dependence on housing benefit. This has had consequences for households on benefit who are affected by means testing and a poverty trap which seriously erodes any financial gains arising through better pay or through obtaining work. For example, cumulative deductions (households eligible for family credit, housing benefit and council tax benefit) from an increase in gross earned income of £1 can leave the family with only three pence and a couple or single person with little more than ten pence (Ford and Wilcox 1994: 80). These calculations take no account of increased transport, child care or other costs associated with work. The lack of net gain in resources acts as a major disincentive and traps the household in their present circumstances. Understanding these processes of exclusion says more about the role of housing and other policy areas than traditional measures of housing poverty can. The coping strategies employed by those in the poverty trap mean that work-experience opportunities are foregone and the chances of future employment or the ability to gain from training are reduced. At the same time such households may be trapped on lower incomes.

Breaking into the housing market: homelessness

Homelessness disrupts education, work and health care. The increased experience of homelessness from the late 1970s onwards has been associated with housing shortages and changes in families and lifestyles. During the period of increased homelessness in the 1980s the use of temporary accommodation increased almost tenfold from 5000 to over 45,000 households in England and Wales between 1985 and 1990 (HMSO 1995). For those who are homeless there are often long periods in temporary accommodation before finding permanent housing solutions. In these periods insecure accommodation and continual movement between temporary accommodation as well as extended periods of living in hostels, hotels and bed and breakfast accommodation has a severe impact. Evidence on access to primary health care suggests that such households have reduced access, which impacts upon their health in later life (Bines 1994).

Edwards (1995) argues that the discussion of the relative economics of private sector lease (PSL) by local authorities in temporarily housing homeless households, tends to focus on the acquisition, management and maintenance costs facing local authorities. Consequently, social and economic costs facing homeless families are often not accounted for when considering the use of temporary accommodation. These costs can be considerable and are often borne by families and social groups (for example, lone parents and minority ethnic groups) already marginalized in the housing market. For example, Edwards (1995) found that while ethnic minorities comprise less than one in five of all households in London, they represent more than two in five homeless families. Furthermore, 60 per cent of homeless families with four or more children are Asian households, and it is large families of this type that are housed for the longest periods in temporary accommodation awaiting rehousing. Edwards also found that a significant proportion of homeless families in London (25 per cent) are placed in temporary housing outside the usual borough of residence. In such situations, large families face social costs associated with their marginalization in the housing system, compounded by social deprivation.

In a report to the Royal College of Physicians of London, Connelly and Crown note how ill health amongst homeless families can limit housing opportunities (Connelly and Crown 1994). Ill health leads to low pay and fewer housing options. Social and financial disadvantage make healthy lifestyles unattainable in most instances, thereby increasing the risk of poor health. Reduced access to social housing through sales and a reduction of the capital programme means that households with poor health cannot guarantee being housed under the medical priority system (MPR). Meanwhile, for homeless families problems of access to primary care persist while increased mental, physical and obstetric ill health increase behavioural problems especially amongst children (Connelly and Crown 1994).

Even where living environments are not unsafe, health and diet are affected. Interruptions to schooling, medical care and work are particularly severe where accommodation is only available at a considerable distance from the previous address. It is a common experience that households in work are unable to sustain work once they become homeless and that it is very difficult to obtain work while living in temporary accommodation. The experience of extended periods of homelessness, insecure accommodation and temporary accommodation is likely to reduce the resources and independence of households. When they do obtain permanent housing they are consequently more likely to be affected by the poverty trap and to be disadvantaged in seeking work.

There are two groups for which the compound effects of housing on health are particularly acute: young people and the elderly. For the growing number of young people leaving the family home the housing options are restricted to poor-quality accommodation often in the private rented sector, or homelessness. Young single homeless people are more likely to have health problems than the general population according to research carried out by the Centre for Housing Policy at the University of York. Bines found in a large-scale study of the health of young single homeless that the risk of mental health problems was eight times greater for young people sleeping rough compared to the general population. When standardized for age and gender the differences are even more acute (Bines 1994).

The effects of housing consumption on health

For elderly people, the home can be more of a threat when combined with poverty; cold houses are a risk to the elderly when linked to fuel poverty (Boardman 1991) as the poorest 30 per cent of households spend twice as much (as a proportion of income) on heating than the remaining 70 per cent (Ineichen 1993). For people living in overcrowded housing or housing with poor amenities the well-documented associations with ill health and educational outcomes continue to affect life chances. Strong influences on mental health and stress-induced morbidity have also been documented (Byrne and Keithley 1993; Kellett 1993). High rates of asthma and respiratory illness especially amongst children are linked to damp housing and the presence of mould. The longer-term implications of such findings are raised by Smith (1989) who notes that frequent or severe bouts of respiratory illness in children affect lung function in adult life.

As basic housing deprivations such as overcrowding, lack of amenities and unfit dwellings declined over the 100-year period to the mid 1970s, so did interest in the linkages between community well-being or public health and housing conditions. However, interest in these linkages has resurfaced because of processes of social polarization and the low replacement rate of the older housing stock together with poor housing design during slum clearance. The revival of interest in the impact of housing on health is also partly due to the wider definitions used, reflecting the relative nature of housing deprivation and a better understanding of the effect of housing on health. Hence, social and psychological effects on health have emerged in the more recent literature, which has emphasized the mental health consequences of bad or poorly-designed housing conditions.

Resistance to existing or traditional policy solutions

Evidence on the compound nature of social exclusion and its connections with a range of policy areas – education, health and employment issues as well as housing – suggests that policies designed to reverse trends which end in people being socially excluded must not rely simply on a traditional departmental and focused intervention. Social exclusion will prove resistant to initiatives that have a single focus and there is increasing recognition, especially in the housing association movement, for locally integrated policies designed at neighbourhood level. The issue of homelessness amongst younger people provides an illustration of how traditional policy measures are resistant to problems of social exclusion and how an integrated approach is slowly emerging which requires increasing emphasis.

Young single homelessness is increasingly a feature of housing exclusion resistant to traditional housing policies as homelessness is defined in such a way that single people are not recognized as having housing rights. In a sense, therefore, homelessness among young people has not so much proved resistant to policy as policy to combat it has been non-existent. In fact, policy has arguably exacerbated the problem. Young people also figure prominently among those adversely affected by changes in the economy and the labour market. For example, over the ten year period 1984–93, long-term unemployment among men aged 16–30 rose both relatively and absolutely from 135,000 (19 per cent) to 187,000 (22 per cent) (HMSO 1995). The prospects for young people entering the labour market is, therefore, very different from 20 or 30 years ago when problems of homelessness in this group were relatively rare and 'most school leavers had no formal qualifications but had access to an employment system in which relatively well paid jobs did not require such qualifications' (Byrne 1995: 110).

The relentless rise in long-term unemployment in Britain and other European Union (EU) countries during the late 1970s and 1980s pointed to a failure of existent employment measures and the need for more innovative approaches. Due to changes in the structure of households (with more single-person households and young people leaving home earlier), youth unemployment, and the compound nature of social exclusion in which interaction with other policy areas is a key process, there has been a growing realization that more innovative polices directed towards young people are needed to combat social exclusion. The development of the 'foyer' system – a concept that originated in France where the establishment of foyer schemes is now widespread – has two aims: meeting the needs of young 16–25-year-old people on their path to independence by providing training, and employment opportunities linked with accommodation at a reasonable price. This reflects a focus not just on labour markets but on the interaction between policy areas, thereby reducing the resistance of compound social exclusion.

Citizenship and social exclusion: the role of housing

In Marshall's model of citizenship, civil and political rights are based on the principle of equality, whereas social rights are distinguished from the other two kinds of right with the legitimation of inequality despite the intervention of the state. In a key phrase Marshall states how 'equality of status is more important than equality of income' (Marshall and Bottomore 1992: 33). While social rights do not alter the principle of inequality of outcomes – due to the ownership of private property, wealth and access to power – the incorporation of social rights into the notion of citizenship implies the erosion of social class divisions. Class-abatement, as Marshall referred to the erosion of social class, '... is no longer content to raise the floor-level in the basement of the social edifice, leaving the superstructure as it was. It has begun to remodel the whole building, and it might even end up converting a skyscraper into a bungalow' (p. 28). Thus, while social *rights* extended common experience and citizenship through the principle of universalism, the *duties* of citizens demanded that they pay their taxes and national insurance contributions. The principle of reciprocity was central in this model of citizenship. Despite the growth of unemployment, it is a principle that has had important implications for present-day policies such as work-fare proposals in the United States and the 'new deal' announced by the Tony Blair's Labour government (Mandelson 1997).

Marshall's incrementalist perspective of citizenship and social rights was predicated on the view that universal services would lead to 'class-abate-ment'. Marshall stressed the importance of extending universal services to achieve equality of status and demonstrated the benefits of universalism with reference to education. A service could be extended universally in a way that created citizenship through a common culture: 'Citizenship requires ... a direct service of community membership based on loyalty to a civilisation which is a common possession' (Marshall and Bottomore 1992: 24). Pre-cedence would be given to collective ideals and the will of the individual would not so much be ignored as relegated. The welfare state, underwritten by full employment and the family and paid for by taxes and national insurance, enshrined these principles.

The role of housing in this model has proved ambivalent. Although the number of council houses built and the proportion of council tenants housed reached unprecedented numbers during the period 1948–60, sales after 1979 have emphasized the limited role of the state in direct housing pro-vision. This is because, as discussed in Chapter 2, housing has never been a central plank of the welfare state in Britain and its status as a service, universally provided and equal to that of education and health, has never been achieved or defended. Slum clearance and the general improvement of housing conditions over the past century have seen the major housing depri-vations decline in significance. The relationship between housing, depri-vation and poverty is typically talked of in terms of the residualization of council housing, the relationship between income poverty and council hous-ing and the narrowing of the social base of that sector.

However, housing deprivation persists and some of its worst aspects persist in the private rented sector where housing conditions are less amen-able to control and regulation. It is precisely because housing has never been a universal service that the main housing tenures are presently characterized by greater differentiation and fragmentation than in the past. Recognizing this differentiation and the interaction between housing and other areas of policy requires different frameworks of analysis such as the focus on social exclusion used in this chapter. It is the interaction between housing and other policy areas that makes the concept of social exclusion relevant to the role of housing.

Use of the term social exclusion in this chapter reflects its linkages with the concept of social citizenship developed in 1990 by the European Commission-funded Observatory on National Policies to Combat Social Exclusion. The Observatory was set up to explore policy issues in the context of exclusion experienced in different member states. Rather than unifying the theme of social exclusion around one policy arena common to all member states, social exclusion was defined by the Observatory with explicit reference to Marshall's concept of citizenship and the extension of social rights. Social exclusion was then defined in terms of '... what social rights the citizen has to employment, housing, health care [and] how effectively national policies enable citizens to secure these rights' (Room 1991: 16–17).

However, a certain degree of ambiguity and a number of interpretations and definitions of social exclusion have emerged. In practical applications of the term, especially because of the attitudes of British and German governments, the term social exclusion has increasingly been associated with (long-term) unemployment, thus implying a relatively narrow view of economic disadvantage. This narrow view of social exclusion has two implications: it links employment 'responsibilities' to social 'rights', and it excludes that part of the population unable to work from policies designed to 'integrate' them.

The case of housing and young people is illustrative of the first implication. Social exclusion among young people involves reinforcing problems associated with housing, education and employment. But, as Jordan (1997: 107) notes, the developing models of social citizenship assume that 'problems of social integration arise because they [young people] are not easily absorbed into the labour market and the social institutions that derive from it'. Policies designed along employment-integrationist lines attempt to define a universal principle of citizenship and lead to two views of how young people can be 'included'. One is through an increase in benefits, training and employment opportunities, while the alternative is to require young people to take up employment through compulsory training and socialization.

In Marshall's model of citizenship reciprocity is being replaced by compulsion. The development of universal principles of social rights is increasingly leading to the linking of responsibilities in one policy arena to 'rights' in another. For example, housing and employment foyer schemes show how the link between housing *rights* and employment *duties* is becoming more explicit; workfare schemes work in a similar way by denying social rights to a minimum income if responsibilities to take up training schemes are not observed. These trends present two dilemmas. First there is a problem of insertion where what is on offer has less attraction than developed forms of behaviour and styles. Insertion is difficult, for example, where 'young people have adapted to their exclusion from labour markets and benefits by seeking other sources of satisfaction, stimulation, meaning and security' (Jordan 1997: 107). In this remark Jordan is not attempting to resurrect the idea of an underclass, but the implication that resistance to social exclusion may be greater when compulsion is employed or, for example, housing rights tied to responsibilities in other spheres of social policy, should not be underestimated.

The second dilemma is that when social exclusion is closely linked to employment rights and duties the focus upon labour markets presents a dichotomy whereby all those outside the labour market are perceived as excluded while those in work are *included* (Levitas 1996). For Ruth Levitas social exclusion has, therefore '. . . become embedded as a crucial element in a new hegemonic discourse. Within this discourse, terms such as social cohesion and solidarity abound, and social exclusion is contrasted not with inclusion but integration, construed as integration into the labour market' (p. 5). Clearly, such a restrictive view of exclusion ignores inequality of income and conditions within the labour market and overlooks other processes of exclusion based on race or gender.

Such a restrictive view of social exclusion does not accord with the increasing spatial focus and the processes which operate to disadvantage not only individuals but also their *communities*. This aspect reflects evidence in Great Britain and Europe of renewed awareness of social and spatial divisions, and this has resulted in a series of policy statements and initiatives which put urban policy at the forefront of tackling social exclusion. The current concern with urban regeneration in England is with holistic approaches. The development of the SRB signalled that urban regeneration was now intended to encompass a range of objectives including housing, transport, training, crime and the environment. In housing, the last Conservative government expressed a renewed concern to tackle the problems of the most deprived council estates and to improve opportunities for the people who live on them: 'Over the next ten years, we will tackle the problems of the most deprived estates . . . Government Offices for the Regions and local authorities will work together to identify the best way of tackling the estates with the worst social, economic and housing problems' (DoE 1995: 35).

In a similar way the report of the Commission on Social Justice stated that: 'In the most disadvantaged parts of the United Kingdom, poverty, unemployment, ill-health and squalor combine to wreck people's chances' (Commission on Social Justice 1994: 50). The report suggested investment through Community Development Trusts in the most disadvantaged areas of the UK.

Conclusion

Housing is central to these debates and the role of urban policy in combating disadvantage and social exclusion connects to housing in a variety of ways. However, housing is not central in existing models of urban policy whether they be proposals to tackle problems on the worst housing estates or area regeneration delivered competitively through the SRB. Implicit assumptions are often made about housing which at worst can stereotype images of disadvantage and exclusion related to housing. In this sense, housing tenure is often used as an indicator of disadvantage – for the worst *estates* read council housing estates – but ignores elements of deprivation or exclusion which surface in other sectors. In the case of urban policies such as the SRB where the competitive process is paramount, the centrality of housing is at best incidental, with increasing evidence that housing budgets have declined or been absorbed into other headings (Nevin *et al.* 1996; Beazley *et al.* 1997). Emphasizing the role that housing plays in social exclusion means that the concept of social exclusion needs to move beyond the restrictive labour-market oriented definitions identified by Levitas (1996) and show how housing rights are central to the combating of social exclusion.

References

Beazley, M., Hall, S., Lee, P., Loftman, P. and Nevin, B. (1997) *Housing and the Single Regeneration Budget in London and The West Midlands*. Birmingham: School of Public Policy, The University of Birmingham.

Bines, W. (1994) *The Health of Single Homeless People*. York: Centre for Housing Policy.

Boardman, B. (1991) *Fuel Poverty: From Cold Homes to Affordable Warmth*. London: Belhaven.

Byrne, D. (1995) Deindustrialisation and dispossession: an examination of social division in the industrial city. *Sociology*, 29(1): 95–115.

Byrne, D. and Keithley, J. (1993) Housing and health in the community, in R. Burridge and D. Ormandy (eds) *Unhealthy Housing: Research, Remedies and Reform*. London: Chapman and Hall.

Castillo, I. (1994) A comparative approach to social exclusion: lessons from Belgium and France. *International Labour Review*, 133(5–6): 613–33.

Commission on Social Justice (1994) *Social Justice: Strategies for National Renewal, The Report of the Commission on Social Justice*. London: Vintage.

Connelly, J. and Crown, J. (eds) (1994) *Homelessness and Ill Health: Report of a Working Party of the Royal College of Physicians*. London: Royal College of Physicians of London.

Dale, A., Williams, M. and Dodgeon, B. (1996) *Housing Deprivation and Social Change*, series LS no. 8. Office for National Statistics, London: HMSO.

DoE (1995) *Our Future Homes: Opportunities, Choices and Responsibilities. The*

Government's Housing Policies for England and Wales, Cm. 2901. London: HMSO.

DoE (1997) *Regeneration Challenge Fund to Be Targeted At Areas of Need Says Regions Minister*, Department of the Environment, Transport & the Regions press release 258 (fax), 7 July. Also at http://www.coi.gov.uk/coi/depts/GTE/coi0385c.ok

DSS (1993) *Households Below Average Income 1979–1990/91*. London: HMSO.

Edwards, R. (1995) Making temporary accommodation permanent: the cost for homeless families. *Critical Social Policy*, 15: 60–75.

Esping-Andersen, G. (1990) *The Three Worlds of Welfare Capitalism*. Cambridge: Polity Press.

Ford, J. and Wilcox, S. (1994) *Affordable Housing, Low Incomes and the Flexible Labour Market*, NFHA Research Report no. 22. London: National Federation of Housing Associations.

Forrest, R. and Murie, A. (1988) *Selling the Welfare State*. London: Routledge.

Hills, J. (1995) *Joseph Rowntree Foundation Inquiry into Income and Wealth*, vol. 2. York: Joseph Rowntree Foundation.

HMSO (1983) *Family Expenditure Survey*. London: HMSO.

HMSO (1992) *Social Trends*, no. 22. London: HMSO.

HMSO (1993) *Households Below Average Incomes: A Statistical Analysis 1979–1992/3*. London: HMSO.

HMSO (1995) *Social Trends*, no. 25. London: HMSO.

Ineichen, B. (1993) *Homes and Health: How Housing and Health Interact*. London: Spon.

Jordan, B. (1997) *A Theory of Poverty and Social Exclusion*. Cambridge: Polity Press.

Kellett, J.M. (1993) Crowding and mortality in London boroughs, in R. Burridge and D. Ormandy (eds) *Unhealthy Housing: Research, Remedies and Reform*. London: Chapman and Hall.

Kennett, P. (1994) Models of regulation and the urban poor. *Urban Studies*, 31: 1017–31.

Kerr, M. (1988) *The Right to Buy: A National Survey of Tenants and Buyers of Council Homes*. London: HMSO.

Leather, P. and Morrison, T. (1997) *The State of UK Housing*. Bristol: Policy Press.

Lee, P. and Murie, A. (1997) *Poverty, Housing Tenure and Social Exclusion*. Bristol: Policy Press.

Lee, P., Murie, A. and Gordon, D. (1995) *Area Measures of Deprivation: A Study of Current Methods and Best Practices in the Identification of Poor Areas in Great Britain*. Birmingham: Centre for Urban and Regional Studies, the University of Birmingham.

Levitas, R. (1996) The concept of social exclusion and the new Durkheimian hegemony. *Critical Social Policy*, 16: 5–20.

Mack, J. and Lansley, S. (1985) *Poor Britain*. London: Allen & Unwin.

Mandelson, P. (1997) *Labour's Next Steps: Tackling Social Exclusion*. London: Fabian Society.

Marshall, T.H. and Bottomore, T. (1992) *Citizenship and Social Class*. London: Pluto.

Murie, A. (1983) *Housing Inequality and Deprivation*. London: Heinemann.

Murray, C. (1990) *The Emerging British Underclass*. London: Institute of Economic Affairs.

Nevin, B., Lee, P. and Murie, A. (1996) *London in Need: Regeneration, Housing and Deprivation in the Capital*. Birmingham: School of Public Policy, The University of Birmingham.

OPCS (1991a) *Population Census: Local Base Statistics*. London: OPCS.

OPCS (1991b) *Population Census: Sample of Anonymised Records*. London: OPCS.

Page, D. (1993) *Building for Communities*. York: Joseph Rowntree Foundation.

Prescott-Clarke, P., Allen, P. and Morrissey, C. (1988) *Queuing for Housing: A Study of Council Housing Waiting Lists*. London: HMSO.

Prescott-Clarke, P., Clemens, S. and Park, A. (1994) *Routes into Local Authority Housing*. London: HMSO.

Room, G. (1991) *National Policies to Combat Social Exclusion: First Annual Report of the EC Observatory*. Bath: University of Bath.

Room, G. (ed.) (1995a) *Beyond the Threshold: The Measurement and Analysis of Social Exclusion*. Bristol: Policy Press.

Room, G. (1995b) Poverty in Europe: competing paradigms of analysis, *Policy and Politics*, 23: 103–13.

Smith, S. (1989) *Housing and Health: A Review and Research Agenda*, Discussion Paper no. 27. Glasgow: Centre for Housing Research, Glasgow University.

Townsend, P. (1979) *Poverty in the UK*. London: Penguin.

Walker, R. (1995) The dynamics of poverty and social exclusion, in G. Room (ed.) *Beyond the Threshold: The Measurement and Analysis of Social Exclusion*. Bristol: Policy Press.

Wilson, W.J. (1987) *The Truly Disadvantaged: the Inner City, the Underclass, and Public Policy*. Chicago: University of Chicago Press.

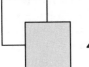

4

Secure and contented citizens?
Home ownership in Britain

Alan Murie

Introduction

In recent years within the housing debate it is home ownership that has been most often associated with notions of citizenship, choice and individual control. The high ground of the housing debate has been taken by home ownership, with the rhetoric equating this tenure with all that is best for independent citizens in a modern economy. The focus of housing policy debate has shifted away from concern with housing shortages and housing condition problems and with delivering quality of shelter to households, to concern with the form of ownership and control. Perhaps the assumption has been that the quality of shelter flowed automatically from the form of tenure, or perhaps the assumption was that housing quality and condition and housing shortages had been solved and the focus could now be on the higher realms of housing autonomy and ontological security.

Although the term 'property-owning democracy' was not initially coined to relate to housing and home ownership, it had increasingly become associated with the widespread individual ownership of houses by the people that live in them. There was a shift from an emphasis on material rights towards individual property rights. Home ownership created and reflected good citizenship and those who were not home owners were increasingly seen as damaged citizens.

This chapter seeks to explore these issues further. It provides a background to the development of home ownership as a mass tenure in Britain and argues that through the period of the growth of home ownership, there were pragmatic reasons for focusing upon this tenure. However, over time, these pragmatic and short-term considerations were translated into a deep-rooted ideological commitment to home ownership as a superior form of tenure. On this basis, governments actively promoted home ownership and encouraged people through a range of incentives to become homeowners. One of the key examples of this encouragement, the Right to Buy, is discussed in some detail, and this chapter also reflects upon the experience of the growth of home ownership and the problems and issues surrounding the tenure. Finally conclusions are drawn about the significance of the tenure in debates about citizenship, choice and individual control.

The origins of home ownership

The nineteenth-century man of property did not own his own home. The Victorian middle and upper classes, as well as those with low income, were renters. Britain, at the turn of the century, was a nation of tenants and this applied to rural and urban areas and to the rich and the poor. Home ownership should not therefore be viewed as the natural tenure – mass home ownership is a product of post-war history.

There is a wide literature which discusses how the nature of housing and its high cost requires separate financial arrangements to be put in place from those that are required for the production of many other goods. The mechanism which worked in the nineteenth century was one through which speculators built and developed housing and sold it to (or converted themselves into) landlords, who charged a rent sufficient to service the debt associated with the development and to make a reasonable return on the capital. In nineteenth-century Britain the rate of return that could be made from house property was sufficiently high to make this a viable proposition. In the absence of controls over the quality and standards of housing, this was in some cases at the expense of the people who lived in the properties, but for households with cash – for the middle class affluent household in Victorian Britain – there was no shortage of good quality rented housing and there was no reason to take on the burden of indebtedness associated with individual house purchase. Only when people hit hard times was the rented sector deficient. The emergence of home ownership as a significant tenure was associated with the shortcomings of provision through private rental.

These shortcomings were evident in a number of ways. First of all, there was a failure to provide good quality affordable housing to lower income groups and the increasingly evident problem of slums and poor housing. Accounts of housing reforms in the nineteenth century provide ample evidence of the failure of the private rented sector to deliver the housing that was needed for this section of the community (see, for example, Gauldie 1974; Merrett 1979). Persistent and repeated failure led policymakers to look for other solutions, from 5 per cent philanthropy to the introduction of state housing. Politicians were reluctant to take steps which abandoned the dependence on private sector provision through the private landlord but the increasingly apparent discontent in British cities required some response. The housing legislation after the First World War had its origins in a longer-term build-up of discontent about urban housing conditions and the organization of the emergent Labour Party was strongly rooted in campaigns to improve housing (see Pooley 1993). The private landlord did not provide housing fit for *citizens* to live in and, with the demand for homes fit for *heroes* to live in, the abandonment of reliance on private renting was unavoidable.

A second factor contributed to this development: the withdrawal of investment in the provision of private rented housing. Again there is an ample literature which demonstrates that in the period from the turn of the century up to the First World War there was a significant decline in investment. This was partly associated with the increasing pressure that landlords were put under to meet public health, planning and other standards, but more fundamentally it was to do with the higher rates of return that could be gained through investment in other parts of the global economy. The flight of capital from housing was not fundamentally a product of state intervention but rather of the way in which the international economy and opportunities for investment had expanded. The introduction of rent controls in 1915 added a further major problem for landlords' profitability but it is inaccurate to regard the demise of private renting as initiated by this late act in controlling the sector.

If these two factors explain why an increasing crisis emerged in the existing form of housing provision and created an opportunity for the development of alternative tenures, they do not in themselves explain the growth of owner occupation specifically. A third factor is more directly associated with the growth of home ownership.

Alongside the provision of rented housing from the eighteenth century onwards, there had been, especially amongst working-class groups, the development of self-help housing, associated with the provision of lending through building societies. Again there is a wide literature which describes the origins of terminating building societies as mutual organizations to enable their members in turn to build houses for themselves to live in (see, for example, Boddy 1980; Merrett 1982; Boleat and Coles 1987). These societies later changed into permanent societies which provided a retail banking service and lent principally for house purchase. They were essentially banks aimed at the mass of the population in a period in which the high-street banks were upper class business institutions who did not open their doors to the small saver. By 1919 it is usually argued that around 10 per cent of the population was in home ownership but there were enormous variations in the levels of home ownership in different parts of the country. Where the tradition of working-class home ownership funded through building society loans was best developed, home ownership was at very much higher levels (Forrest *et al.* 1990; Pooley 1993).

By 1919 British housing had reached a turning point. The dominant providers of housing were failing to deliver in terms of the quantity and quality of housing and politically, with fears of public disorder very prominent in the minds of politicians. At the same time there were two alternative forms of tenure which had gone through a formative phase. Public sector housing had developed on a small scale and the experience of providing housing through local authorities was established. Home ownership was supported by a set of financial institutions and this tradition was well-established in some localities. It is against this backdrop that most accounts of housing in Britain refer to a major shift in policy. If much of the emphasis is placed upon the introduction of the exchequer subsidies to enable the growth of council housing, this should at least be balanced by reference to the increasing promotion of home ownership. The early housing legislation after 1918 provided the possibility of subsidies for building in the private sector but the lack of political support and sympathy for private landlords was apparent in the absence of strong advocacy for leaving the housing task to this part of the community.

Increasingly, the alternative to state provision was seen as home ownership. The most quoted phrase in this literature is the reference to home ownership as a 'bulwark against Bolshevism'. The private landlord was not likely to be a bulwark against Bolshevism. Indeed the failings of private landlordism contributed to the new demands and organization of the urban working class. State housing was not likely to be a bulwark against Bolshevism as there was a danger identified by some that it would encourage the growth of demands for collective and state action. It was home ownership that offered the alternative and its most prominent advocates emphasized individual rights and responsibilities. The promotion and growth of home ownership in the inter-war period can be seen to be the product of a number of contingent factors and as a pragmatic response to a series of crises and problems. It was, nevertheless, embraced enthusiastically, especially in the political community and certain attributes of the tenure were increasingly identified as if they were inherent to it and were the underlying reason for its promotion. However reluctant they had been initially, the housing modernizers of the 1920s began to articulate the merits of home ownership and associate these with individual rights and enhanced citizenship.

Merrett (1982: 5) argues that the Housing Act 1923 introduced by Neville Chamberlain, the Conservative minister of health, and so often quoted because it reduced the subsidies available for local authority housing, was 'the most important legislative measure specifically concerned with home-ownership before the Second World War. It made producer subsidies and house purchase finance a central part of the state's policy'. The Act's central objective was to promote speculative building of small working-class houses, either for sale or rental. Merrett argues that Chamberlain believed that the age of the small investor in houses had passed and regarded building for sale as more realistic. In fact the great majority of dwellings were built for sale. Lump-sum subsidies were payable to builders on dwellings completed before October 1925. Local authority mortgage provision was extended and local authorities were empowered to guarantee building society advances. Finally, local authorities were able to lend money directly to builders to construct modest dwellings.

The effects of these measures were considerable. Local authority mortgage loans accelerated to a peak of almost £10 million in 1926–7 and although loans available to builders were relatively small, they peaked at £4 million in 1925 and 1926. Councils guaranteed some 2000 building society loans each year from 1924–5 onwards. Merrett's estimate is that around 18 per cent of the total number of completions for private owners in 1926–7 were financed by local authority loans. The direct encouragement of home ownership was significant and an important part of policy. Merrett (1982: 6) argues that the ideological purposes of these developments in policy were becoming clear. He quotes Chamberlain's view that 'every spadeful of manure dug in, every fruit tree planted, converted a potential revolutionary into a citizen'.

This sentiment is one which is associated with a wide range of advocates for home ownership in the period. Perhaps the most well used quote is from Harold Bellman, a leading building-society figure, who stated:

> the man who has something to protect and improve – a stake of some sort in the country – naturally turns his thoughts in the direction of sane, ordered, and perforce economical government. The thrifty is seldom or never an extremist agitator. To him revolution is anathema; and, as in the earliest days Building Societies acted as a stabilising force, so today they stand, in the words of the Rt. Hon. G.N. Barnes, as 'a bulwark against Bolshevism and all that Bolshevism stands for'.
>
> (Bellman 1927: 54)

At this point it would appear that although the debate was conducted in terms of the behaviour or loyalty of citizens the advocates of home ownership were not arguing that the tenure was associated with a different pattern of rights, nor were they emphasizing choice, or control by the resident, but possibly and indirectly control by the state. They were referring to the probable political behaviour of citizens who were also homeowners. They were referring to a stake in the system and its impact on the likelihood of people being agitators or upsetting the stability of society. It was not the benefits to the individual that were being emphasized but rather the benefits to the polity which would flow from individuals being homeowners. Harold Bellman (1927: 53–4) stated:

the home owner takes a justifiable pride in his property, and is ever conscious of the fact that all he spends in money and labour thereon serves but to bind him more closely to the home of his choice. The working-man who is merely a tenant has no real anchorage, no permanent abiding place and in certain circumstances is fair prey for breeders of faction and revolutionaries of every sort and condition. Home-ownership is a civic and national asset. The sense of citizenship is more keenly felt and appreciated, and personal independence opens up many an avenue of wider responsibility and usefulness.

Although home ownership delivered things for the individual owner, it delivered more for society as a whole and the political appeal was less in terms of direct benefits in relation to housing but rather in terms of the indirect benefits of social stability.

These comments also indicate another feature of the debate about home ownership: the tendency to develop a confused causal analysis which can be described as follows. There is an observation that more affluent, stable and secure households become homeowners in circumstances where the quality of service provided in that sector is greater than available elsewhere. This association however becomes converted into a view that it is home owner-ship which creates affluent, stable and secure households. Home ownership is increasingly equated with stability, a stake in the system and subsequently choice. As this convenient proposition becomes repeated, in order to high-light its significance the assertion begins to be made that rented properties are less likely to be regarded as a home and do not provide the same attachment to place, locality and family. At this point the fact that the evidence on household behaviour does not conform is completely ignored.

Promoting home ownership

The promotion of home ownership in the inter-war years has already been referred to. The development of building societies and their capacity to provide mortgage finance is a key component in the subsequent account. Other legislation including the Land Registration Act of 1924 which simpli-fied and cheapened the process of conveying land and encouraged the development of the sector. The private house-building boom of the 1930s was predominantly building for sale and was facilitated by building societies and their links with the private building industry. By 1938 some two thirds of civil servants, local government officials and teachers were recorded as being homeowners, as were almost one in five of insured workers in urban areas (i.e. manual workers and non-manual workers with incomes of up to £250 per year) (Merrett 1982: 15).

In the period 1939 to 1951 the enthusiasm for the development of home ownership was dampened. The cessation of building during the war years and the priority given by the post-war Labour government to building for rent, meant that the home ownership sector lost ground. However its advocates did not alter their views and after the Second World War the Conservative Party in opposition strengthened its commitment to a property-owning democracy (Harris 1973), and the party leadership adopted the slogan of 'property-owning democracy'. While the Conservative Party did not have generalized policies to offset the relative concentration of ownership and wealth in society, the restricted application of this slogan to home ownership came to symbolize the Conservative Party's alternative to Labour's programme of public and social ownership. The immediate plan was to increase home owning as part of their plan to create a property-owning democracy, widening the scope for the private builder and lowering costs (Hoffman 1964).

'Private property was an equipoise to political power' (MacLeod and Maude 1950) and the Conservative Party's publication *The Right Road for Britain* in 1949 stated: 'people find satisfaction and stability in the ownership of property, especially of their homes and gardens'. Harold Macmillan, the new minister of housing and local government in 1951 stated: 'Since it is part of our philosophy that a wide distribution of property rather (than) its concentration makes for a sound community, we shall pursue this aim wherever it is appropriate and can be done with due regard to the interests of those who live in rented houses' (*Hansard* 1951a). He went on:

> We think that, of all forms of property suitable for such distribution house property is one of the best. Of course, we recognise that perhaps for many years the majority of families will want houses to rent, but, whenever it suits them better or satisfies some deep desire in their hearts, we mean to see that as many as possible get a chance to own their houses.
>
> (*Hansard* 1951b)

These sentiments provided the background to the relaxation of licensing for private building, its abolition in 1954, the removal of controls on the selling prices of post-war dwellings, the general encouragement of home ownership, and a policy to allow the sale of council houses.

Increasingly, the local authority's role was seen as a residual one directed at clearing the slums, while general housing needs were best met through the expansion of home ownership. With the failure of the attempt to revive the private rented sector in the late 1950s, the Conservative Party chose to make a virtue of necessity and to refer to the expansion of owner occupation as evidence that 'we are the party of owner occupation' (see Murie 1975: 18). In 1958 the Rt. Hon. Henry Brooke, the minister of housing and local government stated that: 'The home owner can get his roots down and get his roses planted. Ownership and responsibility advance hand in hand' (quoted in Samuel *et al.* 1962). The emphasis continued to be upon behaviour rather than choice, citizenship or control. It is also worthwhile reflecting upon the targets for this appeal. Home ownership in the early post-war period grew most rapidly among higher and middle income groups. It is only later that it began to move down the income scale to a considerable extent. Harris (1973: 172–3, 179) argues that the approaches adopted to the property-owning democracy were not in stark contrast with the status quo:

> They did not constitute a coherent and conscious pursuit of a plan to redistribute property ownership and wealth. Indeed, expansion of home ownership occurred most rapidly amongst those who were already propertied, amongst industrialists, financiers and the middle classes ... The ideals remained either as a summation of what was felt to exist already or were simply decorative. They served their main function when the party was in opposition. It was assumed that in so far as the property owning democracy did not already exist, it would evolve out of society without state intervention.

By the 1970s this position had changed, particularly because of an increasingly vocal opposition within the Conservative Party to municipal ownership of housing. 'The prime threat to a Tory society was in the extension of state monopoly landlordism' and 'there was too much emphasis on the needs side, giving to each according to his needs and far too little on the side of incentive and reward for effort' (MacGregor 1965). It is against this background that home ownership was presented as an alternative to council housing and the message of the property-owning democracy needed to be made attractive to those who previously had not been receiving it. In particular the message needed to reach the expanded population who had found good quality housing in the local authority sector and for whom the state rather than the market had provided opportunity and choice. By the 1970s the continued growth and expansion of the property-owning democracy could no longer be sustained at the expense of private renting and came up against the continuing expansion of council housing. One of them had to give. It was at this point that there was a second major shift in the housing policy debate.

By the mid 1970s the major problems associated with post-war housing – those of slums, overcrowding, unfitness for habitation and housing shortages – had been dramatically reduced. There was a general view that the national housing problem had been solved and what remained was a series of local problems, requiring local responses. In a period of increasing concern about fiscal pressures, housing was an easy target for reduced public expenditure. Housing was also an area where the non-state sector could be pointed to as one of success. Leaving aside the extent to which it had benefited from public sector promotion and from financial privileges (see, for example, Nevitt 1966), the quality and levels of satisfaction associated with home ownership was generally high. In retrospect it is clear that there was insufficient analysis of what actually made home ownership successful. There was a tendency to revert back to incautious causal analyses suggesting that the success of home ownership must be because of some inherent attribute of the tenure and that further expansion of the tenure would inevitably mean further expansion of the same successful model.

The alternative view is that home ownership, in the mid-1970s, was marked by a series of characteristics which were peculiar to that point in time: it had expanded amongst younger households and in a period of full employment; it had not been faced either with households affected by interrupted earnings or those with low incomes in retirement; the sector was propped up by a generous welfare state regime which involved full employment and benefits which reduced the risk to homeowners; the sector consisted of a high proportion of newly built dwellings and the images of home ownership were often constructed around newly built estates, where problems of disrepair and maintenance had yet to emerge.

In practice what was already apparent was that the home ownership market was becoming less homogeneous. The literature on housing from the mid-1970s includes accounts of problems in the home ownership sector, especially in inner-city areas where properties had been transferred from private landlords who had failed to maintain them to an adequate standard and where home ownership expanded among ethnic minority and other lower income groups with inadequate resources to maintain and improve properties and who were often exposed to unfavourable lending regimes.

However, at this stage in the history of housing policy it is clear that neither of the major political parties was concerned to take stock of these issues. Both the Labour and Conservative Parties in opposition and in government competed to be the best promoters of home ownership. Neville Chamberlain had seen home ownership as 'a revolution which of necessity enlisted all those who were affected by it on the side of law and order and enrolled them in a great army of good citizens' (quoted in Merrett 1982: 268). The 1953 White Paper *Houses: The Next Step* (MHLG 1953: para 7), in discussing the role of owner occupation, argued: 'Of all forms of ownership this is one of the most satisfying to the individual and the most beneficial to the nation'. John Dunham, chairman of the BSA (Building Societies Association) argued in 1964 that home ownership:

> ... is an essential part of one's life. It satisfies a basic human need to surround oneself with something that is absolutely personal and private between members of one's family. When one talks about it becoming the background of family life, one thinks of it as an anchorage or

harbour from which one emerges each day. Night after night one returns and becomes part of the family again.

(Dunham quoted in Merrett 1982: 270)

By the 1970s there was a more aggressive, assertive tone to these statements. The romantic imagery of gardens and harbours was tinged with a stronger advocacy of the superiority of home ownership over other tenures. Home ownership was no longer seen to simply affect the behaviour of people in society in a way which was beneficial to the rest of society, but was now regarded as more compatible with family life and the natural aspirations of ambitious and responsible citizens.

In the 1971 White Paper *Fair Deal for Housing*, the Conservative government stated:

Home ownership is the most rewarding form of housing tenure. It satisfies a deep natural desire on the part of the householder to have independent control of the home that shelters him and his family. It gives him the greatest possible security against the loss of his home: and particularly against the price changes that may threaten his ability to keep it. If the householder buys his house on mortgage he builds up by steady saving a capital asset for himself and his dependants.

(DoE 1971: 4)

The Labour government's 1977 Housing Policy Review stated:

A preference for home ownership is sometimes explained on the grounds that potential home owners believe that it will bring them financial advantage. A far more likely reason for the secular trend towards home ownership is the sense of general personal independence that it brings. For most people owning ones home is a basic and natural desire ... The widening of entry into home ownership for people with modest incomes will help solve housing problems which used to be faced by the public sector, as well as satisfying deep seated social aspirations.

(Quoted in Merrett 1982: 269)

In 1980 the new Conservative Secretary of State for the Environment, Michael Heseltine, stated that:

There is in this country a deeply ingrained desire for home ownership. The government believes that this spirit should be fostered. It reflects the wishes of the people, ensures the wide spread of wealth through society, encourages personal desire to improve and modernise one's home, enables people to accrue wealth for their children, and stimulates the attitudes of independence and self-reliance that are the bedrock of a free society.

(*Hansard* 1980)

Polarizing housing tenures

Debates about housing in the period leading up to 1979 increasingly posited the two dominant tenures– council housing and home ownership – in opposition to one another. There is an increasingly ideological debate about the strengths and weaknesses of each. From 1919 to the early 1970s both tenures had expanded, admittedly with different degrees of advocacy and support from different groups. By the mid-1970s the support for council housing was severely restricted. The manifesto of the Conservative Party which came into government in 1979 had placed considerable emphasis on housing. Under the heading of 'Helping the Family', housing received one and a half pages – more than social security, health and welfare, or education. (Conservative Party 1979). The emphasis in the manifesto was on home ownership, tax cuts, lower mortgage rates and special schemes to make purchase easier. More prominent than anything else in this approach was the sale of council houses and the commitment to provide a legal right to buy, backed by larger discounts to reduce purchase price and mortgages to enable such purchases to go ahead.

On taking office the government quickly set about applying these manifesto commitments. New housing legislation in 1980 introduced the Right to Buy and changed the rights of council tenants in other ways. It revised the subsidy system for council housing but did not attempt a more general rationalization of housing finance. Subsequent legislation in 1984, 1986 and 1988 was designed to make the Right to Buy more attractive and reduce the scope for local variation in implementation. Other measures were developed to expand low cost home ownership and from the mid-1980s onwards government embarked upon programmes to transfer local authority housing stock to housing associations or other private landlords. The promotion of home ownership was now part of a wider attack upon municipal ownership and not just a good thing in its own right.

In the context of the discussion in this chapter it is worthwhile reflecting more fully upon the Right to Buy and the policy to sell council houses. Council house sales policies had matured over a long period and grown out of local government expertise and practice, especially since the 1960s. They were not the product of new-right thinking but rather of the long Conservative experience in local and central government. The pioneers of council house sales were in the big cities – in Birmingham and Greater London Council in particular (see Murie 1975) – and the advocacy of selling council houses had grown alongside the more vigorous promotion of the idea of a property-owning democracy. Margaret Thatcher, as the new prime minister in 1979, stated:

Thousands of people in council houses and new towns came out to support us for the first time because they wanted a chance to buy their own homes. We will give to every council tenant the right to purchase his own home at a substantial discount on the market price and with 100 per cent mortgages for those who need them. This will be a giant stride towards making a reality of Anthony Eden's dream of a property-owning democracy. It will do something else – it will give to more of our people the prospect of handing something on to their children and grandchildren which owner occupation provides.

(*Hansard* 1979a)

The Secretary of State, Michael Heseltine, explained: 'We intend to provide as far as possible the housing policies that the British people want ... we propose to create a climate in which those who are able can prosper, choose their own priorities and seek the rewards and satisfactions that relate to themselves, their families and their communities' (*Hansard* 1979b).

The shift towards a greater emphasis upon individual choice and the advantages to the individual through home ownership are apparent in these and other statements of the time. The contradiction is that the policy devices then adopted by the government were determinedly concerned to distort these choices. Rather than leaving the market to operate, the Right to Buy involved massive discounts on the valuation of property. By 1986 discounts on market values started in a house at 32 per cent after two years tenancy. For someone living in a flat they started at 44 per cent after two years and could rise to as high as 70 per cent after only fifteen years tenancy. For those in houses the process of discount was slower by 1 per cent a year up to a maximum of 60 per cent after thirty years. In both cases the policy was designed not to expose people to the risks and choices associated with the market but rather to encourage them to exit from the public sector and to access private ownership through an enormously subsidized route. By 1995 some 1.5 million people had bought council houses under the Right to Buy.

Because of the beneficial terms under which purchasers bought, the experience of purchase under the Right to Buy has generally been a good one. Purchasers have bought the best council properties with large discounts and have rarely experienced problems associated with taking on too large an initial mortgage burden. In general purchasers have been more affluent tenants who already had bargaining power and could often have bought low priced houses elsewhere. Problems have been associated with subsequent borrowing or with changes in employment and marital circumstances. Purchasers who bought in the early 1980s have seen these properties appreciate in value to a considerable extent. Where they bought in relatively high price areas, the asset value of their property provides them with an opportunity to move and a choice within the housing market that would rarely have existed for them otherwise. In contrast the range of choice for new applicants for council housing or for existing tenants in less desirable dwellings has decreased with the loss of the best council stock to home ownership. Increased choice always involves winners and losers.

Although the Right to Buy has not benefited the lowest income sections of council tenants, it has contributed to the changing social profile of the home ownership sector. At the same time there is no doubt that it has changed that sector in other ways. In the early years of the Right to Buy some people bought dwellings which were subsequently deemed to be defective and government sought to deal with these problems by providing special financial and policy support to this group. However, a more substantial problem has arisen with households who have purchased flats, where continuing issues associated with service charges and in some cases – admittedly a very small number – with unsaleable properties, have emerged. More general concern is expressed about the maintenance and repair of properties in this sector.

Finally, it is clear that former local authority dwellings will very rarely cease to be associated with the local authority sector. Where dwellings are on council estates, although they are owner occupied, they will still be seen to be former council dwellings and the price differential will often remain. The Right to Buy has contributed to changing the profile and nature of the home ownership sector and to developing new distinctive segments within the market which may only be absorbed very slowly over a long period of time. While the Right to Buy has not destabilized the home ownership sector it has formed a very significant part of the process of expansion of that sector, and with expansion has brought change in the nature and image of the tenure and its uniformity.

Failing promises

Home ownership continued to grow rapidly while council housing contracted in Britain in the 1980s and 1990s. This balance was affected by the injection of stock transfers from the local authority sector and the dominance of new building for sale in the absence of any programme of council-house building. From being remarkable for its level of state housing provision, Britain began to become remarkable for its level of home ownership. It has a much higher level of home ownership at the end of the 1990s than many other advanced industrial economies, especially those in Europe and North America. Home ownership has expanded down the income scale to embrace skilled, semi-skilled and lower-paid workers. It has also matured with the early cohorts of homeowners now in older age, sometimes with low incomes in retirement.

As home ownership has expanded and matured so it has become more differentiated (Forrest et al. 1990). Part of the differentiation of the sector has been the end of the honeymoon with home ownership, in which passage to home ownership appeared to mean the end of housing problems. The figures relating to homeowners with problems have remained at a high level throughout the 1990s. Issues associated with mortgage arrears and repossessions, negative equity, and problems of disrepair and expenditure on maintenance, have become normal features of the housing policy debate. The housing boom of 1986–9 gave way to an unprecedented recession, perhaps crisis, in the home ownership sector, and many commentators do not regard it as likely that home ownership will ever begin to produce the promises that were associated with it at earlier stages. Mass home ownership has different attributes to its predecessors.

Both the changing economic context and the different social profile of homeowners have left the home ownership sector with features not evident in the past. These in particular relate to high levels of mortgage arrears, repossessions, negative equity and a substantial house condition and house repair problem. These issues are discussed in greater detail elsewhere (Wilcox 1997; Williams 1997) and the intention here is to refer to them only very briefly.

In relation to arrears and repossessions the traditional stance of the home ownership industry was to emphasize the very low level of problems of this type. Mortgage arrears and repossessions by building societies were regarded as extremely low in relation to the volume of business undertaken. Although there was evidence that there were problems at the bottom end of the market (Karn 1979), the building society movement tended to argue that these were minimal and mainly associated with marital breakdown. Data for four large building societies with almost 1.5 million mortgages showed that in 1976 only 6215 households had arrears of five months or more and the number of repossession cases in the year was only 1224. In 1979 out of 5.25 million loans outstanding at the end of the year, 0.16 per cent were between six and twelve months in arrears and 0.048 per cent of properties (2530) had been repossessed in the year before. But these figures relate to the phase before changes in housing and the economy, and the declining rates of inflation, put home ownership at greater risk.

By 1985 the number of repossessed properties had risen to 16,590 and 60,000 properties had arrears of six months or more. The biggest surge in arrears and repossessions was associated with the change from boom to bust between 1989 and 1990. (see, for example, Forrest and Murie 1994; Maclennan 1997; Wilcox 1997). Table 4.1 provides some figures on the number of mortgages, repossessions and arrears in the period 1986–96. Figures for repossessions peaked in 1991. However the level they were at in 1996 was still higher than at any time before 1990. In relation to arrears and repossessions the market seemed to have entered an extended if not permanent stage of insecurity. The number of property transactions fell from a peak for England and Wales of 2.1 million in 1988 to 1.6 million in 1989, 1.4 million in 1990, 1.3 million in 1991 and 1.1 million in 1992. For the next four years transactions remained at below 1.3 million. Problems of selling houses made it more difficult to escape arrears difficulties and both factors were associated with falling real house prices and the emergence of a situation in which the value of properties fell below the outstanding loan on the property – negative equity. House prices fell in cash terms in 1992, and while Scotland and Northern Ireland largely escaped declining house prices, the effects were felt most severely in particular regions and in particular parts of the market. Prices fell from a peak in 1989 and had not recovered their previous level by 1996. They were farthest adrift in East Anglia, Greater London and the rest of the South East. Negative equity grew rapidly after 1989. In the United Kingdom 230,000 households were estimated to be in negative equity in 1989 and this rose to 1.8 million in 1992. By 1996 465,000 households were still estimated to be in negative equity and these continued to be concentrated in the South of England.

While the initial reaction may have been to see such developments as a short-term blip reflecting an unusual economic situation, they are now more generally regarded as evidence of a new housing market which reflects different economic realities. 'Housing is now a risky investment. There is no longer the virtual guarantee that prices will rise in nominal terms while the mortgage debt stays fixed' (Boleat 1997: 60). Housing is now purchased as a consumer good, rather than as an investment. It is no longer seen as being imperative to purchase housing at the earliest possible age, with the largest mortgage that one can afford. Rather than being a symbol of status and achievement, ownership could now indicate an unbalanced pattern of investment, unreasonable exposure to risk and a lack of wisdom in investment behaviour. Even the building society movement is no longer so pre-occupied with the expansion of home ownership, being itself more willing to

Table 4.1   Mortgage arrears, repossessions and negative equity, 1989–96

	Number of mortgages (000s)	Mortgage arrears 12+ months	Repossessions during year	Negative equity (000s)
1989	9125	13840	15810	230
1990	9415	36100	43890	564
1991	9815	91740	75540	776
1992	9922	147040	68540	1768
1993	10137	151810	58540	1388
1994	10410	117110	49190	1267
1995	10521	85200	49410	1163
1996	10637	67020	42560	465

Source: Wilcox 1997: 126–7.

fund rented housing. The rush to change from mutual status in the mid-1990s further shows that the building society industry has changed along with the market it grew up with and served.

The new debate, since the mid-1990s, has been about sustainable home ownership. Lenders are no longer so confident of the market and much more reference is made to labour market flexibility and the implications of this for the traditional mortgage market. Reduced job and income security, increased part-time and self-employment and other elements of flexibility are less compatible with the traditional mortgage system. At the same time changes in household structures and the prevalence of one income and one parent households raises new issues. Although it is clear that the home ownership market has moved away from the position where females found it difficult to obtain loans and home ownership was associated with male headed households, changes in the structure of the labour market are regarded as posing threats to lenders. It is widely assumed that financial institutions will be more selective in who they lend to and the best packages will go to those in the most secure sectors of the economy. Those with less earning and bargaining power are likely only to be able to access more expensive loans from less understanding lenders. If the risks in the sector are generally greater, they are most likely to be experienced by groups with lower incomes and in less secure employment.

The government's concern about sustainable home ownership and the more frequent comments on whether the level of home ownership achieved by the mid-1990s is sustainable, should not be overstated. There is little evidence that there is a generally held view that problems will necessitate government intervention. Indeed the opposite has been the case and government has been withdrawing its safety nets (income support for mortgage interest) and other support (tax relief) for home ownership. Rather, what we have is a major exercise to increase the awareness of the risks associated with home ownership and modify the assumption of its intrinsic advantages in terms of choice, control and citizenship.

One final element in the changing nature of home ownership that deserves separate comment concerns house condition problems. These cannot be regarded as the product of short-term economic changes. While they are partly associated with the movement of home ownership down market to income groups with limited capacity to maintain properties, they are also associated with the ageing of the population in home ownership. For lower income households in different groups the costs of home ownership in use – the costs of maintenance and repair – impose considerable burdens on household budgets. In 1991 some 81 per cent of occupied dwellings in England, Scotland and Northern Ireland with urgent repair costs in excess of £1000 were privately owned (Leather and Mackintosh 1997).

Again, government has withdrawn its major financial programmes, which had minimized these problems. The modification to repair- and improvement-grant systems represents a major withdrawal of financial support to deal with these house condition problems. Low income home ownership, poorly maintained home ownership, home owners who are asset rich but income poor and therefore cannot maintain properties, are all now recognized features of the market. As the early employed entrants to the home ownership system have aged and the sector has matured with a more balanced demographic and social profile, so the presence of these problems has become more apparent. If the level of home ownership is sustainable the quality of the sector appears not to be. The home ownership sector can no longer be assumed to deliver the social rights associated with high-standard housing throughout the lifetime of all home owners. The size and share of the housing market in home ownership is likely to increase and be sustained but the housing rights and qualities once associated with home ownership are less likely to be sustained.

In this later phase of home ownership, sponsorship and promotion by government has been reduced. Mortgage interest tax relief, which had been the most generous buttress for the growth of home ownership among middle and higher income groups began to be withdrawn just as it became more important for lower income groups. The initial steps to remove higher rates of tax relief removed the enhanced advantage for higher tax payers and higher income groups. From 1992 onwards the chancellor of the exchequer began to reduce the value of tax reliefs available to basic-rate taxpayers. While this pattern of change was entirely justified in the broader terms of tax policy and equity, the impact on homeowners was substantial. Home ownership no longer meant accessing such a privileged financial position. For the new cohort of homeowners, unless they purchased under the Right to Buy, neither the process of entry nor the certainties associated with becoming a homeowner could be relied upon. Increased risks in the labour market, both from unemployment and the development of part-time and flexible working reduced security for mortgage borrowing. The homeowner was therefore more exposed to risk, and the withdrawal of government financial support through income-support mortgage interest payments removed protection for that risk. With fewer people with the security of jobs for life, fewer could be sure that they would support a mortgage for life. Without the certainty of appreciating values of property, the homeowner in the 1990s was in a more precarious and powerless position than at any stage since the 1950s.

Contingent conclusions

How far has and does home ownership provide a key element in choice, control and citizenship? The account of the development of policy and debate about home ownership in Britain in this chapter has emphasized the changing nature of home ownership and the world about it. Its attributes are contingent. If the golden age of home ownership was one in which the sector was expanding most rapidly because of demographic and demand factors, and properties were appreciating in value (again because of these factors and rising affluence), it is also important to recognize that underpinning this golden age were generous tax relief, financial privileges and a safety net, both in terms of the social security system and the availability of good-quality council housing. These factors meant that the home ownership sector and homeowners themselves were not fully exposed to risk. After the golden age the safety nets were withdrawn. The alternative tenures are much less attractive, the financial privileges are less and the economic and social context leaves people much more exposed to risk. It is not home ownership *per se* that has changed but the contingent factors associated with it.

Against this background many of the assertions about home ownership now appear to be rather dubious. The academic literature on home owner-ship has indulged in an elaborate display which has sought on the one side to imply that home ownership is a natural demand-led product associated with ontological security and on the other side that it represents manipulation of the masses through false consciousness. Neither stance is very convincing. The home ownership sector has proved attractive and satisfactory for house-holds because of the contingent factors referred to and because: it has provided a better standard of housing at affordable prices than was available in the private rented sector; it has provided different routes of access to housing than were provided in the council housing sector; and latterly a better range of choice and quality than in the council sector. The reasons for the attractiveness and high levels of satisfaction in the owner-occupied sector do not require the exploration of biological and ontological dimen-sions. They are much more straightforward and because of this, home-owners are likely to survive some of the changes which have been described above. Although the homeowner is more exposed to risk, the range of properties and the quality of properties available in the home ownership sector are very different to those available either in the private or social rented sector. Consequently people will still choose to buy properties. The material circumstances which can be achieved through home ownership remain superior. It may be that because of the greater exposure to risk there will, over time, be an incremental change in this pattern but it will take decades before the changed context and contingencies of home owner-ship result in different patterns of choice and preference.

The implications of all of these points are that we should exercise great caution in assuming that different tenures are universally or exclusively associated with different choices, different rights and different citizenship status. While there may be a greater likelihood of certain conditions apply-ing in particular tenures, there is no guarantee of these circumstances. There are variations between social groups spatially and there are changes which occur over time. The features which have dominated the experience of one cohort in one context, in one phase of the growth of home ownership, are not likely to hold true for all time and for all groups.

Throughout the period of the development of home ownership and through the different claims made for it at different stages, reference to citizenship has been frequent. Different commentators have made different claims related to citizenship. Although it is now clear that home ownership does not guarantee citizenship, control and choice, it has been associated with these elements at different stages. Although it has not been the source of these securities, the political debates around housing tenure have tended to attribute these qualities to home ownership, rather than to other tenures. References to citizenship in the past were rarely references to the social rights of citizenship in a Marshallian sense but were rather about the behaviour or obligations of citizens. Over time, perhaps as political concerns about the threats of Bolshevism and revolution receded, the idea of ownership of property as citizenship associated with the behaviour and obligations of citizens gave way to an argument about owner-occupiers as more *complete* citizens.

With the decline of private renting and the damaged status of council housing, the status and reputation of home ownership in terms of the housing debate had reached its peak by the 1980s. The most unqualified assertions about the merits, qualities and rights associated with that tenure appeared in that period. However in more recent years it would appear that there has been a further redefinition of the ideas of citizenship associated with owner occupation. Homeowners are clearly no longer a uniform group (if they ever were) and they do not universally benefit from the highest standards of housing. Nor are they any longer secure and contented citizens insulated against market forces and without risk of been deprived of their housing, their wealth, their citizenship or their status as a result of changed economic circumstances or the actions of financial institutions.

The rights and status of the homeowner are no longer intrinsic in the 1990s and the concern of policy makers and the policy debate is to *sustain* home ownership. If at one stage the view was that the tenure itself was indicator of rights, independence and security and a route to success, the implications of the debates in the 1990s are that being a homeowner is no longer a sufficient guarantee, and sustainable home ownership requires continued policy intervention.

References

Bellman, H. (1927) *The Building Society Movement*. London: Methuen.
Boddy, M. (1980) *The Building Societies*. London: Macmillan.
Boleat, M. (1997) The politics of home ownership, in P. Williams (ed.) *Directions in*

Housing Policy: Towards Sustainable Housing Policies for the UK. London: Paul Chapman Publishing.

Boleat, M. and Coles, A. (1987) *The Mortgage Market.* London: Allen & Unwin.

Conservative Party (1949) *The Right Road for Britain.* London: Conservative Central Office.

Conservative Party (1979) *The Conservative Party Manifesto.* London: Conservative Central Office.

DoE (1971) *Fair Deal for Housing,* Cmnd 6851. London: HMSO.

Forrest, R. and Murie, A. (1994) Home ownership in recession. *Housing Studies,* 9: 55–74.

Forrest, R., Murie, A. and Williams, P. (1990) *Home Ownership: Differentiation and Fragmentation.* London: Unwin Hyman.

Gauldie, E. (1974) *Cruel Habitations.* London: George Allen & Unwin.

Hansard (1951a) vol. 493, cols 846–7, 13 November. London: HMSO.

Hansard (1951b) vol. 495, cols 2251–2, 4 December. London: HMSO.

Hansard (1979a) vol. 967, cols 79–80, 15 May. London: HMSO.

Hansard (1979b) vol. 967, col. 407, 15 May. London: HMSO.

Hansard (1980) vol. 976, col. 1445, 15 January. London: HMSO.

Harris, N. (1973) *Competition and the Corporate Society.* London: Methuen.

Hoffman, J.D. (1964) *The Conservative Party in Opposition 1945–51.* London: MacGibbon & Kee.

Leather, P. and Mackintosh, S. (1997) Towards sustainable policies for housing renewal in the private sector, in P. Williams (ed.) *Directions in Housing Policy: Towards Sustainable Housing Policies for the UK.* London: Paul Chapman Publishing.

MacGregor, J. (1965) Strategy for housing, in *The Conservative Opportunity.* London: Batsford.

Maclennan, D. (1997) The UK housing market: up, down and where next?, in P. Williams (ed.) *Directions in Housing Policy: Towards Sustainable Housing Policies for the UK.* London: Paul Chapman Publishing.

MacLeod, I. and Maude, A. (1950) *One Nation.* London: Conservative Political Centre.

Merrett, S. (1979) *State Housing in Britain.* London: Routledge and Kegan Paul.

Merrett, S. (1982) *Owner Occupation in Britain.* London: Routledge and Kegan Paul.

Ministry of Housing and Local Government (1953) *Houses: The Next Step,* Cmd 8996.

Murie, A. (1975) *The Sale of Council Houses.* Birmingham: Centre for Urban and Regional Studies, University of Birmingham.

Nevitt, A.A. (1966) *Housing Finance, Taxation and Subsidies.* London: Nelson.

Pooley, C. (ed.) (1993) *Housing Strategies in Europe 1880–1930.* Leicester: Leicester University Press.

Samuel, R., Kincaid, J. and Slater, E. (1962) But nothing happens. *New Left Review,* 13–14.

Wilcox, S. (1997) *Housing Finance Review 1997/98.* York: Joseph Rowntree Foundation.

Williams, P. (ed.) (1997) *Directions in Housing Policy: Towards Sustainable Housing Policies for the UK.* London: Paul Chapman Publishing.

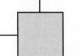

5

Expanding private renting: flexibility at a price?

Alex Marsh and Moyra Riseborough

Introduction

The role that the private rented sector plays in housing British households has changed dramatically during the twentieth century. In 1938 more than half the dwellings in England and Wales were in the private rented sector, whereas by 1988 the sector had declined such that it accounted for only 8.7 per cent of the housing stock (Kemp 1997). The causes and consequences of this decline have been much debated. In the context of both wider economic and labour market change and the specific problems encountered by owner-occupiers in the late 1980s and early 1990s, the decline of private renting, and the search for appropriate remedies, has taken on increased significance.

This chapter has two aims. It seeks to examine the changes that have occurred in policy towards the sector and to explore the experience of those living in the sector. The themes of citizenship, choice and control provide a valuable aid to thinking about the private rented sector: they are central to debates on the changing role and future of the sector, even if such debates are not always explicitly conducted in these terms.

Understanding change in the private rented sector

In thinking about change in the private rented sector we can consider three distinct features of housing as a commodity. First, there are the physical characteristics of the structure (number of rooms, heating, location etc.), second, there are considerations of security of occupancy, and third, there are issues of cost. When considering the physical characteristics of a dwelling the quality and not just the nature of those characteristics plays an important part in housing consumption decisions. Further, there may be a trade-off between the quality of a dwelling and its environment. That is, some households may be willing to consume relatively poor-quality accommodation in order to reside in a location which has features they find particularly desirable, or to avoid locations perceived to be undesirable. Each of the three features of housing may be examined at a more abstract level by considering the set of rights attached to housing. Let us consider rights in relation to each of the three features in turn.

Rights accruing to housing consumers can be considered to be of two types: 'use rights' and 'exchange rights'. Two particular use rights are the right to alter the physical structure or appearance of a property and the right to enjoy the consumption of the commodity, undisturbed, for a particular period of time (security of tenure). These use rights are conditional, regardless of whether a household rents a property or is purchasing it with a mortgage. However, private tenants experience this conditionality more directly: legislation has repeatedly altered the rights to which both landlord and tenant are entitled once they enter into a rental agreement.

Renters in Britain are typically constrained by their rental agreement not to alter the physical structure or decoration of the property that they are renting. Rights in these areas are retained by the landlord, with the tenant making a contribution to the upkeep of the dwelling through rental payments. In Britain, therefore, private tenants have choice over the level and nature of housing they consume only prior to deciding to rent a particular property, which they may have selected after comparison with a number of others. Once a rental agreement has been entered into it is the landlord who controls the characteristics of the housing consumed by the tenant. If a landlord fails to carry out urgent repairs then tenants have legal rights to compel the landlord to act, but whether these rights are meaningful in practice is a question we will return to below. If a landlord's inaction means that a dwelling poses a threat to the health of the tenants or others, the state – in the form of environmental health officers – may override concerns about private property rights and intervene directly in the landlord-tenant relationship. This distribution of rights between landlord and tenant has remained largely unchanged over time and has not been the most prominent feature in debates about private renting in Britain. It is important to recognize, however, that this distribution of rights is by no means 'natural' and could be contested.

Rights to security of tenure, in contrast to rights to alter the physical character of properties, have been of considerable importance in debates about private renting. At the beginning of the century tenants had very limited rights and landlords could remove them from a property with as little as a week's notice. Subsequent legislation increased security of tenure and during certain periods it was difficult, if not impossible, for the landlord legally to regain possession of the property as long as the tenant kept paying the rent. Over time the formal balance of power and the level of control over housing consumption has shifted back and forth between landlord and tenant. Yet to focus upon formal legal rights alone would be to miss crucial aspects of the operation of the private rented sector and the experience of living in private rented accommodation. As we explore further below, security of tenure and the extent of tenants' rights have been seen as central policy concerns.

Equally significant in debates about the private rented sector is the issue of control over rent levels. Should they be determined by 'the market' or in some other way? There are at least four possible alternatives to determination by the market: first, rents could be determined directly by legislation; second, rent-setting could involve imposition of 'floors', 'ceilings' or maximum rates of increase on the rents for different types of property; third, rents could be determined by a public-sector agent on the basis of some criteria – such as 'fairness' – which market-based determination might fail to take into account; fourth, governments could intervene indirectly by manipulating subsidy systems to help low-income households pay their rents. In this way the government may effectively establish the 'going rate' for properties in those segments of the market catering for low-income households. The past and present system in Britain has displayed many features of this sort of indirect regulation.

When rent regulation suppresses rents below market levels then security of tenure becomes an issue. If a landlord can see an opportunity either to let a property on an unregulated rent or to sell the property at a profit once an existing regulated tenant leaves, then this can lead to harassment and illegal eviction. Whether landlords have the incentive to take these sorts of action depends on a number of factors including the nature and scope of the rent regulations imposed, the price that an untenanted property could fetch, the demand for such property, and the landlords' perceptions of the chances of being prosecuted for their actions. These factors in turn are shaped by wider policy agendas, subsidy systems and economic conditions.

We begin our examination of these issues by outlining the changing role of the private rented sector in Britain. We then examine policy change. The focus of our discussion then shifts towards the way in which the private rented sector operates at micro-level. We conclude by reflecting upon the experience of the private rented sector in Britain in the light of the three themes of this book: citizenship, choice and control.

The changing role of private renting

From its position as the majority tenure at the start of the twentieth century, the private rented sector declined such that by 1989 it accounted for only 9.1

per cent of dwellings (see Table 5.1). Between the First and the Second World Wars the sector declined steadily. It was in the 30 years following the outbreak of the Second World War that the sector went into rapid decline. The decline continued into the late 1980s. From 1989 onward the sector appeared to be reviving: by 1995 10 per cent of dwellings in Great Britain were privately rented. This represents 319,000 more dwellings than in 1989 (Wilcox 1997: Table 16c).

A range of factors have been identified as responsible for this decline (see Kemp 1988a; 1993). Key factors in housing finance policy include the relatively favourable tax treatment of owner occupation, the lack of depreciation allowances for landlords (in contrast to other types of investor), and the direct subsidy for development of local authority housing. The development of a housing finance system built on retail savings institutions (the building societies) providing long term mortgage finance meant that alternatives to private renting became accessible to consumers. The

Table 5.1   Housing tenure in Great Britain, 1914–95 (percentage of all dwellings)

Year	Homeowner	Local authority	Private rented	Other/housing association[1]
1914	10.0	1.0	80.0	9.0
1938	25.0	10.0	56.0	9.0
1945	26.0	12.0	54.0	8.0
1951	29.0	18.0	45.0	8.0
1961	43.0	27.0	25.0	6.0
1966	47.1	28.7	18.8	5.4
1970	50.0	30.4	14.9	5.1
1981	56.4	30.3	11.1	2.2
1982	57.7	29.1	10.9	2.3
1983	58.7	28.1	10.8	2.3
1984	59.6	27.4	10.6	2.4
1985	60.5	26.6	10.4	2.5
1986	61.5	25.9	10.0	2.6
1987	62.6	25.1	9.6	2.6
1988	64.0	24.0	9.2	2.7
1989	65.2	22.8	9.1	2.9
1990	65.8	21.9	9.3	3.1
1991	66.0	21.2	9.6	3.2
1992	66.1	20.6	9.8	3.4
1993	66.4	20.1	9.8	3.7
1994	66.8	19.5	9.9	4.0
1995	66.7	18.9	10.0	4.1

[1] From 1981 figures are for housing associations only.
Source: Forrest *et al.* 1990, Table 3.1; Wilcox 1997, Table 16d.

development of investment opportunities other than residential property gave small investors alternative, more liquid, vehicles for their investment.

The exodus of investors from the sector was spurred by the negative image of the private landlord which was reinforced by the 1960s case of Peter Rachman, the West London landlord whose name came to symbolize bad management, poor living conditions and exploitation of tenants (see Kemp 1992). The stigma that became attached to private landlordism in the post-war period reduced further its appeal to 'respectable' investors.

On the demand side, wider economic factors such as increasing employment stability and rising real incomes for many households made owner occupation both attractive and attainable. High general inflation coupled with a house price boom in the 1970s further enhanced the appeal of owner occupation to those who could gain access to mortgage finance.

Rising real incomes in the post-war period did not touch everyone and many of those seeking accommodation in the private rented sector remained on relatively low incomes. They were therefore not in a position to pay rents which provided landlords with a competitive rate of return. This has been described as the 'central dilemma' of the sector (HCEC 1982).

The imposition of rent control reduced further the return on investment that landlords could obtain. If rents are artificially suppressed below those which landlords would otherwise wish to charge then, it is argued, landlords' will either let the quality of the property decline so that the controlled rent becomes an acceptable rate of return on the property or sell up and get out of private landlordism. Rent control legislation has covered the private rented stock to a greater or lesser extent almost continuously in Britain since it was first imposed during the First World War.

Strong demand for owner occupation coupled with the relatively low returns available to landlords meant that there was a strong incentive for landlords to move out of the sector. It has been estimated that 2.6 million private rented dwellings were sold to owner occupation between 1938 and 1975 (DoE 1977b: 39). During this period more than a million privately rented dwellings were demolished through slum clearance.

The apparent recovery of the sector during the early 1990s is also intimately linked with owner occupation. Recent research suggests that around 10 per cent of lettings in the early 1990s can be accounted for by owner-occupiers who were unable to sell their dwelling and consequently let the property, waiting for the market to recover (Crook and Kemp 1996: 58). Another factor in the revival of the sector was the use of the Business Expansion Scheme (BES) for residential property. The scheme provided favourable tax treatment for investors in private rented property during the period 1988–93 (see Crook et al. 1991) and evidence suggests that many of the investors who entered the market exited again once the favourable treatment was no longer available. A third factor, identified by Mullins et al. (1997), also relates to the slump in owner occupation. Some landlords were attracted back into the sector in the mid-1990s by a combination of low purchase prices, low mortgage interest rates and the relatively high rents that could be covered by housing benefit. Entry costs and the cost of capital were low and the rate of return was relatively healthy. However, subsequent rises in house prices and interest rates, coupled with restrictions on housing benefit in 1995 and 1996 mean that such reinvestment is likely to appear less attractive in the current environment. All the indications are that unless the policy framework or the economic fundamentals alter significantly the mid-1990s revival of renting is likely to be a temporary pause in the longer-term decline.

Current debates regarding the sector have largely focused on the issue of economic fundamentals, labour markets and the changing nature of work. These point to the conclusion that the previous reliance upon owner occu-pation and social housing is not an appropriate strategy. While the decline of the sector generated little concern for much of the twentieth century, there has been considerably more interest during the last decade and the idea that the sector serves a valuable function in a modern economy has become more widely accepted. Nonetheless, some commentators have noted that using the private sector to house poorer households is likely to be poor value for public money where rents are high and tenants rely on housing benefit.

The rehabilitation of the reputation of the sector started with the recog-nition that the remaining private rented sector plays an important role in catering for particular sectors of society. In particular, four distinct subsec-tors have been identified (Bovaird *et al.* 1985):

1 A declining traditional sub-sector which contains mainly older people who have regarded private renting as their lifetime tenure.
2 A sub-sector providing easy access short-term accommodation for young and mobile households.
3 A sub-sector in which accommodation is rented with a job or business.
4 A residual sub-sector which houses those who live in the private rented sector because they are unable to obtain accommodation in one of the majority tenures.

The traditional sub-sector can be considered simply to be a legacy of a previous era and accommodation rented with a job or business is provided on a basis without direct connection to the broader dynamics of the housing market, but the sub-sector providing for young and mobile households and the residual sub-sector are of continued and ongoing importance to the operation of the housing market. Much attention has recently focused on the role that private renting plays in catering for those households who are unwilling or unable to become owner-occupiers.

The sector has always accommodated young mobile households, but, whereas in the 1980s younger groups may have moved out of the sector into owner occupation at the earliest opportunity, in the 1990s circumstances have changed. Having witnessing the experiences of many owner-occupiers in the early 1990s – of falling house prices, negative equity and repossessions – younger households may now postpone entry into owner occupation. This will in turn increase overall demand for privately rented accommodation. Changes to the contemporary labour market – with an increase in temporary, contract and casual labour – could hamper the ability of some households to access owner occupation, even if they might wish to. Similarly the deregulation of labour markets and increases in low-paid employment point to the need for more affordable rented accommodation. Current policy priorities suggest it will have to come from the private sector.

Assuming these labour market changes persist or intensify then it will be necessary to have a housing system which can accommodate an increasing number of households in insecure employment. Such a system cannot rely so heavily on owner occupation as has been the case in the past and is therefore likely to require a functioning private rented sector (Ford and Wilcox 1994; Maclennan 1994). But even though private rented housing may have a particular role to play in ensuring the British economy is competitive, it does not imply that the sector need grow in size. When the expansion of 'the private rented sector' is discussed it is typically the expansion of one or more sub-sectors that is being considered. Even if the sub-sector catering for the young and mobile and the residual sub-sector expand, older people will be leaving the traditional sub-sector and therefore the sector overall may not grow markedly.

The residual sub-sector is inhabited by households who are unable to access other tenures. This can be because they have insufficient income to enter owner occupation or because they do not qualify for social housing because they do not satisfy rules regarding length of residence (immigrant households) or are not considered in sufficient need (e.g. single people without children). Those living in the residual sub-sector are likely to be on low incomes, often reliant on housing benefit to assist them to meet their housing costs, and would probably not choose to reside in the sector given the opportunity to do otherwise.

A final component in the re-evaluation of the private rented sector is the reconfiguration of social housing and local authority duties to house homeless households. For at least two decades many local authorities have placed households in private rented accommodation on a more or less temporary basis while, for example, claims for unintentional homelessness are investigated. The move to an enabling role for local authorities and towards the use of a range of local providers of housing for homeless households saw governments place increased emphasis upon the use of the private rented sector in the mid-1990s (DoE 1994; Walker *et al.* forthcoming). The distinction between the circumstances of those who find accommodation through their local authority and those who find private solutions through the residual sub-sector of the private rented sector becomes increasingly blurred. If this trend continues then it may reinforce the need for private rented housing for low-income households in particular localities.

Changing policy towards the private rented sector

Policy until the late 1970s

The first major government intervention in the housing market which didn't draw its justification from public health concerns occurred when the government introduced rent control and security of tenure into the private sector through the 1915 Increase of Rents and Mortgage Interest (War Restrictions) Act. This intervention has been interpreted as either an attempt to stop landlords exploiting wartime housing shortages in areas of high demand or as the culmination of a lengthy period of unrest about the behaviour of landlords towards tenants. Regardless of its origins, the 1915 Act was accompanied by political debate regarding the appropriateness of rent control. Following the Act the decline of the sector began: debate regarding the contribution of rent control and security of tenure to the decline has recurred ever since. The debate is a classic example of Hirschman's (1991) 'perversity thesis' in action. Those who wish citizens to have access to secure affordable private rented accommodation argue that rent control is the only way to curb the worst instincts of the private landlord. This is countered with the argument that even if we all agree that secure affordable accommodation is desirable, rent control is a perverse means to use to attain it – by stopping landlords earning a satisfactory rate of return, rent control will reduce both the number and the quality of private rented units, which in turn makes it harder to achieve the objective.

There was little consensus between the major political parties about what, if anything, should be done about the decline of private renting in the post-Second World War period. The main political parties took different views regarding the import of the decline in private renting. The Conservative Party typically viewed it as an undesirable development, whereas the Labour Party took a much more negative view of private landlordism and consequently viewed the decline with equanimity.

As a consequence of the differing perspectives on decline, the evolution of legislation has involved switching between attempts to increase the scope and strength of regulation and attempts to deregulate rents and reduce security of tenure. Perhaps the starkest example of this divergence of views occurred in the decade from 1955 to 1965 (see Banting 1979). Kemp (1997) notes the strongly ideological tone of political debate about the sector during this period. The 1957 Rent Act introduced by the Conservatives raised controlled rents, deregulated rents on higher-value properties and introduced deregulation of re-letting. Tenants who were in the deregulated sector would have no security of tenure other than a month's notice. This Act was followed by Labour's 1965 Rent Act which introduced the concept of the 'regulated' tenancy for unfurnished properties: the rent on such tenancies would be controlled through being set and registered at the 'fair rent' and they would have the same security of tenure as under earlier controlled tenancies.

The legal rights of tenants were strengthened by the 1964 Protection from Eviction Act, and the 1972 Housing Finance Act introduced a national scheme of rent allowances for tenants of unfurnished lets. Both fair rents and rent allowances were extended to cover furnished dwellings in 1974.

Although the position of tenants appeared to have been strengthened as a result, during the 1970s it became clear that legislation may have established regulation and control over large parts of the private rented sector but landlords were able to find loopholes in the law which allowed them to let properties outside the provision of the 1965 and 1974 Rent Acts with very limited security of tenure (DoE 1977a, 1977b, 1977c). Many tenancies that were covered by the Rent Act were being let at a rent other than the registered rent. During this period there was a sense in which the legislative framework was increasingly out of step with the functioning of the market in particular localities. Properties were being let at higher rents than dictated by the Rent Acts and with less security of tenure than was considered desirable by government. This situation was in part a function of the land-lords' perceptions of the likelihood that any action would be taken against them for breaching the regulations. It was also a function of the fact that there was demand for the sort of accommodation that could be offered by the private rented sector. Some consumers were willing to forego their formal rights in order to secure accommodation. Later in the chapter we consider why that might be.

The major review of housing policy undertaken by the Labour govern-ment of the mid-1970s (see DoE 1977a) encompassed all tenures and included a detailed examination of the private rented sector (see DoE 1977c). The Labour government was aware that in other countries the tax treatment of private rented housing made landlordism more attractive, but introducing such a scheme in Britain did not fit with contemporary policy priorities (Holmans 1991: 211). In the mid-1970s the possible disappear-ance of the private landlord was not viewed as a cause for serious concern by government. Some commentators felt able to declare with enthusiasm that private landlordism was dead (e.g. Finnis 1977). Yet at the same time the political right continued to argue that rent deregulation and reductions in security of tenure would revive the tenure and were therefore valuable components of housing policy (e.g. Hayek 1975; Conservative Central Office 1976). Nonetheless, despite the parties' differences, the fate of private renting was not a central concern because owner occupation and local authority renting were being championed as more suitable and desirable tenures.

Policy towards private renting in the early Thatcher years

The major political parties approached the 1979 general election using very different rhetoric regarding the private rented sector. The Labour Party adopted a position which continued its long-standing antipathy towards the private landlord. The rhetoric was oriented towards the interests of tenants and extending the bundle of rights that came with a tenancy. The Labour election manifesto stated that 'private renting has entered an irreversible decline' (Labour Party 1979: 19). It went on to affirm the principles of security of tenure and rent regulation and to state that if re-elected it would legislate to close loopholes in the Rent Acts. The manifesto stated that it would be made easier for tenants to force their landlord to undertake necessary repairs and that the party would continue to encourage 'socially-accountable landlords' to take over privately-rented property, except when let by a resident landlord.

The Conservative Party had been discussing policies of a very different type for a number of years (Conservative Central Office 1976; Holmans 1991: 207). The principal housing policy in the 1979 manifesto was the proposal for 'the right to buy' for council tenants. Even though it dealt with the private rented sector relatively briefly, it clearly took a very different tone to Labour. It focused on the disincentives to landlords to let property, caused by the contemporary legal framework. To encourage the revival of the sector it proposed introducing a system of shorthold tenure which would allow short fixed-term lets. This section of the manifesto finished by seeking to reassure readers that the proposed changes would not affect existing tenants and asserted that 'we must try to achieve a greater take-up in rent allowances for poorer tenants' (Conservative Party 1979: 24). The manifesto attempted to counter the long-standing concern that removing rent regulation would lead to rapidly increasing rents and unreasonable demands being placed on poorer households. Even at this stage, however, the commitment to ensuring poorer tenants were protected by rent allowances was perhaps less than emphatic.

The change of government in 1979 thus brought to power a government which saw, rhetorically at least, the decline of the private rented sector in terms of ill-advised legislation regulating the sector. The Conservatives saw a key role for the sector in catering for 'those who are mobile, those who want accommodation for a short period of time ... people who may be saving up to buy sooner, or later, who may have relatively low incomes at this particular time but can see income growth coming' (J. Stanley, minister for housing and construction quoted in Kemp 1993: 63). The party envisaged a future of 'creeping decontrol' of new lettings.

One of the first things that the Conservative government did on its election in 1979 was to begin dismantling the provisions of the Rent Acts. The 1980 Housing Act introduced a range of measures affecting the private rented sector including two new types of tenancy which would apply to new lettings: the protected shorthold tenancy and the assured tenancy. Shorthold tenancies circumscribed the security of tenure available to tenants, whereas assured tenancies deregulated rents in an attempt to attract landlords with the possibility of charging higher rents. Shorthold tenancies were for a fixed term of between one and five years. During the tenancy the tenant would have the same security as under a regulated tenancy, but the landlord had no obligation to renew the tenancy when the fixed term ended. The rents for shorthold lets were determined according to the same rules as for regulated tenancies. Assured tenancies only applied to properties which were newly-built or substantially renovated after the 1980 Act came into force and which were owned by a body approved by the Secretary of State for the Environment. Rents were agreed between landlord and tenant. Along with assured tenancies came the right to extend the tenancy at a market rent unless the landlord could demonstrate to a court that such an extension was inappropriate on one or more of a number of specific grounds. When the assured tenancy scheme was announced the Secretary of State reported that he had in mind bodies such as financial institutions or building societies as the new approved landlords (Kemp 1988b: 81).

Soon after the 1980 Act became law the House of Commons Environment Committee undertook an examination of the private rented sector (HCEC, 1982). The report reaffirmed some key issues noted in the earlier housing policy review (DoE, 1977a, 1977b). In particular it noted that during the 1970s a large proportion of lets were occurring outside of the Rent Acts on unregulated rents and with limited security of tenure. If rent control was not effective in practice, then removing it was not in itself likely to lead to the revival of the sector. The committee felt that the impact of the provisions of the 1980 Act were therefore unlikely to make a substantial contribution to stemming the decline of the sector. This analysis was confirmed by later research which showed that the overall impact of the initiatives contained in the 1980 Act was limited, even with the additional short-lived incentives to landlords introduced by the chancellor in 1982 but withdrawn two years later (see Kemp 1988b). The number of new tenancies created nationally numbered in the hundreds, rather than thousands.

For the 1983 general election the Conservative government contented itself with drawing attention to the wrong-headedness of the Labour Party's position on the private rented sector and to the innovations it had already made in the 1980 Act. The Labour Party restated its position that the sector was in decline, that tenants rights should be strengthened and that socially responsible landlords should supersede the private landlord. In 1985 the Conservatives considered removing rent controls on new lets but, partly as a result of concerns regarding the impact of rising rents on the cost of housing benefit, did not pursue this line further. The government did, however, introduce a range of initiatives which could be seen as paving the way for new private investment in rented housing (see Kemp 1993: 65–6).

Outside the party-political arena commentators were giving the private rented sector increased attention. For example, the first Duke of Edinburgh's Inquiry into British Housing (1985) accepted the continuing value of the private rented sector and considered the issue of declining investment in the sector. It made proposals regarding what might be considered appropriate rates of return to encourage further investment.

Promoting private renting

It is widely accepted that the 1987 Housing White Paper represents a significant shift in the then Conservative government's policy stance. The government moved away from the single-minded promotion of owner occupation towards the idea that a more balanced tenure structure, specifically one with a more prominent role for the private rented sector, would be appropriate. This reorientation came at a time when some economists were forcefully arguing that rigidities in the housing market were impeding the performance of the economy (Minford *et al.* 1987). Not only did the government apparently shift its position but so did the Labour Party. For example, the Labour manifesto for the 1987 election dropped the party's overtly hostile attitude towards the sector.

Although the White Paper has been interpreted as a change in policy stance, Boleat (1997) has recently offered a dissenting view. He suggests that the 1987 White Paper and the subsequent 1988 Act need to be related to the 1980 Act as part of a longer-term strategy: thus the two Acts could be interpreted as flowing from a single policy stance. He argues that the 1980 Act was a symbolic policy to overcome opposition to deregulation, without the expectation that it would have dramatic outcomes. It could then be argued that when the significant change in policy occurred in 1987 the battle had already been won at a rhetorical level.

Boleat's (1997) contribution does not, we would argue, present a compelling case for this alternative interpretation of policy development. Nonetheless it clearly illustrates the difficulties the policy analyst faces in attempting to disentangle and identify policy objectives and policy change, as noted in Chapter 1.

Although the Housing Bill which followed the White Paper was criticized at the time by some right-wing commentators for failing to take reforms far enough (e.g. Coleman 1990), the 1988 Housing Act which followed has resulted in significant changes in social relations within the private sector, even though it has not resulted in quite the dramatic increase in the number of private lets some might have hoped for.

The 1988 Act ended the possibility of creating new regulated tenancies, except in very specific circumstances. From 1989 new tenancies would normally be on either an assured or an assured shorthold basis. An assured shorthold tenancy is a letting for a term of at least six months with the rent agreed between landlord and tenant. The tenant has a right to apply for a rent determination by a rent assessment committee where it appears that the rent they are being asked to pay is significantly higher than rents for similar tenancies locally. During the term of the tenancy a landlord can seek repossession on one of a number of specified bases, but after the term ends the landlord is *entitled* to possession, hence security of tenure is strictly limited. An element of this legislation that was to prove important was that in order to create an assured shorthold tenancy the landlord had to follow specific procedures before the tenancy commenced. If the procedures were not followed then the tenancy would be deemed to be an assured tenancy, which gave the tenant greater security.

Given earlier concerns regarding the possibility of deregulation leading to rents increasing rapidly, the government felt it appropriate to attempt to curb the impact of rent deregulation on the public purse. So from 1989 when a tenant wished to claim housing benefit to assist with their housing costs the rent was referred to the rent officer to determine whether the rent was 'reasonable' and whether the dwelling was larger than was required to meet the tenant's 'reasonable needs'. If the rent officer determined that the rent was unreasonable then that reduced the subsidy which the local authority received in order to cover the housing benefit payment. However if the rent was considered unreasonable there was no obligation on the landlord to reduce it. A local authority had the discretion to fund the difference between benefit entitlement and subsidy receipt from its own funds and it might well do so given its responsibilities to consider hardship, but if it chose not to then the tenant would either have to fund the increased proportion of the rent from their own pocket or attempt to renegotiate the rent.

This policy change is significant because it means that effectively, although the rhetoric was of deregulation and withdrawal from direct interference with the market, the government at the same time introduced indirect control over rent levels for a significant portion of the market through capping tenants' subsidy-assisted ability to pay.

The other significant policy innovation during this period was, as noted earlier, the use of the BES for investment in private rented accommodation (see Crook *et al.* 1991). The scheme provided tax relief to those who purchased shares in BES companies and exempted the sale of the shares from capital gains tax as long as they were held for at least five years. The project was intended to 'kick-start' investment in the sector rather than demonstrate the need for subsidies in order to make investment competitive

(Kemp 1993). Yet the fact that most investors sold their shares as soon as they qualified for exemption from capital gains tax suggests that the principal lesson to be drawn from this experiment is precisely that subsidies are needed to make investment competitive.

Policy towards the private rented sector in the 1990s

During the 1990s it is has become possible for some commentators to talk of a consensus about the future of private renting (e.g. Best *et al.* 1992). Perhaps the most notable development has been the continued thawing of the Labour Party's position towards the sector. Its position has moved to such an extent that in the run-up to the 1997 general election, Labour could assert that a thriving private rented sector was a desirable feature of a modern economy. The emergence of this consensus has been strongly influenced by the growing acceptance on all sides of the arguments linking the performance of the economy with the need for a flexible housing market, as discussed above. The sector has a role in housing those who do not wish to buy, for whatever reason, and because social housing is unlikely to expand it will continue to play a role in housing those who cannot gain access to social housing or buy.

If the private rented sector is to play its role in providing acceptable quality accommodation to households who might previously have chosen to own, then the relevant sub-sector needs to both expand in scale and to upgrade the average quality of its housing stock. Most commentators accept that this will require the entry into the market of institutional investors with the necessary financial muscle. This would represent a move away from the traditional structure of private landlordism in Britain which has largely been based on very small-scale landlords (Crook *et al.* 1995). The search for a means to tempt investors into the sector, which saw the innovative use of the BES has continued with the more recent proposals to set up housing investment trusts.

One of the features of the system under the 1988 Housing Act was that, typically because of a failure to understand the provisions of the Act properly, many landlords inadvertently created assured tenancies instead of assured shorthold tenancies and therefore gave their tenants greater security of tenure than the landlord might have wished. Given that much of the current concern is with removing disincentives to investment by private landlords, the 1996 Housing Act made an important modification to the system by making the default tenure the assured shorthold rather than the assured. Thus, landlord and tenant have to agree explicitly to enter into an agreement granting the tenant more rights than those of an assured shorthold.

Moves of this nature might suggest that the progress of deregulation continues. But the use of indirect regulation through the subsidy system has if anything been strengthened by the introduction of 'local reference rents' in the calculation of housing benefit subsidies. Indeed the housing benefit system has perhaps taken on a more general importance. In 1996 the Conservative government modified the housing benefit rules such that single people under 25 can only claim housing benefit on non-self contained property: 'the single room rent' (Zebedee and Ward 1996). Thus if such households rely on housing benefit in order to secure accommodation then they are being filtered towards houses in multiple occupation (HMOs), and these form the part of the sector suffering from particular problems of quality and safety. More broadly, this change was linked to the government's rhetoric regarding the importance of family values and the intention behind the change was to discourage low income individuals from forming separate households. Although commentators have argued that this is likely to have a significant effect upon household formation, there is little systematic evidence so far to show what has occurred in practice.

There now appears to be broad agreement at the political level regarding the need for the private rented sector, but it is important to note that the political parties are not in complete accord. Prior to the 1997 election the then Labour housing spokesman distinguished between the two parts of the private rented sector and suggested that they should be treated differently. While the part of the rented sector which caters for those households who can secure accommodation on an unsubsidised market basis might properly be left to continue on that basis, he felt that there was a need to regulate closely the part of the sector which caters for low income households who rely on public subsidy. More recently it appears that the government is developing proposals to regulate and licence HMOs (*Housing Today* 1997).

The experience of private renting

Kemp (1990, 1997) draws on Hindess (1987) to argue that much of the debate around private renting has been conducted in idealized and essentialist terms. Those who advocate deregulation and free-market solutions work on the basis of a model of the way in which perfect markets function, and this abstracts from the complexities and imperfections of real-world markets as social institutions. Those who seek the demise of private landlords as a housing provider often do so on the basis of a portrayal of landlords as rapacious and unscrupulous individuals. While there are undoubtedly landlords who fit this description, to start from the assumption that these are the defining characteristics of the private landlord is inappropriate. Evidence suggests that many landlords do not attempt to maximize rents or set market rents; indeed many are not aware what the market rent for their property might be (Crook *et al.* 1995).

The 1980s legislation which reduced security of tenure and deregulated rents is also based on an idealized conception of the landlord-tenant relationship. It sees them as freely entering a contract together as equal parties. On the basis of this conception, market rents can be viewed as the product of a process of negotiation between the two parties. The thinking behind this legislation suffers from the same deficiency as much microeconomic theory. When markets are perfectly competitive there are a large number of well-informed buyers and sellers and no seller has the power to affect price. If such a situation obtained in the private rented sector then neither landlord nor tenant could exert any power over the other party. If tenants do not like the accommodation offered by a landlord then there is plenty of alternative accommodation on offer. A landlord need not be concerned if a particular tenant does not wish to pay for the accommodation on offer because there are many other tenants seeking accommodation. The key to the model is choice: what Hirschman (1970) termed the power of 'exit'. It is only when there are equally good alternatives on offer to each party that transactions between them can be seen as voluntary and mutually beneficial exchanges.

This conception of market exchange can be criticized because it ignores issues of power and control which are evident in many real-world economic relationships. Where there is market disequilibrium then the alternatives available to some market participants are reduced and that curtails the power of exit. If, for example, supply is insufficient to meet demand then consumers must compete to secure a share of the available supply and some will inevitably go without, in the short term at least. In this situation suppliers are on the 'short side' of the market and find themselves with a degree of power over consumers. Some economists have gone further and suggested that even in fully competitive markets in equilibrium there are still good reasons for seeing power as an important element of exchange (Bowles and Gintis 1993a, 1993b).

The deregulation and reduced security of tenure introduced in the 1980s were intended to encourage landlords to increase the supply of privately-rented dwellings, and by implication, this move was attempting to remedy an excess demand for such dwellings. In situations of excess demand landlords will possess a degree of bargaining power over tenants. Indeed it can be argued that because landlords have the option to sell up and invest in something other than rented property, while many tenants have no choice – except homelessness – other than to rent privately, the landlord will always be in a stronger bargaining position. It is here that the legislation exhibits a tension because at the same time as instigating change on the basis of an ideal of voluntary exchange it strengthened legal protection against harassment and illegal eviction, which in effect concedes that landlords are the relatively powerful party.

The balance of power between landlord and tenant is likely to vary with both local market conditions and the segment of the market under consideration. As excess demand increases the shortage of property worsens and power concentrates further in the hands of landlords. Households who are young and mobile may have reasonable incomes and be able to afford alternatives including, if necessary, owner occupation. For such households private renting is 'a tenure of positive choice' (Whitehead *et al.* 1985: 172) and thus the power that landlords can exert over them is moderated. However, for many poorer tenants the private rented sector is a residual tenure in which they reside because they have little alternative, including a lack of access to social housing. They may have limited financial resources of their own and be reliant on the state, through the housing benefit system, to keep a roof over their heads. In this situation landlords' bargaining power increases relative to that of tenants. The long-term excess demand that has existed in segments of the private rented sector has direct implications for many tenants' experience of private renting.

Yet, not all poorer households find themselves compelled to live in the sector. In their study of Southend-on-Sea Mullins *et al.* (1997) found households – including older people – who chose to live in less than satisfactory private rented accommodation because it offered access to services, facilities and social networks which they would have found much more difficult to reach had they lived in an alternative tenure, simply because of the location of alternative accommodation, including social housing. Focusing policy on improving the quality of the housing stock by building alternatives to private rented housing may offer the potential for ensuring that the population is adequately housed, but rights to good quality housing need to be set in the context of rights to other services. Better housing which renders households unable to secure rights in other areas may not improve their overall quality of life.

Excess demand in the private rented sector opens up the possibility of landlords discriminating between tenants. If a landlord knows that not letting a property to a particular household will not significantly affect rental income because there is a queue of other potential tenants, then there is considerable scope for direct discrimination. There is extensive evidence that such discrimination against black and minority ethnic households is widespread in the sector (e.g. HCEC 1982; LARH 1988; MacEwen 1991). As previously noted, in the past it has been possible in certain circumstances to inadvertently create a secure tenancy. This led landlords to discriminate against families and to favour letting to young mobile households who were unlikely to stay even if the tenancy was secure.

Similarly, an ability to fill vacancies without difficulty means that landlords can stipulate that they will not, for example, house those in receipt of housing benefit, although such stipulations can equally be seen as a screening device which signals that the landlord is attempting to cater for a different segment of the market, or may indicate that the landlord has concerns about the administration of the housing benefit system (Bevan *et al.* 1995) rather than about the tenants themselves.

A centrally important concern in the private sector is the quality of accommodation. Where there is an acute shortage of private rented accommodation landlords will always be able to let their property to *someone* and so have little incentive to provide accommodation of a satisfactory standard. Although the quality of the private rented stock has been improving over time, in 1991 some 20.5 per cent of private rented dwellings in England were unfit. This compares with only 5.5 per cent of owner-occupied dwellings, 6.9 per cent of local authority dwellings and 6.7 per cent of dwellings owned by housing associations (Leather and Morrison 1997: 32). Although not strictly comparable due to differences in definition, levels of unfitness in the private rented sector in both Wales and Northern Ireland appear somewhat higher than in England, and in Scotland 15 per cent of private rented dwellings were below tolerable standard in 1991. Thus, if we consider that citizens' rights include the right to good quality accommodation then it is in the private rented sector that this right has the highest probability of being denied.

One of the key 'use rights' to housing, identified at the start of the chapter, was the right to enjoy the consumption of the commodity, undisturbed, for the full length of an agreed tenancy (security of tenure). Throughout the post-war period concerns regarding the harassment or illegal eviction of tenants have been a recurrent feature of those demanding regulation or the demise of the private landlord.

The most recent survey of private renting in England (Carey 1995) gives some insight into the current state of the relationship between tenants and landlords. It suggests that while 77 per cent of tenants are on good terms with their landlord and a further 18 per cent have a fairly neutral relationship, some 5 per cent of tenants – equivalent to over 100,000 households – felt that they were on poor terms with their landlord (Carey 1995: Table A6.11). The survey suggests that the vast majority of those on poor terms with their landlord are renting from private individuals, but that tenants of property companies are more *likely* to be on poor terms with their landlord than those renting from other types of landlord.

There are a range of reasons why the relationship between landlord and tenant might not be positive, not all of which point to overt harassment. For example, a third of tenants who stated that they were not on good terms indicated this was because the landlord was hard to contact. The single most common reason for being on poor terms was stated to be conflict about repairs, cited by 58 per cent of those on poor terms (Carey 1995: Table A6.13). Although 5 per cent of tenants overall felt they had a poor relationship with their landlord this figure increased to 9 per cent for those living in accommodation which needed some kind of repair, compared to only 1 per cent for those living in accommodation which did not need repairing. Clearly, the magnitude of this difference cannot be accounted for by conflict over repairs alone, but suggests that disrepair acts as a good indicator of potential landlord-tenant difficulties. Four out of ten tenants on poor terms with their landlord felt that their landlord was unpleasant, untrustworthy or difficult. Some 18 per cent reported that their landlord was trying to evict them which, even if it sours relations, may of course not be illegal. More seriously, 17 per cent of tenants on poor terms with their landlord – which represents some 13,000 households – stated that their landlord used threats or intimidating behaviour. If one of key 'use rights' of housing is undisturbed consumption then this right is in question for the 7 per cent of tenants on poor terms with their landlord who reported that their landlord entered the premises without permission.

The survey of private renting also indicates that fears about the harassment of tenants with regulated tenancies by landlords wishing to secure vacant possession in order to sell or re-let on a shorthold tenancy are not without foundation. The percentage of tenants reporting that their landlord had asked them to leave or had done something to make them feel uncomfortable or want to leave declined along with security of tenure. While some 14 per cent of those on regulated tenancies reported being in this position only 9 per cent of those on assured tenancies found themselves similarly placed. This figure declined to only 6 per cent among those on assured shorthold tenancies (Carey 1995: Table A6.15). As might be expected, in situations where a landlord can legally regain possession within six months the incentive to harass tenants is weakened.

Given that the bargaining power of tenants in market exchange is limited, an alternative remedy for the problems of disrepair, harassment and illegal eviction is to put in place legislation making landlords' responsibilities and rights clear. As was noted at the beginning of this chapter, obligations to repair have been placed on landlords so tenants have legal rights to compel landlords to rectify serious deficiencies. Similarly, deregulation and reduced security of tenure were accompanied by a clarifying and strengthening of tenants' rights with regard to harassment and eviction during the term of the tenancy. While tenants may formally possess such rights, it is important to investigate whether they are effective.

There are four concerns which affect whether these rights are effective, but at source they all relate to the possibility of tenants seeking legal remedy without fear of reprisals. The first is a tenant's security of occupancy, the second is the state of the market, the third is securing housing in the future, and the fourth is the cost, complexity and timeliness of enforcing legal rights and, where they have been breached, of gaining redress. If a tenant has limited security of tenure or security of tenure for only a limited period then that may mitigate against pressing a landlord to act upon disrepair because the landlord can either rid themself of the tenant or simply wait for a tenancy to expire and not renew it. This strategy becomes even more likely when there is excess demand because the landlord can quickly fill any vacancy while the tenant may have more difficulty finding alternative accommodation. If a tenant has to rely on a reference from their landlord to secure such alternative accommodation then the necessity of not 'making waves' increases. Finally, although legislation has recently strengthened tenants' rights, they are required to pursue their case through courts which can be extremely costly and complex, and the time it can take is such that a tenant may well have had to leave a property because a tenancy has expired before a resolution is reached in the courts. Research which has attempted to assess the effectiveness of methods of enforcing tenants' rights under the current legislation (e.g. Burrows and Hunter 1990; Jew 1994) found that despite harassment apparently being common only a very small number of cases ever come to court. Further, when a landlord is found to be at fault the penalties incurred are extremely modest – hence the current system is therefore likely to be ineffective.

During the early 1980s there was considerable support for the idea of a housing court or tribunal which could act more quickly, simply and cheaply on housing matters (HCEC 1982; Whitehead and Kleinman 1986). Indeed the Labour Party included a proposal to set up a housing tribunal in both its 1979 and 1983 manifestos. Nonetheless, nothing came of this idea. More important in contemporary debate is the role of preventative measures in the form of 'tenancy relations advisors'. Where these have existed for some time they have been able to intercede between landlord and tenant, to clarify rights and point out responsibilities. This can go some way to defusing potentially difficult situations and disputes. While some local authorities have been running such services for some time, the 1996 Housing Act placed the requirement to operate some form of housing advice service directed towards homelessness on all authorities. Some practitioners have detected increasing use of such services by tenants during 1997.

It has long been recognized that an adequate understanding of the private rented sector – or indeed any market – needs to incorporate consideration of the way in which market conditions affect the provider-consumer relationship (DoE 1977c; HCEC 1982; Whitehead and Kleinman 1986). To understand the experience of private renting, therefore, it must be recognized that in real, rather than textbook, markets, the issue of bargaining power plays a fundamental role. The balance of power can shift as a result of local market conditions, but in the widespread condition of excess demand the landlord possesses the advantage. This opens the possibility for a whole range of less desirable practices and outcomes. One possibility for mitigating these problems is to increase supply and therefore provide tenants with more choice and the opportunity to exercise the power of exit. Yet some of the problems of the sector would remain even if excess demand were not an issue (Whitehead and Kleinman 1986). Changes in the market institutions – particularly legal rules and regulations – can shape the way in which markets function and can help to ensure that tenants' experience of housing is satisfactory, but only if they are enforceable and enforced.

Conclusion

Policy change in the private rented sector during the 1980s was intimately linked with issues of citizenship, choice and control at both the level of policy debate and in terms of policy outcomes. The Conservative governments spoke of removing unnecessary regulation from landlords and giving them greater control over their assets. This would lead to a greater willingness on the part of landlords to invest. The aim of the policy was to shift the balance of power in the landlord-tenant relationship in favour of landlords. Critics of this approach argue that it erodes the protection that tenants require in order to counterbalance the power of landlords and ensure that tenants experience the peaceful enjoyment of a good quality, secure, affordable home to which all citizens are entitled.

Perhaps the most interesting element of the policy debate since 1980 has been the dramatic repositioning of the Labour Party. In the early 1980s the Labour Party viewed the Conservative moves to deregulate the sector as an erosion of the rights of social citizenship and advocated extending the rights of tenants and the eventual demise of the private rented sector. Yet by the 1990s the party had shifted from implacable opposition to the sector to accepting that a thriving private rented sector is a valuable element of the housing system. It is thus possible for some commentators to talk of consensus in policy.

As an indicator of the success of the Conservative policy in achieving its object, Crook *et al.* (1995) found that over a half of the landlords they surveyed felt that the situation had changed to the advantage of landlords since 1988, whereas a quarter felt that it had not. Almost half of those who felt that things had improved cited easier repossessions and a third mentioned the ability to charge market rents. Nominal market rents rose by over 80 per cent between 1989 and 1996, while nominal fair rents more than doubled (from £24.38 per week to £49.90 per week). Figure 5.1 indicates that the price of rented housing was rising well ahead of inflation over the period. The increase in the housing benefit bill which accompanied these rent rises indicates that the central dilemma of the sector remains.

Among those landlords who felt that things had got worse, the reasons for this change were more diffuse. The most frequently cited reasons were: difficulty in letting properties because of increased competition or because tenants were demanding higher standards (17 per cent); the law being too much in tenants' favour (14 per cent); economic recession (13 per cent); and difficulty in repossessing or in court procedures and costs (11 per cent) (Crook *et al.* 1995: 13). Thus while the key factors making the environment more positive related to the legalisation, the negative factors were mixed: economic factors were as prominent as government action.

In the light of our discussion of the experience of private renting, the finding that some landlords were having difficulty in letting properties either

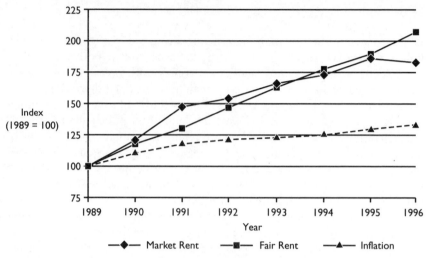

Figure 5.1   Increase in market and fair rents in England, 1989–96

Note: market rents are those determined by the rent officer for housing benefit purposes
Source: Authors' calculations based on figures drawn from Wilcox 1997.

because of increased competition or because tenants were demanding higher standards is particularly interesting. It could be interpreted as indicating that the power which landlords have had by virtue of operating in an environment of excess demand may have been eroded in certain localities. Greater competition would mean that tenants are being offered more choice and the fact that tenants felt able to demand higher standards may be a product of this. As we argued above, many of the problems in the private sector can be traced to the lack of incentives for landlords to address the inadequacy of the service they offer. It would be inappropriate to place too much weight on the findings presented by Crook *et al.* (1995) because further work looking at the operation of specific local housing markets is needed, but it may indicate that some landlords are starting to perceive that their environment is now presenting them with incentives to provide a good quality service which may not have been there previously.

Despite the political debate and legislative action since 1980 relating to the private rented sector it appears that much of its revival in the 1990s has been due to stagnation in the related (owner-occupied) market. Given the reasons for the decline of the sector it can be seen that, even though the legislation of the 1980s altered the social relations of private renting at the micro-level, in terms of the relative balance of influences on housing processes it is broader, economic, demographic and social forces which have been central to determining the role the sector plays in the contemporary housing market. The experience of private renting provides a good example of the way in which policy can attempt to stipulate the formal rights of citizens but, unless there are credible ways of enforcing those rights, it is economic and social factors that will determine the reality of many tenants' experience.

Yet, it would be inappropriate to suggest that policy is entirely ineffective in influencing the way in which the sector operates. Many landlords may not have complied with legislation on standards, rents or tenants' rights, but the issue of housing benefit has a considerable impact upon landlords' behaviour and willingness to cater for particular groups of households. In those parts of the sector in which benefit recipients reside it is questionable whether it is sensible to talk in terms of 'a market' for private rented housing, even though rents are formally deregulated and set at market levels. Where the majority of tenants rely on housing benefit to secure their accommodation the prevailing rent levels are inextricably bound to the administrative rules and rent determination procedures that govern housing benefit. In particular localities the private rented sector may depart even further from the market model because a large proportion of the sector is controlled through local authority contracts with landlords to provide for homeless households (see Walker *et al.* 1997).

While it may have withdrawn from blanket regulation, government has not disengaged from significant sections of the private rented sector. It could be argued that in the setting of housing benefit entitlements it has in fact found a means of regulating the sector which is considerably more difficult for the landlords of low income tenants to ignore. To the extent that this is more effective in influencing rent levels than direct control of rents, it may mean that policy will play a larger part in determining the future of the sector than it did in the past.

References

Banting, K. (1979) *Poverty, Politics and Policy*. London: Macmillan.

Best, R., Kemp, P., Coleman, D., Merrett, S. and Crook, T. (1992) *The Future of Private Renting: Consensus and Action*. York: Joseph Rowntree Foundation.

Bevan, M., Kemp, P. and Rhodes, D. (1995) *Private Landlords and Housing Benefit*, Centre for Housing Policy Research report. York: University of York.

Boleat, M. (1997) The politics of home ownership, in P. Williams (ed.) *Directions in Housing Policy: Towards Sustainable Housing Policies for the UK*. London: Paul Chapman Publishing.

Bovaird, A., Harloe, M. and Whitehead, C.M.E. (1985) Private rented housing: its current role. *Journal of Social Policy*, 14: 1–23.

Bowles, S. and Gintis, H. (1993a) Power and wealth in the competitive capitalist economy. *Philosophy and Public Affairs*, 21: 324–53.

Bowles, S. and Gintis, H. (1993b) The revenge of Homo Economicus: contested exchange and the revival of political economy. *Journal of Economic Perspectives*, 7: 83–102.

Burrows, L. and Hunter, N. (1990) *Forced Out!* London: Shelter Publications.

Carey, S. (1995) *Private Renting in England 1993/94*. London: HMSO.

Coleman, D. (1990) The new housing policy: a critique. *Housing Studies*, 4: 44–57.

Conservative Central Office (1976) *The Right Approach: A Statement of Conservative Aims*. London: CCO.

Conservative Party (1979) *Conservative Party Manifesto*. London: CCO.

Crook, A.D.H. and Kemp, P.A. (1996) The revival of private rented housing in Britain. *Housing Studies*, 11: 51–68.

Crook, A.D.H., Kemp, P.A., Anderson, I. and Bowman, S. (1991) *Tax Incentives and the Revival of Private Renting*. York: Cloister Press.

Crook, A.D.H., Hughes, J. and Kemp, P.A. (1995) *The Supply of Privately Rented Homes*. York: Joseph Rowntree Foundation.

DoE (1977a) *Housing Policy: A Consultative Document*. Cmnd. 6851. London: HMSO.

DoE (1977b) *Housing Policy: Technical Volume*, part I. London: HMSO.

DoE (1977c) *Housing Policy: Technical Volume*, part III. London: HMSO.

DoE (1994) *Access to Local Authority and Housing Association Tenancies: A Consultation Paper*. London: HMSO.

Finnis, N. (1977) The private landlord is dead but he won't lie down. *Roof*, July: 109–12.

Ford, J. and Wilcox, S. (1994) *Affordable Housing, Low Incomes, and the Flexible Housing Market*, NFHA Report 22. London: National Federation of Housing Associations.

Forrest, R., Murie, A. and Williams, P. (1990) *Home Ownership; Differentiation and Fragmentation*. London: Unwin Hyman.

Hayek, F.A. (1975) *Rent Control, a Popular Paradox: Evidence on the Economic Effects of Rent Control*. Vancouver: Fraser Institute.

HCEC (1982) *The Private Rented Sector*, first report from the House of Commons Environment Committee, session 1981–2. London: HMSO.

Hindess, B. (1987) *Freedom, Equality and the Market*. London: Tavistock.

Hirschman, A.O. (1970) *Exit, Voice and Loyalty*. Cambridge, MA: Harvard University Press.

Hirschman, A.O. (1991) *The Rhetoric of Reaction: Perversity, Futility, Jeopardy*. Cambridge, MA: Belknap Press.

Holmans, A. (1991) The 1977 National Housing Policy Review in retrospect. *Housing Studies*, 6: 206–19.

Housing Today (1997) HMOs 'will be regulated', 23 October: 3.

Inquiry into British Housing (1985) *Report*. London: NFHA.

Jew, P. (1994) *Law and Order in Private Rented Housing: Tackling Harassment and Illegal Eviction*. London: Campaign for Bedsit Rights.

Kemp, P. (1988a) Private renting: an overview, in P. Kemp (ed.) *The Private Provision of Rented Housing*. Aldershot: Avebury.

Kemp, P. (1988b) The impact of the assured tenancy scheme, 1980–1986, in P. Kemp (ed.) *The Private Provision of Rented Housing*. Aldershot: Avebury.

Kemp, P. (1990) Deregulation, markets and the 1988 Housing Act. *Social Policy & Administration*, 24: 145–55.

Kemp. P. (1992) The ghost of Rachman, in C. Grant (ed.) *Built to last? Reflections on British housing policy*. London: Roof.

Kemp, P. (1993) Rebuilding the private rented sector?, in P. Malpass and R. Means (eds) *Implementing Housing Policy*. Buckingham: Open University Press.

Kemp, P. (1997) Ideology, public policy and private rental housing since the War, in P. Williams (ed.) *Directions in Housing Policy: Towards Sustainable Housing Policies for the UK*. London: Paul Chapman Publishing.

Labour Party (1979) *Labour Party Manifesto*. London: Labour Party Central Office.

LARH (1988) *Anti-Racism for the Private Rented Sector*. London: London Against Racism in Housing.

Leather, P. and Morrison, T. (1997) *The State of UK Housing*. Bristol: Policy Press.

MacEwen, M. (1991) *Housing, Race and Law: The British Experience*. London: Routledge.

Maclennan, D. (1994) *A Competitive UK Economy: The Challenges for Housing Policy*. York: Joseph Rowntree Foundation.

Minford, P., Peel, M., and Ashton, P. (1987) *The Housing Morass*, Hobart Paper 25. London: Institute of Economic Affairs.

Mullins, D., Niner, P. and Riseborough, M. (1997) *Housing Need in Southend-on-Sea*. Birmingham: CURS, The University of Birmingham.

Walker, B., Marsh, A. and Watt, P. (forthcoming) *Local Authority Use of the Private Rented Sector*.

Whitehead, C.M.E. and Kleinman, M.P. (1986) *Private Renting in the 1980s and 1990s*, Occasional Paper 17, Department of Land Economy. Cambridge: Granta Editions.

Whitehead, C.M.E., Harloe, M. and Bovaird, A. (1985) Prospects and strategies for housing in the private rented sector. *Journal of Social Policy*, 14: 151–74.

Wilcox, S. (1997) *Housing Finance Review 1997/98*. York: Joseph Rowntree Foundation.

Zebedee, J. and Ward, M. (1996) *Guide to Housing Benefit and Council Tax Benefit*. London: Shelter/CIOH.

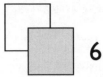

6

More choice in social rented housing?

David Mullins

> Social rented housing does not need to be provided exclusively in the
> public sector.
>
> (DoE 1995: 1)

Introduction

Having examined change in owner-occupied housing (Chapter 4) and the
private rented sector (Chapter 5) we now turn to consider the remainder of
the rented housing sector. 'Social rented housing' is a relatively recent term
generally used to refer to housing with public subsidy provided for low-
income groups on a not-for-profit basis by local government and by
voluntary sector organizations. The provision and form of such housing
has been contested over a long period, but particularly since the mid-1970s.
The quotation at the start of this chapter is drawn from a consultation paper
entitled *More Choice in the Social Rented Sector* (DoE 1995) which heralded the latest instalment in the story. A key theme of this chapter is to
establish: more choice for whom? The quotation captures succinctly an
underlying policy aim of the Conservative governments in the 1980s and
1990s. However, this aim was only partially achieved in practice, and the
provision of social rented housing continues to be closely associated with a
distinctive group of not-for-profit landlords.

Nevertheless, there has been a considerable blurring of the boundaries
between the public and private sectors in social housing provision and a
significant redistribution of stock from local government to other non-profit
landlords. Also between 1988 and 1995, there was an important shift in

public subsidy from capital subsidies to landlords to personal subsidies to tenants, intended at least in part to shift provision for low income groups from the non-profit to the private sector (see Chapter 7). Some acceleration of this shift was attempted in the 1996 Housing Act by increasing the role of private landlords in housing homeless people (see Chapter 8). On the other hand the long-standing principle of not providing capital subsidy to profit-distributing providers of rented housing remains unbreached. Proposals in the 1995 Housing White Paper and associated consultation papers to allow profit distributing interests to compete for capital subsidies were dropped by the time the resulting legislation was drafted.

To provide a context in which these changes can be understood we begin by considering the term 'social rented housing', and the recent restructuring of the sectors with which this term has been most closely associated. We consider the main initiatives which have produced 'more choice' for, or rather control by, the agencies responsible for channelling state subsidies into social housing; the Department of Environment Transport and the Regions (DETR), the Housing Corporation and local authorities. We then introduce a number of explanatory frameworks which may be used to understand this restructuring. The relevance of these frameworks is explored through the discussion of a case study of stock transfers from local authorities to housing associations. The chapter concludes by reflecting on the implications of the restructuring of the social rented housing sector for citizenship, choice and control.

What is 'social rented housing'?

This chapter employs the term most widely used in the 1990s to discuss non-market rented housing in the UK. Cole and Furbey (1994:120) note that the category 'social rented housing' has been used in recent years to combine council housing, housing association, cooperative and charitable trust accommodation. They cite the Inquiry into British Housing (1990) which referred to housing provision where the underlying purposes were social rather than commercial, allocation was based on need rather than ability to pay, and tenants' interests were uppermost. Bramley (1993a) adopts a similar approach, but also includes low cost home ownership. He defines social housing as 'housing provided for rent (or part-rent/part-buy) at less than full market cost by a socially responsible agency conforming to some form of tenant's charter or guarantee and allocating accommodation on a basis related to need' (p. 155).

The ideological component of the term 'social rented housing' cannot be ignored. While it had been used for a considerable period in a comparatively neutral way in many European housing systems, its belated introduction into the discourse of UK housing policy in the late 1980s was seen by some as controversial. This was largely a result of the political context and its association with the 1988 Housing Act. A Government White Paper (HMSO 1987) and related consultation papers had coined the term 'independent rented sector'[1] to stress proposals to unify the private rented and housing association sectors through common, new deregulated tenancies and rents. While the term 'social rented housing' could be read as oppositional to this privatizing tendency, re-stressing the common features of council and housing association sectors, it was read by some critics in precisely the opposite way. For example Ball (1989: 33) criticized the use of the term as 'an attack on the principle of state provided housing', and as obscuring the aims of increasing rents nearer to market levels and sales of council estates to housing associations and the private sector. In 1994 the pages of the otherwise quiescent trade journal *Housing Association Weekly* witnessed a sharp exchange over the term throughout April 1994, with the editor defending it as a preferable alternative to 'welfare housing' and disgruntled letter writers arguing for 'public housing' or even 'rented housing with choice' as preferable alternatives.

From the above it can be seen that there are a number of ways in which the term social rented housing is currently used. At least three usages can be identified: first, to refer to distinctive aspects of the production and management of housing; second, to indicate its consumption and the profile of its tenants; third, to refer the financial arrangements made to secure access to housing. However, in practice these usages are often combined, as the following discussion indicates.

In the British context considerable emphasis is usually placed on production, with a distinctive group of landlords being characterized as social landlords. These are landlords who operate on a non-profit basis and let properties at sub-market rents or cost rents, and apply distinctive, socially based policies. From this point of view, the fact that in 1980 council housing housed one in seven of the top income decile (Murie 1997: 95) would not have detracted from its status as social housing. This distinctive role for social housing providers was boosted by the 1995 consultation paper cited in the introduction, which talks of the government's commitment to a strong social rented sector in which 'subsidy is given to landlords to provide housing at rents below market levels' (DoE 1995: 1).

The second usage, in contrast, focuses on consumption and the tenant profile. Social housing is increasingly seen as being provided only for those groups who are unable to afford market housing. Such a conception can lead to attention being given to patterns of exit from as well as entry to the sector. Policies concerned with the best use of the housing stock and which actively

---

[1] Interestingly while the term 'independent rented sector' never really caught on in the 1980s, a new term, 'independent social landlords' was to appear after the 1996 Housing Act to cover non-profit landlords registered with the Housing Corporation, thereby excluding both private landlords and local authorities.

encourage tenants with higher incomes to leave the sector, thus accelerating the process of residualization, would be seen as in accord with this usage.

While the increasing concentration of low income households in council housing represents a key element in patterns of urban social stratification (Murie 1997: 93), there is clearly more than one model of social housing provision. Harloe (1995) identifies three structures of social housing provision: the residual, mass, and workers cooperative models. The residual model has been increasingly followed since the 1970s in the six societies studied by Harloe, but earlier periods saw the adoption of mass state housing because the scope for private commodified provision was limited. In the early part of the twentieth century, until the 1930s, council housing was seen as housing 'the respectable skilled working class' (Clapham and Franklin 1997: 13) and as recently as 1980 council housing housed one in three households in the UK (Murie 1997: 95). Thus the identification of social housing by tenant profile is problematic as a result of considerable variations over time and between different states (see Chapter 8 for a more detailed discussion of the changing profile of social housing tenants).

The third usage relates to the provision of state subsidy and sees the main function of social housing as being to meet the gap between the incomes and housing costs of poorer citizens. However, if the primary concern is with the provision of public subsidy it does not necessarily entail the production of an identifiable social housing product. Elsewhere in Europe, in Germany for example, subsidies may be provided to tenants and to private as well as social landlords and there need be no identifiable stock of housing for which subsidy is provided. Where landlords receive subsidy the housing is considered social housing only for the duration of the subsidy, rather than in perpetuity. In Britain between 1988 and 1995 there was a redistribution of subsidy from capital towards personal subsidies (see Chapter 7).

An exclusive focus on subsidy also means that much private rented housing should fall within the definition of social housing. Throughout most of the century the private rented sector has formed an important tenure for low-income households (see Chapter 5). During the 1990s it has enjoyed increasing indirect public subsidy through the housing benefit system. Furthermore, the homes of owner-occupiers in receipt of assistance through Income Support Mortgage Interest (ISMI) might also be considered social housing while the residents remained in that position.

Housing policy debates are often conducted using conflicting conceptions of the term 'social housing' which draw on one – or more often an amalgam – of the above usages. The term carries multiple meanings and these can often embrace hidden policy agendas. Care is therefore needed to clarify meaning when using the term 'social rented sector'. For the purposes of this chapter we argue that it is most useful as a construct in allowing discussion and analysis of not-for-profit housing. This usage was strongly challenged by proposals set out by the last Conservative government in a White Paper and associated consultation papers. However, these proposals were not implemented in the legislation which followed, and all social landlords must still operate on a non-profit distributing basis.

Restructuring social rented housing

Until 1988 local authorities were pre-eminent in the provision and management of social rented housing in Britain. While the local authority stock had already been significantly eroded by Right to Buy sales and a declining level of new building activity, it still accounted for 89 per cent of social rented housing in England, 92 per cent in Wales and 94 per cent in Scotland in 1988. Housing associations were generally seen as complementary to local authorities during this period, and despite their receipt of relatively generous public subsidies after the 1974 Housing Act they were often neglected in discussions of public policy. Thus the terms public housing and council housing were the most commonly used, and social housing policy was almost synonymous with council housing policy.

Deakin (1994: 152) describes a widely held view that 'the 1987 election marks a watershed in the Conservative Government's approach to social policy'. While the Conservative's third-term welfare policy initiatives were not a clean break with earlier approaches, there was a series of new and concerted attempts to introduce a mixed economy of welfare in education, health, social care and housing. Smith and Mallinson (1997: 174) describe these changes as 'the triumph of neo-liberalism over social democracy'. In housing this new agenda was summed up by the secretary of state at the time as designed 'to weaken the almost incestuous relationship between some councils and their tenants' (Ridley 1992: 87). Housing restructuring was particularly concerned with transferring the management of social rented housing to new landlords while maintaining sales of individual properties to sitting tenants under the Right to Buy. The schemes established in the 1988 Housing Act to facilitate stock transfers, Tenants' Choice and Housing Action Trusts (Karn 1993) had relatively little impact. However, responses by local authorities themselves to the policy disincentives for a continued council housing role were much more far reaching. Large Scale Voluntary Transfers (LSVTs) used earlier permissive legislation (the 1985 Housing Act) to become the main mechanism for stock transfer (Mullins *et al.* 1995). Between 1988 and 1996 almost 250,000 homes were transferred from local authorities to housing associations under LSVTs.

By the mid-1990s the balance of social housing provision had begun to change, and it had become increasingly common to use the term social housing to describe local authority and housing association activity. However, this change had been uneven between nations, regions and local authority areas. Local authorities remained the largest social housing landlord but the proportion of social housing provided by other landlords had increased to 21 per cent in England, 18 per cent in Wales and 11 per cent in Scotland (Wilcox 1997). Wholesale transfer of the local authority stock to housing associations had occurred in 55 areas in England, but elsewhere local authorities still accounted for the vast majority of the social housing stock in their area. Nevertheless the relative importance of housing associations was increasing everywhere and the focus of public policy for new housing was on the housing association sector. From the mid-1990s new approaches were being developed to transfer poorer condition urban stock to new landlords, including the provision of a new source of public funding, the Estates Renewal Challenge Fund. Local Housing Companies emerged as an alternative model to housing associations for such transfers (Wilcox 1993; Zitron 1995). However, the new arrangements for registration of social landlords established following the 1996 Housing Act apply the same regulations to new, stock transfer, housing associations as to Local Housing Companies (Housing Corporation 1996a). Provided that they can demonstrate independence from the local authority, and have at least a third of their membership and board made up of independent members, both may in theory have up to 49 per cent tenant or local authority representation on the board.

Changes in ownership were only part of the restructuring process in the social housing sector. New financial regimes for both housing associations (specified in the 1988 Housing Act) and local authorities (outlined in the 1989 Local Government and Housing Act) changed the incentive structure for landlords. There were moves towards higher rents in both sectors, reflecting shifts from producer to consumer subsidies, increased central control of council rents and the need to meet the costs of private borrowing in the housing association sector (see Chapter 7). Other new approaches in the local authority sector included the extension of compulsory competitive tendering to housing management, an increased emphasis on costing and monitoring performance (see Chapter 9), and the development of an enabling role to influence the pattern of local housing provision (Audit Commission 1992; Bramley 1993a; Goodlad 1993). Meanwhile, housing associations were affected by increasing competition for development funding (Best 1997), a regulatory regime with specified performance standards and indicators (Mullins 1997a), and wider influences in management thinking producing 'efficiency drives', 'downsizing' and 'decentralization' (Ferlie et al. 1996; Walker 1998).

All of these changes must be seen in the context of a national housing policy which placed increasing emphasis on private market provision for most needs. Owner occupation expanded rapidly, particularly through sales of council homes to sitting tenants (see Chapter 4). As a result 'in the period 1979 to 1995 the stock of social housing in Britain declined by more than a quarter, contributing nearly half the growth in home ownership' (Malpass 1996: 461).

Meanwhile, there was also some redistribution of state support from the social rented sector to the private rented sector. Direct funding for private renting was still extremely limited; with the exception of the business expansion scheme (1988–93), and the 'Gro-Grant' scheme in Scotland, there were no direct subsidies to landlords. However, indirect support was provided by the encouragement of local authorities to use the private rented sector in discharge of homelessness duties, and by schemes such as Housing Associations as Managing Agents (HAMA) which encouraged landlords to let properties. Moreover, in the early 1990s there were increasing reports of potential tenants refusing social housing offers to take up private tenancies.

More importantly, the shift in subsidies from producers to consumers tended to redistribute these subsidies from social landlords to private landlords. Despite their different trajectories, the private rented sector was still twice as large as the housing association sector in 1996 and 60 per cent of tenants in receipt of rent allowances were in the private rented sector. Average weekly rents for private tenants on benefit were still 12 per cent higher and average benefit payments 15 per cent higher than for housing association tenants on housing benefit (Wilcox 1997). Detailed work by the London Housing Unit (1997) indicates that between 1988/9 and 1998/9 rent allowances to private tenants increased from £1.3 billion to £4 billion, numbers of claimants increased from 650,000 to 1.4 million and benefit per claimant from £1900 a year to £2900 a year at 1996/7 prices. Comparisons between rent allowance expenditure on the private rented sector and overall Housing Revenue Account (HRA) subsidies to the council sector indicate a substantial shift of state support from the latter to the former during the 1990s. Whereas in 1988/9 HRA subsidy per council tenant exceeded rent allowance subsidy per private tenant by 12 per cent, by 1998/9 HRA subsidy per council tenant was just 39 per cent of rent allowance subsidy per private tenant (London Housing Unit 1997). Thus there is some evidence that changes were occurring in the direction envisaged in the 1995 government consultation paper, which stated that 'social rented housing does not need to be provided exclusively in the public sector', albeit without the introduction of capital subsidies for private landlords (DoE 1995: 1).

Interpretations of change

A number of perspectives have been applied to the analysis of the recent restructuring of social rented housing in Britain. Five approaches are summarized in Table 6.1, are briefly reviewed in this section, and are then explored in a case study in the following section.

Table 6.1 Perspectives on restructuring social housing in the 1990s

Privatization	Introduction of market mechanisms into public services, e.g. through load shedding, liberalization, user charges, contracts for service management. Many distinct processes covered by blanket term, but general emphasis on reducing control by public service hierarchies. However, growth in indirect control through regulation often accompanies privatization. Ideology of privatization underpinned by notion of consumer choice.
Quasi-markets	More specific approach substituting contract relationships for hierarchical controls in service delivery. Used in situations where full market provision difficult, Purchaser/provider splits. Emphasis on reducing provider control and increasing control by funders rather than choice by users.
Networks	Emphasis on horizontal links at local level arising from fragmentation of public services rather than either markets or hierarchies. Use of cooperation rather than competition mechanisms, although local partnerships often formed as part of competitive strategies to access funds.
Local Public Spending Bodies	Emphasis on governance changes arising from transfer of functions from state and local state to non-elected bodies. Concept of democratic deficit emphasizes reduction in control by local state. Citizenship issues used to support local regulation of LPSBs.
Third sector	Distinguishes non-profit provision from state and market. Role of value-based organizations. Links to wider citizenship and civil society may be emphasized. Conflicts may arise between strategic responses to competition and internal values and purposes.

Privatization

Privatization is the concept most frequently used to sum up the main changes in direction in social housing policy in the 1980s and 1990s. Forrest and Murie (1988) have described the Right to Buy as the biggest of all privatizations. Meanwhile Randolph (1993) referred to the 're-privatization' of housing associations by a reduction in capital subsidies from the state and the introduction of private finance following the 1988 Housing Act. Similarly the shift of housing outside of the Public Sector Borrowing Requirement (PSBR) through stock transfers to housing associations under LSVT has also been described as privatization (Kleinman 1993). It can be seen therefore that privatization is something of a blanket term referring to a variety of changes including shifts in ownership from local state to individuals, and non-state organizations, changes in management arrangements, and changes in funding mechanisms. To these might be added changes occurring within the public sector as a result of the spread of new public management ideas from the private sector (Stewart and Walsh 1992, Ferlie *et al.* 1996).

The main limitation to the use of the term privatization is the lack of precision introduced by its multiple meanings. This is apparent from the wider literature on privatization, particularly in relation to former nationalized industries and utilities (Beesley and Littlechild 1992). Samson (1994) for example, identifies three faces to privatization – economic, political and ideological – while others have noted the lack of consensus about either the objectives of privatization (Bishop and Kay 1988) or its precise nature (Beesley and Littlechild 1992). Heald (1984) identifies four distinct processes which can be referred to by the term: charging users for services which were formerly collectively funded from taxation; contracting out the management of publicly-owned services; the sale of public assets; and deregulation to allow competition with public service providers.

Turning to consider the use of the term privatization in relation to housing restructuring, Murie (1993) identifies a more comprehensive range of processes which have occurred in the housing sector. Table 6.2 summarizes these processes, which may appear in different combinations in the examples identified. The overall effect has been to further reduce the role of the public sector in housing provision, to shift the burden of cost onto users of these services, and to render alternative modes of provision, both by not-for-profit bodies and the profit distributing private sector more attractive.

It is notable that much of the recent restructuring of social rented housing provision has been a response to accounting conventions (PSBR) and funding regimes which enabled housing associations to escape the constraints placed on local authority landlords in reinvesting in and adding to their housing stock. Alternative proposals have been made to recast definitions of public spending to avoid the substantial transaction costs involved in stock transfer. One proposal was to use a General Government Financial Deficit (GGFD) definition which would exclude borrowing for investment with a trading return from rental income (Hawksworth and Wilcox 1995). This was rejected by the political parties in advance of the 1997 general election, however alternative methods of providing access to private sector borrowing against the asset base and income stream of council housing continued to be explored. While the Private Finance Initiative launched by the Conservative government in the early 1990s was not initially applied to social housing schemes, proposals were being developed by the time of the election. After the election proposals for local housing quasi-corporations began to be developed as a vehicle for local authorities to borrow privately without transferring their stock, however a change of public accounting conventions would still be needed for these proposals to succeed (Weaver 1997: 9).

To date, the bodies used for stock transfers have been almost exclusively not-for-profit organizations. While the introduction of profit distributing

Table 6.2   Forms of housing privatization

Type	Process	Example
Deregulation	Reducing or removing state regulation of private activity	Legislation affecting private renting
Commercialization	Increasing user charges and reducing subsidy and tax finance of state activity	Increased public sector rents and reduced subsidy
Demunicipalization	Reducing municipal ownership and development activity	Transfers of council housing to sitting tenants and to independent organizations. Restricting capacity for new building by local authorities.
Encouragement of privatization	Increasing subsidy, tax finance and legislative provision for private production or consumption	Fiscal arrangements and legislation relating to low-cost home ownership and to private renting
Contracting out	Arrangements for an increased private role in areas which remain the responsibility of state agencies	Developments in competitive tendering for various activities including house building, repairs and management
Incorporation	Embracing quasi-public agencies in the private sector	Changes to the position of housing associations
Preparation for privatization	Preparing the ground for other forms of privatization	Moving council rents towards market levels. Establishing unit costings and estate budgets.

Source: Murie 1993: 155.

competitors for capital subsidy was considered in the run-up to the 1996 Housing Act (DoE 1995), it was not introduced in practice. Thus the extent to which the recent restructuring of ownership of social housing can be seen as privatization depends on how much is made of the distinction between non-profit distributing housing associations and the 'genuine' private sector. This led one Conservative critic to describe stock transfer as 'only in effect moving one block of insulated and subsidised housing stock from the direct public sector to the quasi-public domain of the housing association' (Wandsworth Borough Council 1993: 8). We return to these questions later in our discussion of stock transfers.

Thus privatization is a useful umbrella term which sketches the general direction of social housing policy in the 1980s and 1990s. However, it has been used to cover a wide range of changes, each with potentially very different impacts on patterns of citizenship, choice and control. There are significant differences between the Right to Buy, which in the long run has the effect of exposing former state assets to full market influences, and the third-term initiatives to transfer rented housing stock to new owners and managers, none of whom have so far been profit-distributing companies. Thus more subtle and specific perspectives are required to interpret the full extent of the restructuring of social rented housing. The next four perspectives all contribute to this task.

Quasi-markets

A second and more specific perspective used to analyse recent housing restructuring is quasi-markets. Le Grand and Bartlett (1993) describe a series of radical reforms introduced in the third term of the last Conservative administration involving a decentralization of decision making and the introduction of competition between service providers. According to Le Grand and Bartlett, the key feature of these changes was that 'the state was to become primarily only a purchaser of welfare services, with state provision being systematically replaced by a system of independent providers competing with one another in internal or "quasi"-markets' (p. 3).

Bramley (1993b: 180) argues that 'there is no question that a quasi-market is developing in social housing'. His account describes the arrangements for purchasing and allocating housing association homes in the period after 1987. A distinctive feature of the social housing sector was the co-existence of two sets of purchasers, the Housing Corporation and local authorities. This resulted from the two main funding channels for social housing: the Approved Development Programme allocated by the Housing Corporation direct to housing associations, and the Housing Investment Programme allocated by the Department of the Environment to local authorities, some of which could be used to fund housing associations. In either case there was considerable competition between housing associations for Social Housing Grant, with bids exceeding allocations by a considerable ratio. During this period competition was on the basis of minimizing grant per new letting, and associations were tending to reduce the proportion of scheme costs for which grant funding was sought. The balance of scheme costs was made up from private borrowing, ultimately financed through rental income, and from accumulated reserves, again ultimately derived from rental surpluses.

Bramley distinguishes between the gains in choice experienced by funders from quasi-markets and the more limited gains which accrue to 'individual clients' who still have relatively little choice, particularly those in urgent need such as homeless applicants. This is because 'the local authority (remains) the intermediary rationing agency for most individual households and competition is not translated into much wider choice for individual clients' (1993b: 180). These issues are discussed in more detail in Chapter 8 in relation to Common Housing Registers. Other issues raised by Bramley were the explicit exclusion of rent competition and the 'high rent burdens and poverty traps' which were emerging at the time, and the lack of attention to future management costs in the competition process. Interestingly his account ended by suggesting that the successful operation of this quasi-market in part depends on the goodwill of associations and 'the survival of some of the qualities that stem from their voluntaristic origins' (p. 182). This highlights the limited correspondence between quasi-markets and privatization in social housing restructuring, since the providers involved in competition for funding are exclusively non-profit distributing and have social rather than purely commercial purposes. The implications of this are discussed later in this section.

The arrangements described by Bramley have changed in the period since his account. Most notably, concerns about rising housing benefit expenditure led to the introduction of a form of rent control into the bidding process for Social Housing Grants from 1995 and into the more general regulation of social landlords from 1997. Other changes include the incorporation of some housing funding into more general regeneration programmes through the Single Regeneration Budget (SRB) from 1994/5 with its greater emphasis on partnerships. Further change in the quasi-market structure includes the replacement of the dual purchaser system in Wales, with the abolition of Tai Cymru, the Welsh Housing Corporation, and absorption of its functions into the Welsh Office as part of the regional government changes to be introduced in 1999. However, the dual funding system survived intact in England following the establishment of Government Regional Offices and a five-yearly review of the Housing Corporation in the mid-1990s.

More significant rethinking of the adverse impact of competitive strategies on the ability of local authorities to deliver effective local strategies was also beginning in the late 1990s (Aldbourne Associates 1996; Mullins 1996; Office for Public Management 1997). A reduction in the extent of competition between providers may emerge through longer-term commissioning arrangements being introduced on a pilot basis in 1997/8.

Networks

A third perspective on restructuring places greater emphasis on the extent of cooperative relationships which have developed at the local level in response to the fragmentation and competition outlined above. Reid (1995: 133) has argued that 'local housing services are now planned and provided through networks of organisations, necessitating the development and maintenance of effective cooperative interorganisational relationships'. These networks 'have developed alongside market mechanisms, providing a complementary means of coordinating policy and implementation' (p. 134). They may also be contrasted with hierarchical systems of organization on which many governance and regulation approaches are based.

Examples of local housing networks studied by Reid include barter deals between local authorities and private developers to provide starter homes, the development of public-private partnerships for urban and housing renewal, and joint approaches to service provision by statutory and voluntary agencies in areas such as community care. Another example, discussed in Chapter 9, is the emergence of Common Housing Register partnerships to streamline access to local social housing. The net result of these changes is that 'the housing service in Britain is expanding in the sense that it encompasses a widening range of various types of organisation orientated towards service delivery' and 'local service delivery depends upon the successful formation and operation of interorganisational networks' (Reid 1995: 147).

The network approach is important in understanding the restructuring of social housing because it focuses attention on organizational and interorganizational processes. These processes are frequently neglected in approaches to housing studies which try to read off local outcomes from the national policy framework. Issues such as the propensity of organizations to cooperate, the variety of formal and informal agreements which form the basis of cooperation, the operating arrangements used to undertake joint activities, and the varying perceptions of the task become central to understanding what services are provided and the pattern of choice available at the local level (Reid 1997). However, the term 'partnership' disguises the differing approaches taken by organizations to cooperation. Some organizations take an entrepreneurial and competitive approach, carefully choosing which projects and which organizations to cooperate with in order to promote their strategic objectives. Others are seen as more collaborative, being prepared to commit resources to longer-term relationships, exercising less choice over partners, and working towards more collectively defined goals. Such differences in the ways in which organizations approach interorganizational relationships have important implications not only for the way in which services are provided but also to the nature of the restructuring of social housing. Reid's concept of a 'virtual housing organization', through which consumers now experience local housing services, captures the current importance of horizontal links in comparison with hierarchical links implied by quasi-market and bureaucratic type models.

Local Public Spending Bodies

A fourth perspective on social housing restructuring focuses on another specific aspect of privatization, that of demunicipalization. The transfer of local services from the local state to a variety of alternative bodies, many of them not directly elected, has been one focus of attention of the growing literature on governance. Stoker has defined governance as 'the action, manner or system of governing in which the boundary between organisations and the public and private sectors has become permeable ... The essence of governance is the interactive relationship between and within governmental and non-governmental forces' (Stoker 1995: 1).

Malpass (1997) introduces a collection of articles on changing patterns of ownership, control and accountability in housing by referring to the emergence of a 'new governance of housing'. In relation to social housing Malpass identifies as a key issue whether the fragmentation of governance increases or decreases the scope for local decision making. In his view the suggestion in the networks literature referred to above (Rhodes 1995) that local networks may enjoy a significant degree of freedom from the state is hard to sustain in relation to housing, where the Housing Corporation is seen to exert considerable control over local activity (Malpass 1997: 6).

The concept of Local Public Spending Bodies (LPSBs) was used by the Nolan Committee as the subject of its second report of its work on standards of conduct in public life (Committee on Standards in Public Life 1996). It refers to 'not for profit organisations which are neither fully elected nor appointed by Ministers but which provide public services often delivered at local level which are wholly or largely publicly funded' (p. 5). Housing associations were included within this definition and have been subject to increasing scrutiny as concerns about the probity and accountability of LPSBs have developed. Associations have long been subject to criticism as self-perpetuating oligarchies, but with the increasing interest in LPSBs they were seen as prime examples of the 'democratic deficit' whereby public services were moving away from institutions of democratic control. A former Housing Corporation senior officer saw a danger of 'associations becoming less accountable exactly at a time when local authorities and their successors become more accountable' (NFHA 1995a: 32). This made action to address concerns about association governance and accountability more immediate.

Despite the holding of a governance enquiry by the housing association's trade body (NFHA 1995b) and the adoption of a code of governance (NFHA 1995c), housing associations were still subject to some criticism when the Nolan Committee's second report was published (Committee on Standards in Public Life 1996). In particular, recommendations made reference to the need to enhance tenant involvement, increase accountability through membership schemes and for the regulator to pay particular attention to stewardship of LSVT (stock transfer) associations where near monopolies of local social housing supply had been created. Further pressure for enhanced accountability was created by the election of a Labour government in 1997, and the emergence of new social landlord models for stock transfer. An early response by the National Housing Federation (NHF 1997) was a new guide for independent social landlords setting out good practice on accountability. It emphasized the benefits of open membership, resident involvement and close working relationships with local authorities. Ironically, stock transfer associations, with their constituency approach to representing tenants, local authority and independent interests on their boards, were now seen as a model for social landlords (NHF 1997: xii). Previously, the NFHA governance enquiry had specifically rejected the use of membership and constituency approaches to accountability and Nolan had singled out LSVTs for particular criticism despite their greater representation of local authority and tenant interests than most other housing associations.

The usefulness of the LPSB perspective on social housing restructuring is that it illuminates changing governance arrangements arising from the adoption of privatization and quasi-market policies and the emergence of network forms of service provision. Attention is drawn to the shift from local state to non-elected bodies in patterns of influence over public spending on housing. A closer focus is placed on changes in the relationship between citizens, the institutions they elect, and other institutions which may now control services. However, this perspective shares a limitation with the approaches described earlier, all of which, with the possible exception of the networks approach, tend to represent social housing organizations on a bipolar continuum between the state and the market.

Third sector and civil society

We conclude this discussion by drawing attention to the not-for-profit basis on which social housing organizations operate, discussed earlier. The not-for-profit housing sector includes an increasing proportion of landlords who are neither state nor market based but who operate from a 'third frame of reference' (Mullins 1997b). Like other third-sector organizations these social housing providers may respond to funding and regulatory signals from the state and to financial signals from private funders, but these influences are often mediated by a third influence relating to the values and purposes of the organizations themselves. Housing associations have a variety of origins and purposes and include nineteenth-century philanthropic trusts, 1960s entrepreneurial and social action bodies, 1970s cooperatives and 1990s stock transfer vehicles. However, most would claim to be based on a distinctive set of values and emphasize their social purposes over their business efficiency (Riseborough 1997). Cooperatives provide a special case of often highly value-based organizations, but account for a very small part of third sector housing in Britain (Birchall 1988).

Figure 6.1 illustrates the influence of this third frame of reference. The three sector model has a long pedigree and has been traced back to a visit by Alexis de Tocqueville to the United States in the 1830s, during which he contrasted the activities of government, economic exchange and voluntary

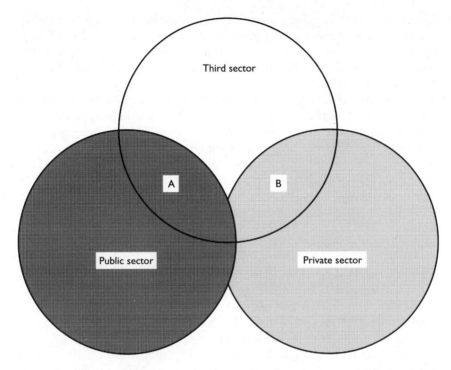

Figure 6.1   Locating housing associations between state, market and third sector

Note: Housing associations have moved between A in (1974–88) and B (1988–96)
Source: Based on Wuthnow 1991.

efforts of citizens (Wuthnow 1991). Here we apply it to the changing position of housing associations, which rather than moving along a continuum between public and private sectors, may instead be depicted as operating on the boundary of three sectors. Interpreting the restructuring of social housing therefore involves exploring the voluntary sector and non-profit influences on organizational change (Mullins and Riseborough 1996).

   Leaving aside the definition of non-profit, this third influence has been the most enduring characteristic of the sector as it has made its pendulum-swings between the public and the private spheres (Spencer *et al.* 1995). For example, 'the message which the NFHA has tried to put over on the movement's behalf is that it is not public sector, nor private sector, but something different' (NFHA 1990: 38). The development of mixed economies of welfare has increasingly involved third sector organizations taking on primary rather than complementary roles internationally (Kramer 1987). There are strong parallels for example between housing associations and not-for-profit foundations in the United States, as well as more obvious comparisons with housing associations elsewhere in Europe (Jensen 1995). Connections with the role and purpose of the non-profit sector have been made by practitioners and policy makers in, for example, studies of the relevance of American community development corporations (SHAPE 1993; Bowman 1996).

Despite this mobilization of value-based third sector characteristics by key actors involved in the restructuring of social housing, this is the most neglected of the five perspectives discussed here within the housing studies literature. The influence of the third sector stance on housing association decision making is still little understood: at worst it is ignored and at best contested. One possible starting point in locating housing associations in relation to the wider field of third sector studies is provided by the growing literature on citizenship and civil society. At the macro-scale Salamon and Anheier (1996) review a number of theoretical perspectives to 'explain the nonprofit sector crossnationally'. One of these, 'social origins theory', draws on Esping-Andersen's (1990) theory of welfare regimes to explore the development and role of the non-profit sector and the embeddedness of non-profit institutions in economic and social structures (liberalism, social democracy, corporatism and statism). Work in progress (Mullins 1997b; Riseborough 1997) is seeking to clarify the role of values and voluntarism in defining the purposes of social landlords.

Preliminary findings from this research indicate that key actors in these organizations place a high degree of importance on having social purposes compared to being efficient businesses. Greater emphasis is placed on independence and ability to set their own priorities than on voluntarism. Of the three most important external influences on recent change in the sector, greatest importance is attached to the influence of private funders, and least to state regulation, with the interests of consumers coming somewhere in between. However, such changes are mediated by internal processes and any attempt to understand the role of the 'third frame of reference' must necessarily consider how strategic choices are made in response to external stimuli. Work in progress seeks to track strategic choices through a long term dialogue with key actors in a sample of housing associations (Mullins and Riseborough 1996).

A third sector perspective on the restructuring of social housing is important since the majority of stock transferred under load-shedding policies has been to non-profit organizations,[2] and the non-profit sector has built all the new homes under quasi-market policies. As Bramley (1993b) acknowledges, the successful operation of quasi-markets in housing may be partly related to the voluntary-sector origins and values of housing associations. The networks literature highlights the importance of understanding the purposes

---

[2] One stock transfer under LSVT was to a non-registered housing association and a number of other transfers, e.g. under Tenants' Choice, involved private-sector interests.

of organizations in order to assess the propensity and form of cooperation. The LPSB literature highlights the importance of accountabilities and links between housing providers and civil society. Moreover, a third sector perspective identifies common threads between UK and European housing, where the existence of a third sector which is neither state nor market but with strong connections to both is a more common form of social housing provision (Harloe 1995).

All five perspectives outlined in this section cast some light on the recent restructuring of social rented housing. Interpretation of their interaction needs to be teased out through detailed case studies.

The case of stock transfers

Stock transfers under LSVT were a central element of the restructuring of social housing between 1988 and the mid-1990s. As Table 6.3 illustrates, LSVT made a significant contribution to demunicipalization and the growth in the housing association sector. Over the period between 1988 and 1997 stock transferred under LSVT was equivalent to about 40 per cent of stock sold under the Right to Buy, and equivalent to over 90 per cent of new housing association homes for rent. However, the impact of LSVT was greatest at the local level where for the first time since the First World War

Table 6.3 Change in social housing stock 1988–95 through LSVT, Right to Buy and new housing association homes

Year	LSVT	Right to Buy	New rented housing association homes[1]
1988/89	11176	128566	13925
1989/90	14405	139722	17728
1990/91	45512	92995	17610
1991/92	10791	51414	21529
1992/93	26325	41445	45278
1993/94	30103	41188	40136
1994/95	40234	44999	40420
1995/96	44871	33960	40583
1996/97	22549	31335	27647
Total	245966	605624	264856
Ratio[2]		40.61	92.87

Notes:
1 Completions less sale, shared ownership, Tenants' Incentive Scheme and short life
2 LSVTs to Right to Buy and new housing association homes
Sources: Wilcox 1997, Housing Corporation 1996b.

over 50 districts no longer had housing stocks owned and managed by local government. In most of these areas new housing associations were set up to receive the transferred stock and enjoy a virtual monopoly in the supply of social rented housing, a factor which sets them apart from other housing associations.

The process of stock transfer and the early impact on tenants, staff, local authorities and the new associations have been evaluated in work commissioned by the Department of the Environment (Mullins *et al.* 1992, 1993, 1995) and in a variety of other research (Gardiner *et al.* 1991; Audit Commission 1993; Kleinman 1993; Birchall *et al.* 1995). Some distinctive features of LSVT were that it was initiated by local authorities themselves and only incorporated into a national programme in 1993. It was geographically concentrated in rural, suburban, and resort areas mostly in the south of England, and in areas where the housing stock was in reasonable repair and outstanding loan debt was relatively low. The new landlords usually employed staff transferred from the local authority, but there was considerable change in the stakeholders involved. Independent management boards, Housing Corporation regulation and covenants to funders constituted important new influences. While accelerated modernization, repairs and new building were usually possible, this resulted in a considerable increase in long-term debt: business plans were drawn up on the basis that 25–30 years were required to complete repayments. The position of tenants was affected by the need to secure a majority vote before transfer to the new landlord could proceed. Five-year rent guarantees were given to tenants at the time of the ballot, but new tenants after transfer were excluded. This resulted in a two-tier rent structure during the early years after transfer.

How can the five perspectives outlined in the previous section help us interpret stock transfer? Stock transfer is a particularly ambiguous process and provides a testing case study. The privatization framework assists in understanding the rationale for the process of stock transfer and the resulting change in interest group representation, but it makes only a limited contribution to understanding the outcome of LSVT. A fuller picture is provided by reference to the alternative perspectives. Consideration of the relationship between local authorities and stock transfer associations provides evidence of both quasi-market and network approaches. Meanwhile the governance arrangements for stock transfers have been important in the LPSB debate over recent years. Finally, differences between LSVT associations and both local authorities and private landlords suggest the relevance of a third frame of reference. Approaches to tenant representation in some cases suggest a building of new citizenship links which did not exist prior to restructuring.

The rationale for stock transfer was quite simple: it provided a mechanism to escape the restrictions placed on local authorities by the public expenditure regime. Specifically, it enabled borrowing for investment in housing repairs and new building to be classified as private sector and thereby be excluded from PSBR definitions. While substantial transaction costs (of about £1000 per home) were involved to achieve transfer, this seemed worthwhile as there was little prospect of changing borrowing conventions in the short term.

The change in interest representation involved a reduction in the role of local authority members and increased the role of the private sector by indirect means. Local authority persons, a category applying to current and recent councillors, were restricted to 20 per cent of the membership and management committee of the new landlords until the 1996 Housing Act. While the Housing Corporation required representation of a range of professional groups such as accountants on boards, the more significant increase in private sector influence was through indebtedness to private funders. In return for loans which averaged 1.5 times the transfer price, funders required regular monitoring of performance against the business plan and covenant agreements on such matters as rent collection and keeping properties occupied. The latent power of funders was revealed in some early transfers where business plan assumptions were not met, for example as a result of higher interest rates or lower Right to Buy sales income than anticipated. One association was forced to make staff reductions, defer improvement programmes and seek permission for voluntary sales of empty properties to satisfy its funders that early income shortfalls could be made up (Mullins *et al.* 1995).

However, while the stock transfer associations were clearly exposed to financial risk, were outside local authority control and could be seen as examples of 'load shedding' privatization (Heald 1984), they retained certain characteristics which had more in common with the public sector. The most important feature was that the new landlords were not able to distribute profits. Second, they continued to be eligible for public subsidy. The new associations sought Social Housing Grant initially from the transferring authority's spending power, and subsequently through competitive bids for Housing Corporation funding to develop elsewhere. Their business plans also relied on the continued flow of personal subsidy through housing benefits. Another influence preserving, and sometimes reinforcing, a public-service orientation in the new landlords was the role of Housing Corporation regulation which included a strong social agenda (e.g. in relation to access to housing, tenant participation and equal opportunities). A final respect in which a quasi-public sector identity was preserved in most associations was in their organizational culture. While the culture became more 'businesslike' than under the local authority, it usually preserved and in some cases reinvigorated a strong commitment to social purposes both at board and staff levels. For all these reasons case studies of stock transfer associations found organizations with far greater similarities to local authorities than to private landlords.

Examining the relationship between stock transfer local authorities and the new associations provides an opportunity to consider the relevance of quasi-market and network interpretations of restructuring. The majority of early stock transfers had generated a substantial capital receipt which left these authorities with options for new investment after setting aside funds to pay off debt. Investment in housing associations was an attractive option as any grant payments were refundable by the Housing Corporation (Housing Corporation 1996b), although thereafter only the interest accruing could be reinvested.

A survey of local authority enabling officers (Mullins 1996) revealed a variety of strategies for spending the capital receipt and variable relationships with the new associations. Some local authorities had clearly been influenced by quasi-market thinking and adopted a competitive strategy towards spending the capital receipt resulting from stock transfer. No guarantees were made to the new association and grant was allocated on the basis of competitive bidding from a range of associations. In other cases there was a much closer partnership with the stock transfer association, with a guaranteed proportion of the spendable receipt made available to provide early development opportunities for the new association. There were dangers in both approaches. Some stock transfer associations were resentful of competitive approaches, which were felt to deprive them of 'their money' and thus undermine their business plans. Local authority representatives on such associations were sometimes perplexed that having set these bodies up, their authorities were now abandoning them to the competitive market. Other local authorities which had guaranteed grant felt that they often got poor value for money from complacent partners, and were particularly upset to find their 'offspring' bidding at lower grant rates in other authorities than on home base (Mullins 1996).

There are clearly conflicts between the underlying assumptions on which these differing post-transfer strategies are based. These assumptions also relate to the governance issues raised in the LPSB literature. Competition-based strategies recognize that stock transfer associations will develop their own interests which may not always coincide with those of the parent authority. For example they may seek development funding in other areas, change their name to downplay ties with the authority, and even change their governance structure to reduce the influence of the authority on their decision making. In the longer term they may enter into mergers with other associations which may reduce the capacity for local influence even further. In such a context the local authority may see greater benefit to the community as a whole from a quasi-market purchaser role, rather than from continuing a special relationship with the association through direct representation of councillors on the board.

On the other hand a strong case can be constructed for partnership-based strategies which seek to enhance the local accountability of services and to exert maximum strategic leverage over a quasi-monopoly social landlord.

The Nolan Committee expressed particular concern about accountability issues in stock transfer authorities because of the near monopoly role of the new landlord (Committee on Standards in Public Life 1996). Ironically, stock transfer associations have a more structured model for representation of local authority members on their board than do the majority of associations. Most early transfers had sought to maximize the representation of councillors on the new board, then limited to 20 per cent under the Local Government and Housing Act. In this model councillor board members could play an important role in delivering their authority's enabling strategy through promoting partnership with the stock transfer association. This approach seems to have been an attraction for some urban authorities planning to transfer stock to Local Housing Companies, particularly after an increase in the level of possible representation to 49 per cent in the 1996 Housing Act (Housing Corporation 1996a).

However, there are a number of problems with strategies to maximize strategic influence through political partnership approaches which tend to limit the influence provided by representation on these LPSBs. First, any increase in councillor representation may be at the expense of tenant representation since the two combined may not exceed two thirds of the membership. Second, despite the increase in possible councillor representation, stock transfer landlords must demonstrate that they are independent of the local authority in order for their borrowing to be excluded from the PSBR. Third, under the regulations which govern the new landlords, board members have an overriding duty to pursue the best interests of the landlord. Fourth, under the national code of local government conduct there may be conflicts of interest for board members also sitting on the local authority committee involved in housing strategy. Finally, there has been very little thought given to the role played by local authority board members in practice (Mullins 1997c). Nevertheless, after the 1997 election increasing concern about the accountability of LPSBs and the wastefulness of excessively competitive approaches appeared to be creating a climate in which these problems might be seriously addressed (Aldbourne Associates 1996; Office for Public Management 1997).

Stock transfer associations have clearly been influenced by market pressures, and by Housing Corporation regulation, and there has been a continued debate as to the capacity of the local state to influence them. Yet there is also evidence to suggest that they are not simply either private or public bodies. Compared to other housing associations they are more affected by private sector influences because of their much greater level of indebtedness in relation to their asset base. Yet their non-profit basis and social purpose distinguishes them from private landlords. At the same time, because of their recent history, transfer of staff, and continued local ties with councillors, they may be more affected by public sector influences than other associations. Also, their attempts to distance themselves to some extent from the local authority through name changes, office moves, and development of separate support services have been sufficient to satisfy the Housing Corporation of their independence from the local authority sector.

Is this ambiguity sufficient evidence to suggest that stock transfer associations are part of a third sector? Their claim to be part of an independent value-based sector is an interesting one since they cannot appropriate the history of voluntarism as easily as other housing associations, some of which may indeed have lengthy third sector pedigree. Indeed it can be argued that the 'voluntary housing movement' has had to make as much adjustment to accommodate stock transfer associations as the new landlords have to become part of the movement. For example, the representative body changed its name (from National Federation of Housing Associations to National Housing Federation) to incorporate organizations other than housing associations, in particular the new stock transfer Local Housing Companies. Recent research on the changing identity of the housing association sector (Mullins 1997b; Riseborough 1997) suggests that stock transfer associations are very much part of current repositioning and emergent identities of independent social landlords.

One chief executive of a stock transfer association saw his role as threefold: 'to make this a proper housing association, to secure its financial and organisational stability and then to take the organisation forward and develop it' (quoted in Mullins 1997b: 66). In the process this organization may be forging a new model for third sector housing through a very high level of emphasis on user involvement. Tenant board members are elected by a ballot of all tenants and election turnouts actually exceed those achieved in local government elections. Another stock transfer association has a majority of board members made up of tenants.

Thus a process which could be interpreted simply as an example of privatization through load-shedding by the local authority may turn out to be providing a new model for opening up social landlords to the influences of citizenship and civil society. In this way these social landlords may succeed in meeting the legitimacy challenges raised by the LPSB debates. While the extent of autonomy from market pressures should not be exaggerated, these examples do indicate the need for a broader interpretative perspective than that provided by privatization. The not-for-profit status and potential for responsiveness to citizenship do provide common ground between stock transfer associations and longer-established voluntary organizations which provide space for expressions of civil society between state and market.

Conclusion

The relationship between social housing provision and citizenship has always been less direct than for other welfare services such as health and education. The recent restructuring of social housing may be seen as a consequence of the relatively weakly established principle of state provision to meet the housing needs of citizens. The scale of demunicipalization since 1980 may be seen to support Harloe's (1995) view that decommodified housing is only provided where adequate provision in a commodified form is not possible.

However, since 1988 a significant element of demuncipalization has consisted of the transfer of stock to other landlords operating on a not-for-profit basis. These landlords have been subject to policies on public subsidy for social housing similar to those in the remaining council sector; i.e. a shift from bricks and mortar to personal subsidies between 1988 and 1995 with an element of retrenchment thereafter. The significant difference has been the treatment of private borrowing on the asset base of these landlords which is excluded from definitions of public spending. While technically transfer of stock to, and private borrowing by, these landlords may be viewed as privatization, the effect has been to support and extend social welfare provision with public subsidies, both through a housing benefit income stream to support private borrowing and through capital grants for new construction, partly supported by privatization receipts, but ultimately funded by the Treasury. To the extent that transfer has allowed landlords to invest in and upgrade their stock, higher quality accommodation has been brought within the reach of a larger number of local people. However, if a dimension of the social rights of citizens is access to accommodation which is affordable then it could be that the extent of reliance of stock transfer associations on private finance has meant rent increases, particularly for new tenants, which could place this right in greater jeopardy than elsewhere, depending on the fate of the housing benefit system. There are still greater similarities between these housing associations and local authorities than with private landlords.

The operation of choice in the restructuring process relates mainly to the establishment of quasi-markets which allow the central and local state to choose between competing housing association providers on the basis of bids for new construction activity. In the context of stock transfers, most transferring authorities have chosen to establish new associations rather than transferring to an existing landlord. However, there has been considerable recent interest in the concept of group structures whereby new local associations of Local Housing Companies may gain financial strength by becoming part of a larger housing association group. Having established a transfer association, authorities have had a second choice of either developing a special relationship with the new landlord or treating them simply as one of a number of competing providers for new development funding. These choices have been affected by political strategies and may relate to decisions on the benefits of local democratic representation on the new landlord body to deal with some of the accountability problems common to LPSBs.

As Chapter 8 demonstrates, quasi-markets for funding new homes have relatively little impact on the choices available to individual housing applicants and tenants. Similarly, the transfer of blocks of social housing from one near monopoly landlord to another does not appear to be a recipe for extending user choice. However, regulations introduced in 1993 requiring larger proposed transfers to split the stock between two or more successor landlords appeared to add to costs without providing any clear benefits to consumers since new landlords still usually had a geographical monopoly in parts of a district. It is possible however that some stock transfer landlords may be providing a significantly greater voice for tenants than was previously experienced, for example through elected representatives on management boards, and more general support for tenant involvement. While new entrants to the voluntary housing sector, stock transfer associations may be developing governance models which will have a wider long-term application in strengthening the independent value base of the third sector (NHF 1997). In this way they may be creating conditions for widening of civil society influence on housing institutions, and widening individual choice.

The impact of restructuring on patterns of control in social housing is the subject of considerable debate. There has clearly been a weakening of the influence of some stakeholders, particularly local authority councillors, and a strengthening of others, particularly private funders and Housing Corporation regulators as a result of stock transfers. Writers such as Malpass have taken the view that the fragmentation of governance in housing has resulted in a centralization of control rather than any extension of local influence. Support for this view is provided by referring to the 'considerable influence over the volume and type of work undertaken at the local level' exerted by the Housing Corporation as funder and regulator (Malpass 1997: 6). However, a key motivation for stock transfers was to escape the draconian central control over local authority borrowing and benefit from the relatively more benign treatment of housing associations. Moreover, the spending power of the capital receipt resulting from transfer has provided local authorities with considerable short term influence which some have chosen to exercise through local quasi-markets while others have preferred strategic alliances with chosen providers. The considerable potential for developing local interorganizational networks by effective enabling strategies in LSVT authorities is also beginning to be more fully recognized (Aldbourne Associates 1996).

References

Aldbourne Associates (1996) *Vision into Reality*. Marlborough: Aldbourne Associates.
Audit Commission (1992) *The Enabling Role of the Local Authority: The Strategic Framework*. London: HMSO.

Audit Commission (1993) *Who wins? Voluntary Housing Transfers*, occasional paper no. 20. London: Audit Commission.

Ball, M. (1989) Saying no! to newspeak. *Roof*, March/April: 33–4.

Beesley, M. and Littlechild, S.C. (1992) *Privatisation, Regulation and Deregulation*. London: Routledge.

Best, R. (1997) Housing associations: the sustainable solution, in P. Williams (ed.) *Directions in Housing Policy: Towards Sustainable Housing Policies for the UK*. London: Paul Chapman Publishing.

Birchall, J. (1988) *Building Communities the Co-operative Way*. London: Routledge.

Birchall, J., Pollitt, C. and Putman, D. (1995) The difference that makes for autonomy: a comparative study of opted out schools, hospitals and housing associations. Conference paper, Housing Studies Association conference, September.

Bishop, M. and Kay, J. (1988) *Does Privatisation Work?* London: London Business School.

Bowman, A. (1996) *Models of Collaboration: The Experience of Neighbourhood Transformation in the USA*. London: West Hampstead Housing Association.

Bramley, G. (1993a) The enabling role for local authorities: a preliminary evaluation, in P. Malpass and R. Means (eds) *Implementing Housing Policy*. Buckingham: Open University Press.

Bramley, G. (1993b) Quasi-markets and social housing, in J. Le Grand and W. Bartlett (eds) *Quasi-Markets and Social Policy*. Basingstoke: Macmillan.

Clapham, D. and Franklin, B. (1997) The social construction of housing management. *Housing Studies*, 12: 7–26.

Cole, I. and Furbey, R. (1994) *The Eclipse of Council Housing*. London: Routledge.

Committee on Standards in Public Life (1996) *Second Report: Local Public Spending Bodies*. London: HMSO.

Deakin, N. (1994) *The Politics of Welfare: Continuities and Change*. Hemel Hempstead: Harvester.

DoE (1995) *More Choice in the Social Rented Sector*. Consultation paper linked to housing White Paper *Our Future Homes*. London: HMSO.

Esping-Andersen, G. (1990) *The Three Worlds of Welfare Capitalism*. Princeton, NJ: Princeton University Press.

Ferlie, E., Ashburner, L., Fitzgerald, L. and Pettigrew, A. (1996) *The New Public Management in Action*. Oxford: Oxford University Press.

Forrest, R. and Murie, A. (1988) *Selling the Welfare State: The Privatisation of Public Housing*. London: Routledge.

Gardiner, K., Hills, J. and Kleinman, M. (1991) *Putting a Price on Council Housing: Valuing Voluntary Transfers*. London School of Economics welfare state programme discussion paper WSP/62. London: LSE.

Goodlad, R. (1993) *The Housing Authority as Enabler*. Coventry: Longman/Institute of Housing.

Harloe, M. (1995) *The People's Home: Social Rented Housing in Europe and America*. Oxford: Blackwell.

Hawksworth, J. and Wilcox, S. (1995) *Challenging the Conventions: Public Borrowing Rules and Housing Investment*. Coventry: Chartered Institute of Housing.

Heald, D. (1984) Privatisation and public money, in D. Steel and D. Heald (eds) *Privatising Public Enterprises*. London: Royal Institute of Public Administration.

HMSO (1987) Housing: the Government's Proposals, Cm. 214. London: HMSO.

Housing Corporation (1996a) *Guidelines for Applicants Seeking to Become Registered Social Landlords: Stock Transfer Applicants.* London: Housing Corporation.

Housing Corporation (1996b) *Investment Report 1996/7.* London: Housing Corporation.

Inquiry into British Housing (1990) *Information Notes.* York: Joseph Rowntree Foundation.

Jensen, L. (1995) Stuck in the middle? The Danish social housing associations between state, market and civil society. Conference paper, IRES Conference, Stockholm, June.

Karn, V. (1993) Remodelling a HAT: the implementation of the Housing Action Trust legislation 1987–92, in P. Malpass and R. Means (eds) *Implementing Housing Policy.* Buckingham: Open University Press.

Kleinman, M. (1993) Large scale transfers of council housing to new landlords: is British social housing becoming more European? *Housing Studies,* 8: 163–78.

Kramer, R. (1987) Voluntary agencies and the personal social services, in W.J. Powell (ed.) *The Non-Profit Sector: A Research Handbook.* New Haven: Yale University Press..

Le Grand, J. and Bartlett, W. (eds) (1993) *Quasi-Markets and Social Policy.* Basingstoke: Macmillan.

London Housing Unit (1997) *Comparing HRA and Rent Allowance Subsidy Levels,* spreadsheets. London: London Housing Unit.

Malpass, P. (1996) The unravelling of housing policy in Britain. *Housing Studies,* 11: 459–70.

Malpass, P. (1997) The local governance of housing, in P. Malpass (ed.) *Ownership, Control and Accountability: The New Governance of Housing.* Coventry: Chartered Institute of Housing.

Mullins, D. (1996) *Us and Them. Report of a Survey of Housing Enabling Officers.* Birmingham: Centre for Urban and Regional Studies, The University of Birmingham.

Mullins, D. (1997a) From regulatory capture to regulated competition: an interest group analysis of the regulation of housing associations in England. *Housing Studies,* 12: 301–19.

Mullins, D. (1997b) Changing with the times: housing association responses to a changing environment, in D. Mullins and M. Riseborough (eds) *Changing with the Times. Critical Interpretations of the Repositioning of Housing Associations,* University of Birmingham Occasional Paper no. 12. Birmingham: University of Birmingham, School of Public Policy.

Mullins, D. (1997c) Stock transfers create conflicts of interest. *Housing Agenda,* July/August: 20–1.

Mullins, D. and Riseborough, M. (1996) Managerial strategy and organisational purpose: how housing associations are responding to their move from margin to mainstream, in D. Mullins and M. Riseborough (eds) *Changing with the Times. Critical Interpretations of the Repositioning of Housing Associations,* University of Birmingham Occasional Paper no. 12. Birmingham: University of Birmingham, School of Public Policy.

Mullins, D., Niner, P. and Riseborough, M. (1992) *Evaluating Large Scale Voluntary Transfers of Local Authority Housing: An Interim Report.* London: HMSO.

Mullins, D., Niner, P. and Riseborough, M. (1993) Large scale voluntary transfers, in P. Malpass and R. Means (eds) *Implementing Housing Policy*. Buckingham: Open University Press.

Mullins, D., Niner, P. and Riseborough, M. (1995) *Evaluating Large Scale Voluntary Transfers of Local Authority Housing*. London: HMSO.

Murie, A. (1993) Privatisation and restructuring public involvement in housing provision in Britain. *Scandinavian Housing and Planning Research*, 10: 145–57.

Murie, A. (1997) Beyond state housing, in P. Williams (ed.) *Directions in Housing Policy: Towards Sustainable Housing Policies for the UK*. London: Paul Chapman Publishing.

NFHA (1990) *Towards 2000. The Housing Association Agenda*. London: NFHA.

NFHA (1995a) *Much in Evidence*. London: NFHA.

NFHA (1995b) *Competence and Accountability. Report of Inquiry into Housing Association Governance*. London: NFHA.

NFHA (1995c) *Code of Governance*. London: NFHA.

NHF (1997) *Action for Accountability: A Guide for Independent Social Landlords*. London: NHF.

Office for Public Management (1997) *Local Housing Strategies*. London: National Housing Federation.

Randolph, B. (1993) The re-privatisation of housing associations, in P. Malpass and R. Means (eds) *Implementing Housing Policy*. Buckingham: Open University Press.

Reid, B. (1995) Interorganisational networks and the delivery of local housing services. *Housing Studies*, 10: 133–50.

Reid, B. (1997) Interorganisational relationships and social housing services, in P. Malpass (ed.) *Ownership, Control and Accountability: The New Governance of Housing*. Coventry: Chartered Institute of Housing.

Rhodes, R. (1995) *The New Governance: Governing Without Government*. Seminar paper, 'The State of Britain' seminars, 11. Swindon: ESRC.

Ridley, N. (1992) *My Style of Government*. London: Fontana.

Riseborough, M. (1997) Private bodies working in the public interest? Housing associations presenting images of self, in D. Mullins and M. Riseborough (eds) *Changing With the Times. Critical Interpretations of the Repositioning of Housing Associations*, University of Birmingham Occasional Paper no. 12. Birmingham: University of Birmingham, School of Public Policy.

SHAPE (1993) *American Community Development Corporations: A Model for UK Housing Associations?* Birmingham: SHAPE Group.

Salamon, L. and Anheier, H.K. (1996) *Social Origins of Civil Society: Explaining the Nonprofit Sector Cross-Nationally*. Johns Hopkins comparative nonprofit sector project working paper no. 22. Baltimore: Johns Hopkins Institute for Policy Studies.

Samson, S. (1994) The three faces of privatisation. *Sociology*, 28: 79–97.

Smith, S. and Mallinson, S. (1997) Housing for health in a post-welfare state. *Housing Studies*, 12: 173–200.

Spencer, K., Mullins, D. and Walker, B. (1995) *Voluntary Housing Today and Tomorrow*. Occasional paper no. 1. Birmingham: School of Public Policy, The University of Birmingham.

Stewart, J. and Walsh, K. (1992) Change in the management of public services. *Public Administration*, 70: 499–518.

Stoker, G. (1995) Public-private partnerships in urban governance. Conference paper, Housing Studies Association conference, Edinburgh, September.

Walker, R.M. (1998) New public management and housing associations: from comfort to competition. *Policy and Politics*, 26(1): 71–87.

Wandsworth Borough Council (1993) *Report by Chairman of Housing Committee.* London: Wandsworth Borough Council.

Weaver, M. (1997) *Housing Today*, 9 October.

Wilcox, S. (1993) *Local Housing Companies.* York: Joseph Rowntree Foundation.

Wilcox, S. (1997) *Housing Review 1997/98.* York: Joseph Rowntree Foundation.

Wuthnow, R. (1991) The voluntary sector: legacy of the past, hope for the future? in R. Wuthnow (ed.) *Between States and Markets: The Voluntary Sector in Comparative Perspective.* Princeton, NJ: Princeton University Press.

Zitron, J. (1995) *Local Housing Companies. A Good Practice Guide.* Coventry: Chartered Institute of Housing.

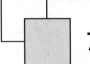

7

Incentives, choice and control in the finance of council housing

Bruce Walker

Introduction

In this chapter we are concerned with the provision of rented housing by local authorities. This restricts our analysis to one subset of the potentially wider group of 'social housing providers'. The other main providers are 'registered social landlords': not-for-profit (NFP) organizations registered with the Housing Corporation. Local authority housing still accounts for 80 per cent of social housing in England and a larger proportion in both Wales and Scotland, and thus continues to be, quantitatively, the most significant direct supplier of existing, as opposed to new, social housing.

The main purpose of this chapter is to consider who it is that pays for council housing. This requires us to examine the changing financial relationship between the various stakeholders. Particular attention is paid to changes in central and locally determined subsidies, especially in respect of the changing use of personal and producer subsidies, and we attempt to trace some of the impact of these changes which in themselves both reflect and reinforce patterns of control. The changes have had variable but significant impacts on the choices available to a range of stakeholders, including central government departments, local authorities, local and national taxpayers and council tenants.

In exploring these issues in both past and current policy it is important to be aware that economic thinking has had a major impact on the form and development of housing policy. It is also important, therefore, to understand the principles which underlie that thinking, particularly those relating to pricing and subsidy options.

Prices, subsidies and the implications for choice: some principles

One of the basic tenets of economic theory is that the price which is set for a good (or service) will bear some relationship, in the long term at least, to the value of the resources used in providing that good. Faced with the good at a particular price, consumers will choose in the light of both their incomes and their preferences for that good how much of it to consume. Consumers are envisaged as making choices across the range of goods available as to which goods and how much of them to consume. Depending how sensitive the demand of an individual consumer, or consumers as a whole, is to changes in price, an increase in the price of a good will in general lead to a fall in demand, while a decrease in price will lead to an increase in the amount demanded.

Changes in prices will also affect the behaviour of profit-seeking producers. An increase in price caused by an increase in demand will encourage them to supply more of the good by allocating more resources to its provision. Simultaneously, the higher price will 'ration' available supplies among consumers, essentially by allocating the good to those willing and able to pay the higher price. Conversely, a fall in price caused by a fall in demand will tend to encourage producers to produce less and, thus, use fewer resources. In this simple world, resources are allocated to the provision of different goods by fluctuations in the prices and profitability of different lines of production as reflected in the price of those goods, while consumers exercise their choice among goods in the light of those prices by changing their patterns of consumption. An efficient allocation of resources, it follows, is therefore one under which resources are placed in those lines of production in which they are most valued by consumers as demonstrated by the consumers' willingness to pay for the goods produced.

The significance of this brief description of the market model of production, consumption and resource allocation, for our purposes, is to suggest that both producers and consumers will tend to react to price changes in a predictable manner. Thus, if we wish at least some people to consume more housing, in the sense of better housing, than they otherwise would at existing prices, one possibility is to lower the price (rent) of housing to them. They will then choose to consume more housing at the lower price.

A logically prior consideration is, of course, *why* we should seek to affect people's housing consumption. This is fairly well-worn ground (see, for example, Maclennan 1982: 154–62; Hills 1992, ch. 2). Briefly, subsidies intended to increase the housing consumption of particular social groups can be justified on the grounds that poor-quality housing has effects on health, on the occupants' expectations, attitudes and subsequent behaviour, and on the broader sensibilities of society as a whole. None of this is uncontroversial, but the argument is that, since all of these factors materially affect the wider population, the wider population benefits from increases in the amount of housing consumed by groups who would otherwise be disadvantaged. These benefits are reflected in the value of the subsidies that society grants to these groups.

The manner in which consumers should be subsidized brings in another set of considerations. There are basically three alternatives. First, consumers can be helped to purchase more housing at market prices by increasing their ability to pay through a personal subsidy in the form of an income (cash) supplement. Recipients could then exercise their freedom and purchase more goods and services, including more housing, at existing prices from their enhanced incomes. A well-known drawback to this policy is that there is no guarantee that the additional income will be spent on housing, which is the purpose of the subsidy in the first place.

Second, the subsidy could be paid to consumers in a form which is tied to housing consumption so that they cannot spend the subsidy other than on housing. Such a subsidy can be targeted directly to the intended recipients who can then be allowed to exercise their own choice among the different amounts (types, sizes, quality, location) of housing provided by private producers at existing prices. A problem with this policy is that if the supply of housing in the short term is not very sensitive to price the extra purchasing power granted to consumers participating in the programme may simply be absorbed in higher prices. The effect on the housing consumption of the subsidized group may in these circumstances be minimal. If these conditions do obtain on the supply side, some combination of this and either price control and/or provision by NFP producers may be required to ensure that housing is not priced beyond the willingness or ability to pay of the subsidized group.

Third, the subsidy could be paid to producers. However, if one of the major objectives of housing producers is to make profits, extra monitoring costs will be incurred as a result of the need to ensure that the subsidy is passed on to the appropriate consumers in the form of lower prices and is not absorbed in profits. Such problems may help to explain the apparent reluctance of UK governments, certainly in recent years, to provide producer subsidies to profit-making rather than NFP landlords. Paying the subsidy to an NFP landlord therefore has its attractions, although caution must be exercised here since such producers may have a strong interest in accumulating surpluses and may monitor costs less well than profit-oriented suppliers.

In considering the effects of consumer and producer subsidies it is important to bear in mind that the subsidies themselves have to be paid for by someone. The ultimate provider of such subsidies is, usually, although not always, the taxpayer. A subsidy programme which gives households the freedom to consume as much housing as they wish, or gives providers the freedom to engage in 'excessive' subsidized production, is unlikely to be popular with subsidy providers. The ideal subsidy programme from the taxpayers' viewpoint is one which achieves the desired result at minimum cost in tax revenues. Consequently, we would expect that subsidies to consumers would exist alongside controls on how much subsidized housing programme participants are permitted to consume, while producer subsidies would be controlled by regulations as to the cost and type of the housing provided. In both cases, the freedom of choice that producers and consumers have to produce and consume in the light of the subsidies is constrained.

Applying the principles to council housing

When we examine the history of subsidized housing provided by the public sector in the UK many of the features outlined above become apparent. Hence, such housing has at different times been financed mainly through consumer subsidies or mainly through producer subsidies, and at other times through a mixture of the two. Similarly, new housing has been provided on an NFP basis by local authorities, although often physically constructed by private-sector builders. In some periods such housing was provided for the 'working classes' generally, at others for those previously inhabiting slums or for other households exhibiting particular needs.

It is possible to argue, as do Cole and Furbey (1994: 45 *et seq.*), that for much of the period from its first effective introduction under the Housing and Town Planning Act (the Addison Act) of 1919, council housing was by its nature emergency housing. Put in terms of the simple model of market operation outlined above, council housing was provided essentially to supplement the market or to partially offset perceived failures in market provision. These perceived market failures after the First World War, for example, included the problems of an inadequate or constrained supply-side response and poor quality provision, and were certainly seen as severe enough to pose the danger of civil unrest (Merrett 1979, ch. 2) and, therefore, to warrant incurring of new state responsibilities and funding.

Vesting powers to provide housing with local councils can be seen as central government '... declining itself to accept full direct responsibility' for public housing (Cole and Furbey 1994: 51). The public housing service could have been organized along similar lines to, for example, the current social security system (or the previous organization of state housing in many Eastern and Central European countries) where the service is a national responsibility delivered at the local level. However, there are strong reasons of efficiency and accountability for lodging such responsibilities for local housing at the local level, not least because a variety of housing legislation since 1919 has required local taxpayers to contribute to the finance of the public housing provided in their areas. Such a contribution can be taken to reflect the sort of benefits noted above which accrue to local taxpayers from the provision of additional, higher quality housing in the locality, with national taxpayers' contributions reflecting the supra-local benefits and potentially improved welfare distribution that such housing can generate.

Whether in practice the actual local-national funding arrangements mirrored the local-national distribution of benefits in any systematic way is, of course, an entirely different matter. Nevertheless, an important feature of the UK housing system from 1919 until 1989 was that various housing acts placed a requirement upon local authorities, or granted them permissive powers, to draw on local tax funds to support their council housing.

However, the fact that the public housing service became a local responsibility in this fashion can itself be problematic, given that central government also has a legitimate interest in the provision of such housing. Clearly, the priorities and preferences of a local government in respect of housing provision need not reflect those of central government. Consequently, throughout the history of council housing, central government has used a mixture of financial incentives and disincentives – and, occasionally, the force of law – in an attempt to encourage local authorities to pursue the policies at the local level that central government believes to be in the national interest. These financial (dis)incentives, which are the main concern of this chapter, are essentially a way of altering the prices facing local authorities as providers and tenants as consumers, and hence altering their behaviour as providers and consumers.

Thus, for example, if through a subsidy central government lowers the costs of housing provision for local authorities, at least some authorities might be expected to respond by providing more housing. Others may not react in this way, of course, if, in the light of local electoral/political preferences or available local tax revenues, such housing provision is still not an attractive proposition despite the subsidy offered. Further, in authorities which are receiving subsidy, central government has, arguably, both a right and a responsibility to ensure that the subsidy is used efficiently, while local authorities have both rights and responsibilities to manage their housing provision in the light of local priorities. This potential for discord may explain why the housing field has been one of the arenas in which tensions in the central-local government relationship, particularly in recent years, have been most visible.

The era of producer subsidies in council housing, 1919–72

The origins of the growth of local authority housing have been discussed extensively (see, for example, Malpass 1990, especially ch. 2; Malpass and Murie 1994, ch. 3) and the details do not concern us here. However, there are a number of features of the subsidy systems employed between the 1919 Addison Act and the Housing Finance Act of 1972 that relate to the issues of choice and control. First, consider the implications that different forms of subsidy have for the relative powers of central and local government to influence the level and type of new housing provision undertaken.

One of the key features of central government ('exchequer') subsidies for housing during the whole of the period up until 1972 was that they were investment-based producer subsidies, i.e. they were 'bricks and mortar' subsidies paid to local authorities as the providers of housing. The intention of the subsidies was to assist authorities in meeting the costs of the long-term loans taken out to finance construction. Thus, the Addison Act, for example, offered local authorities a subsidy per new dwelling for 20 years on approved projects equal to any deficit incurred minus the product of a penny rate; the 1967 Housing Subsidies Act explicitly tied the subsidy to the costs of financing new housing by granting a subsidy equal to the difference between the rate of interest actually paid by authorities and a notional 4 per cent rate.

The impact of producer subsidies

As would be expected on the basis of the economic principles discussed earlier, variations in the generosity, as perceived by local authorities, in the level of these producer subsidies influenced the level and quality of output of new council housing. Thus, the increased subsidies offered by central government under Wheatley's 1924 Housing (Financial Provisions) Act heralded in a period under which council house completions more than doubled between 1924/5 and 1925/6 and increased to a pre-1939 peak of 104,000 p.a. in 1927/8 (Holmans 1987: 66). The 1952 Housing Subsidies Act substantially raised both exchequer and rate fund contributions which significantly contributed to a public sector output of 939,000 dwellings over the period 1952–6. Clearly, these subsidies proved a comparatively powerful incentive to local authorities to provide more council housing.

The subsidy systems also acted as an incentive in respect of the form of the new housing and the broader function which it was intended to fulfil. In respect of physical form, the 1956 Housing Subsidies Act, which paid authorities a higher subsidy per dwelling (flat) the higher that they built, contributed to the high-rise boom of the late 1950s and 1960s. This has, perhaps, provided the inhabitants of British cities with one of the most striking examples of the physical impact of a particular subsidy arrangement on the urban environment.

The function of the housing built during this period also varied and thus influenced directly the types of household who were housed. The legislation enacted between 1919 and 1930, and between 1946 and 1954, was primarily intended to encourage additions to the stock of housing, i.e. it was housing for 'general needs' at times of perceived housing shortage. During the earlier of these two periods, the rent levels charged were related to the controlled private sector rents obtaining in the area concerned plus an allowance for the higher quality of public sector dwellings. This quality effect was sufficient to put the housing beyond the means of many of the poorest households. Consequently, the earliest occupants of council housing were in general not those with the lowest incomes and, thus, were not necessarily those who had been occupying the lowest quality private sector dwellings (see, for example, Dresser 1984: 197).

The change from subsidies for general needs towards those intended to encourage local authorities to clear and replace slum housing which occurred, for example, in 1930, under Greenwood's Housing Act, and in 1954, under the Housing Repairs and Rents Act, directly affected the types of household gaining access to council housing. In this way, a more explicit 'welfare' role for council housing was defined. Indeed, in the 1930s there were clear concerns about the likely behaviour of those housed as a result of slum clearance and about their ability to treat their new municipal housing in an 'appropriate' manner (see, for example, Harloe 1995: 189 *et seq.*).

In contrast, the dropping of the word 'working classes' from the title of the 1949 Housing Act on its second reading in March of that year could be seen as a rejection of that welfare role. The minister of health, Aneurin Bevan, argued in respect of the occupancy of local authority housing that:

> ... if we are to enable citizens to lead a full life, if they are each to be aware of the problems of their neighbours, then they should be all drawn from different sections of the community ... I believe it leads to the enrichment of every member of the community to live in communities of that sort. Therefore, we are sweeping away all references to 'housing of the working classes'.
>
> (*Hansard* 1949)

The continuing problem faced by local authorities throughout this period was that of reconciling the costs of the provision and operation of their public housing functions with both the willingness of local and national taxpayers and the ability of tenants themselves to meet those costs. A greater willingness by taxpayers' elected representatives to subsidize the costs of provision meant that tenants as a group were required to pay lower rents. However, the supply-side nature of the subsidies meant that, in the absence of action to the contrary, there was no necessary relation between the rents charged and the ability of individual tenants to pay. The financial commitment of the exchequer was fixed by the announcement of the subsidies to be made available under a particular act and local authorities then had the freedom to determine the balance of local taxes and rents which would make up the remainder of the housing income required.

This freedom could be more illusory than real, given the competing claims on local tax revenues, which themselves were subject to fluctuation according to local economic conditions and political decisions as to tax rates. The fact that council tenants themselves were, and are, local taxpayers and that the value of new council houses for tax purposes could be relatively high – adding 50–55 per cent to the rents in County Durham in the late 1920s, for example (Ryder 1984: 83) – compounded the problem of providing public housing which was both affordable to the tenants for whom it was intended and, from the local authority's standpoint, financially viable. Further, until 1935, authorities were required to keep separate accounts, managed on a NFP basis, for each act under which their dwellings had been constructed. This arrangement could lead to wide differentials in the rents of otherwise similar housing built by an authority under different acts and to the possibility of surpluses arising on some accounts, with consequent rent reductions being permitted only on the housing included within those accounts (Holmans 1987: 312).

Producer subsidies and rents: rebate schemes and pooling

Central government's response to both the danger of pricing certain households out of the sector and the distributive effects of the subsidy arrangements took a form which, though again initiated in the 1930s, was to affect profoundly the finance of council housing for the remainder of the century.

First, in 1930, central government clarified local authorities' rights to grant rent rebates to those households whose rents were high relative to their incomes (Daunton 1984: 22). While these could be funded from existing exchequer subsidies, no financial incentive in the form of additional subsidy from central government was offered. Hence, local authorities which chose to introduce rebate schemes had to finance them from a combination of higher rents paid by those tenants not eligible for rebates and from additional contributions from ratepayers. The difficulties of financing such schemes and the political difficulties of charging different tenants different rents for similar housing while determining rebates through means testing are described in the case of Leeds, for example, by Finnigan (1984: 116 et seq.). Such difficulties may explain why by 1938 there were only an estimated 122 rebate schemes in English and Welsh authorities (Daunton 1984: 23).

Indeed, exhortation remained the primary form of encouragement that central government gave to local rebate schemes until 1972. A Ministry of Housing and Local Government circular in 1967, for example, urged that: 'subsidies should not be used wholly or even mainly to keep general rent levels low. Help for those who most need it can be given only if the subsidies are in large part used to provide rebates for tenants whose means are small' (quoted in Holmans 1987: 342). However, while the same circular provided a model rebate scheme for guidance, the precise form of the schemes used in the 60 per cent of authorities employing them by the early 1970s (Malpass 1990: 67) remained a matter for local discretion until 1972.

As Holmans (1987: 342 *et seq.*) and Malpass (1990: 66–7) observe, before the 1972 Act, exchequer subsidies were still formally paid on a per dwelling basis. However, in practice the subsidies could be used flexibly in that the aggregate sum received could be used either to lower all rents or, through the locally-determined rebate schemes, directed primarily at lower-income tenants. The ability of local authorities to use supply-side subsidies – in the form of a subsidy to specific tenants – to ameliorate the differential rents that resulted from the diverse subsidy arrangements built into successive legislation was facilitated by what might seem at first glance to be an arcane change in accounting requirements from 1935 onwards. The then minister of health argued that the result of the arrangements requiring separate accounts for housing built under separate acts '. . . has been a great wastage of effort and of efficiency' (*Hansard* 1935). From that date onwards authorities were required to group or 'pool' all expenditure on, and income from, council housing into a single Housing Revenue Account (HRA).

This meant that, although authorities continued to receive subsidies from the exchequer based upon their entitlements specified in the acts under which they had built their housing, the subsidies received did not have to be directed towards the financing of the specific dwellings giving rise to those subsidies. This also allowed local authorities to pool rents, in that the subsidies could now be used to lower the relatively high rents which would otherwise be associated with the higher costs of (predominantly) newer housing, and raise rents on older, lower cost housing on which much of the debt would already have been amortized. The impact of pooling became particularly important when new building was being undertaken during inflationary times, such as in the late 1950s and early 1960s (Malpass 1990: 66–7: Harloe 1995: 184). The 'surplus' on older houses could be used to finance new construction at a lower level of exchequer subsidy than would otherwise have been possible.

The effects of pooling on the rents faced by tenants in an individual authority, though difficult to estimate precisely, can be dramatic. Walker *et al.* (1991: 61–3), for example, suggest that the average rents set on a relatively new estate in the Birmingham area in 1990/1 covered approximately 41 per cent of current and historic costs, while the average rents on an estate completed 26 years previously were some 22 per cent greater than those costs.

Rent setting policies under producer subsidies

The introduction of pooling also had the effect of liberating local authorities' rent setting policies from direct government control. The Addison Act of 1919, for example, had been accompanied by quite detailed guidance on rent setting while the 1924 Wheatley Act required rents to be set at the 'appropriate normal rent', which was the average rent charged for pre-1914 working-class houses. The effective separation after 1935 of the subsidies from the dwellings to which they had originally applied meant that authorities were free to decide to distribute the rent income which they needed to raise across their housing stock in a different manner if they so wished. Government guidance in the 1935 Act, for example, simply required local authorities to make 'reasonable charges' and to: '... take into consideration the rents ordinarily payable by persons of the working classes in their locality ... [and] from time to time review rents and make such changes, either of rents generally or of particular rents ... as circumstances might require' (quoted in Holmans 1987: 313).

Central government might urge authorities to set, for example, 'realistic rents', as the Conservative government did in 1955, or freeze all rent increases, as the Labour government did for a period during 1966. However, the general requirement simply to make reasonable charges and to review them as necessary still remains in force, and has done since 1935, with the exception of 1972–75. Local authorities freedom of choice in the setting of rents is thus a long-established tradition.

The main method used by authorities to set the rent of individual dwellings for almost 40 years after 1935 was by reference to the gross value of each dwelling, i.e. its rateable value plus an allowance for repairs and maintenance. At the time of their determination, these values were intended to be broadly equivalent to rents in the private sector. The relative rents of council houses, one to another, would thus bear the same relation to each other as relativities in the private sector. Whether this was ever the case is debatable, and because gross values were not systematically updated over time it became increasingly unlikely (see Walker and Marsh, 1995: 40–1 for a brief discussion). Nevertheless, the principle that rent relativities in the public sector should reflect those in the private sector, implicit in the use of the basic gross value method, was one to which the government returned explicitly in 1989, as we discuss below.

Given both the centrally-imposed restrictions on rent increases as part of the prices and incomes policy introduced in 1966 and the rising interest rates and capital costs of new building, local authorities were, by the end of the 1960s, experiencing particularly acute pressure on rent levels and thus on rate fund contributions. The costs of new construction in turn had serious implications for national economic management as they fed through to claims for exchequer subsidy. Further, there were significant variations in the rents faced by otherwise identical tenants in similar dwellings rented from different local authorities. Such variations arose because of the differences between authorities in their past and contemporary building programmes and their individual decisions as to the use of additional rate fund contributions, both of which directly affected different authorities' total income. The comparative freedom that local authorities had been given to use exchequer subsidies and their effective autonomy in determining the rents of individual dwellings added to this variation in rents between authorities.

Rent setting: issues of equity and efficiency

In one sense, the variation in rent levels across local housing authorities could be seen as a 'natural' and even a beneficial outcome of the system, given that it could be taken to reflect the choices made by democratically accountable bodies in the light of local needs and preferences. Conversely, the potential inequities generated as between one tenant and another as a result of rents primarily reflecting '... historic accidents which ... determined the composition of each local authority's housing stock' (HMSO 1971: para. 6) can be argued to be one significant drawback of the system as it existed by 1972.

In addition to inequities between tenants, a further argument concerned the implications of the pre-1972 system for allocative efficiency, although this needs treating with some care. While it is doubtless the case that rents frequently did not reflect the current value of the resources embodied in the dwellings in any consistent way, this is hardly surprising given the historic cost basis of housing (and most other local authority) accounting and, possibly as important, given that local authorities had not been required to set rents in a manner that reflected such values. As we shall discuss further below, the idea that rents reflecting such values would affect household choices as between dwellings within the public sector is open to dispute. Further, the misallocation of resources that was likely to be brought about between authorities as a result of tenants attempting to move across local authority boundaries due to 'arbitrary' inter-authority differences in rent was unlikely to be significant because of the tight constraints on the inter-authority mobility of publicly renting households.

Perhaps the strongest argument for the allocative inefficiency of the pre-1972 system lay in the distortions it brought about in resource allocation and choice between the private and public rented sectors. To the extent that households were attracted to the local authority sector by non-market pricing, the resultant excess demand for council dwellings would attract resources to the public sector from the private sector, or at least lead to demands that resources be so reallocated. A counter argument might be that rents in the private sector were themselves so distorted as a result of a history of regulation, deregulation and 'reregulation' as to render the impact of inter-sectoral rent differentials on the allocation of both households and resources at best highly uncertain. This contention is somewhat weakened by 1965 legislation making possible the setting of 'fair rents' in the unfurnished private rented sector. Increasing consistency in rent setting in the sector with which it was 'competing' could be argued to make the case for greater consistency in rent setting in the public sector.

Irrespective of the strength of these particular arguments, the government argued in 1971 that there was a matter of principle at stake – namely that it was right: 'first to determine a rent which is reasonable for the dwelling and then to consider whether the tenant needs help towards the rent. Any rent subsidy should be directed to the tenant rather than the house' (HMSO 1971: para. 20).

While it may appear that this was no more than a restatement of the need to set reasonable rents and a reiteration of the encouragement to use existing subsidies for rebates rather than rents in general, the 1972 Housing Finance Act which enshrined these principles represented a radical departure from what had gone before.

Consumer subsidies: the significance of the Housing Finance Act 1972

The details of the 1972 Act have been extensively discussed elsewhere (see, for example, Holmans 1987: 349 *et seq.*) and do not require repetition here. For our purposes, the system introduced by that legislation had a number of important features relating to issues of choice and control. First, it decoupled council rents from the historic and current costs of the housing itself by requiring that the rents of individual dwellings should move rapidly to the fair rent levels obtaining under rent registration regulations in the private sector.

Second, since the rent income accruing to an authority's HRA was now to be determined without reference to existing expenditure on that account, a new subsidy system was required to ensure that expenditure could be met. Briefly, this took the form of a series of subsidies intended to make up any deficit arising on the account as a result of a shortfall in rent income. It was envisaged that this subsidy and its associated mandatory rate fund contribution would rapidly fall to zero for most authorities as rents increased.

Third, the Act set up a mandatory rent rebate scheme, which was to be funded 90 per cent by the exchequer and 10 per cent from the rate fund in its first year, changing to 75 per cent and 25 per cent respectively by 1975/6. Local authorities had the freedom to introduce a more favourable scheme for their tenants if they chose to do so, but any resulting additional expenditure had to be met by the authority itself from the rate fund or from any HRA surplus.

In these three ways the 1972 Act redefined the relationships between the local authority, its housing stock (and hence its tenants), and central government. The freedom for local authorities to determine their own rent levels was replaced by a requirement to move to the prices prevailing in the regulated private sector. General subsidies were determined according to, effectively, the total revenue costs of an authority's housing in relation to the income from gross rents. The previous NFP basis of the HRA was replaced by an expectation that surpluses were to be made, albeit still retained within the public sector. Surpluses exceeding a defined working balance were to be returned to central government and used to offset exchequer expenditure on rent allowances for private sector tenants, or, if the surpluses were larger even than this sum, half of the remainder was to be returned to the rate fund and half retained by the exchequer. Tenants in such high surplus authorities, therefore, could be argued to be subsidizing first, low income private sector tenants and, second, their own rebates through their 'contributions' to the exchequer and the rate fund.

The rent rebate scheme itself is arguably the 1972 Act's most lasting memorial. In many ways it was a logical corollary to the removal of authorities' independence in rent setting and the drive to higher rents, and had the benefit in terms of equity in offering tenants of similar means a consistent level of help. However, bearing in mind the envisaged temporary nature of the deficit subsidy to the HRA, its significance for our purposes is that it explicitly made the subsidizing of people, not dwellings, the main focus of the subsidy system. Tenants were expected to face market-related rents, and to be assisted through a means-tested personal subsidy tied to housing consumption only if their circumstances warranted it. Putting the opposition view, Anthony Crosland attacked this explicit introduction of market principles into public housing, arguing that: 'Surely this is wrong in principle – to set rents at a level which the majority of tenants cannot pay without a rebate ... The only fair principle is to set rents at a level which the majority can pay without rebate ... and, as a Tory Government should want, standing on their own two feet' (*Hansard* 1971a).

While in practice a strict majority of tenants did not qualify for a rebate, by 1976 around 945,000 – 44 per cent of all council tenants – did qualify, an increase of 675,000 since 1972 (Malpass and Murie 1994: 82). Further, the subtle cross-subsidy effects of the use of HRA surpluses, as they affected local taxpayers, public tenants paying full and rebated rents, and private tenants receiving rent allowances, can be criticized on the grounds of equity. To quote Anthony Crosland again: 'Poverty and low incomes are not the responsibility of council tenants but of the State and of the central Government. Why should council tenants be made to pay rebates? ... It should be the clear responsibility of the national taxpayer and the central Government' (*Hansard* 1971b).

In has been argued that in some respects the system proposed in the Act 'was likely to be allocatively more efficient within and between rental sectors' (Maclennan 1982: 251). Others saw the Act as opening up 'the prospect of a much more residualised public sector, as higher rents drove out the better off and rebates made council housing more affordable for the least well off' (Malpass 1990: 124). The first of these views highlights the economic efficiency in targeting public subsidy under the Act, although we have some doubts about this which we have expressed above. Malpass, however, draws attention to the wider implications of such policies, including a weakening of citizenship bonds through social fragmentation and residualization. Such concerns have become increasingly central to discussions of social housing generally in the UK and elsewhere as the social base of the sector has narrowed and principles of economic efficiency have reduced the attractiveness of such housing as a 'prize of citizenship' (see Chapter 8).

Either way, the material point here is not the fact that the Housing Finance Act, rescinded in 1975, was a failure in own terms. Rather, the significance of the Act was that it was the first clearly to establish the principles that in public housing people, not investment, should be subsidized, that tenants themselves should make a contribution to that subsidy and that the rents set for council housing should in some way be related to market rents. All of these principles were to make a reappearance in 1980s' housing legislation.

The era of consumer subsidies in council housing: 1980–95

The significance of the 1980 Housing Act

The 1980 Housing Act introduced by the first Thatcher administration is undoubtedly best remembered for its provisions concerning the rights of local authority tenants to buy their council dwellings on very favourable terms, rather than the arrangements it made for the pricing and subsidizing of the housing that was to remain within the public sector. Yet, the implications of the new arrangements for, in particular, the rents of council housing were to prove an important element in encouraging tenants to purchase their dwellings. Council tenants were faced with a financial disincentive, in the form of higher rents, to remain renting in the sector while simultaneously the price of buying was significantly reduced. Further, as the 1980s progressed, the prospect of an increasingly high level of council house rents could also be seen to act as an incentive to tenants to consider changing their landlords under the Tenants' Choice and Large Scale Voluntary Transfer (LSVT) schemes.

In 1980, the Right to Buy was so central to the government's housing policy and to the Act itself that, as Malpass (1990: 137–8) has also observed, virtually no attention was paid to its implications for council rents and subsidies during the Bill's second and third readings. In the Commons debate, the Secretary of State simply said of the new system that it was: '... designed to offer a sensible and fair deal as between central Government and the housing authorities and between council tenants, ratepayers and taxpayers' (*Hansard* 1980a).

The Act retained both a national rent rebate system (later, in 1982, to be incorporated into the new Housing Benefit – HB – arrangements) and the freedom of local authorities to determine the rents of individual dwellings as they saw fit, as the 1975 Housing Rents and Subsidies Act had reintroduced. However, the Act returned to the principle of deficit funding in determining exchequer subsidy.

Under the subsidy system the exchequer contribution amounted, broadly, to a sum necessary for an authority to balance its HRA. The minimum sum that an authority could receive as a result of this calculation was set at zero – i.e. there were no negative subsidy entitlements. The drawback in its operation from the local authorities' point of view was that the increases in costs and rent income were as determined, on an annual basis, by the Secretary of State. The opposition spokesman on the environment, Roy Hattersley, commented during the Bill's second reading that the powers granted under the legislation amounted to: '... enabling the Secretary of State to do what he chooses ... The Secretary of State chooses the rents. The Secretary of State chooses the subsidies ... I regard it as deeply unhealthy ... [to] pass a Bill which enables one Minister to behave in that way' (*Hansard* 1980b).

In practice the subsequent determinations of the Secretary of State meant that in each year rent income was assumed to be increasing at a faster rate than HRA expenditure. Hence, the subsidy entitlement of the great majority of authorities fell, year on year. It is important to stress that local authorities did not have to follow the Secretary of State's assumptions about the annual increase in rents and costs which made up their subsidy entitlement. To that extent, housing authorities retained their freedom to set rents and to run their financial arrangements as they saw fit. However, given the requirement to balance the HRA, local authorities failing to follow the direction indicated by the assumed increases in rents and costs found themselves with only four real options. They could reduce their housing expenditure, increase their rents, realize more housing assets through council house sales (thus lowering outstanding debt or increasing the interest received, as income to the HRA, from capital receipts) or draw upon local tax funds.

In, respectively, reducing public expenditure, raising average rents and encouraging the privatization of the stock, the first three of these options were in complete accord with government policy. The fourth was an option which was became increasingly expensive for many local authorities during the 1980s because of the operation of the broader local authority funding mechanisms (see Bailey 1985 for a contemporary discussion). Consequently, in the early years of the Act's currency at least, the subsidy system enabled central government to determine to a large extent the housing operations of local government.

With subsidy entitlements in general falling year by year, the percentage of income accruing to the combined HRA of English and Welsh authorities from the exchequer fell from 31 per cent in 1980/1 to 5 per cent in 1988/9. In contrast, the amount received in income from HB in the combined account over the same period rose from 8 per cent to 33 per cent. These last two outcomes show very clearly that the key change in the 1980s was not so much the reintroduction of 1972-style deficit subsidies *per se*, but rather the quite dramatic change from producer subsidies to council housing to a system of personal subsidies for council tenants. The HB system was increasingly bearing the costs of the higher rents set for those remaining in the public sector.

However, as has been discussed elsewhere (for example, Walker and Marsh 1997), the declining subsidy received by local authorities posed a problem of control for central government. By the end of the 1980s the great majority of authorities outside London had zero exchequer subsidy entitlements. Thus, there was much less need for such authorities to follow government assumptions concerning housing income and expenditure upon which the subsidy calculation was based. This freedom was, of necessity, constrained by the difficulty authorities faced in attempting to manage their financial operations in the absence of general subsidy. Nevertheless, central government had much less leverage over their revenue-related activities, and in particular the rents set, than previously. Further, it was possible for some authorities to be in notional deficit and so receive subsidy but to be in actual surplus. Malpass (1990: 157), for example, estimates that around one third of authorities receiving subsidy were in this position in 1988/9. Such surpluses could be used to keep down rent increases or, of greater concern to the government, transferred to the local tax fund. Even where authorities were not in receipt of exchequer subsidy, but were receiving income through their tenants' HB entitlements, it was possible for them to generate a surplus on the HRA and to use it in this way. This became one of the arguments used to justify a change in the subsidy system in the 1989 Local Government and Housing Act.

Reasserting control: the 1989 Local Government and Housing Act

The provisions of the 1989 Act have been discussed by a number of writers (e.g. Gibb and Munro 1991, ch. 4; Hills 1992, ch. 7) and have been summarized by Walker and Marsh (1995: 3–4). For our purposes, the main features of the legislation can be briefly described as follows.

First, the Act 'ring fenced' the HRA by effectively proscribing transfers to the account from local tax funds and from the account to those funds. Second, 'guideline' rent increases were to be announced annually for each authority, these increases being targeted according to the capital values of an authority's dwellings as indicated by the pre-discount prices of dwellings sold under the Right To Buy. The total rent income which would be generated within an authority by increasing rents in this manner compared with that authority's expenditure as assumed by central government determined the notional deficit or surplus on the authority's HRA. Third, the exchequer subsidy implied as a result of this calculation, whether positive or negative, was added to the authority's actual HB entitlement to form the new, combined HRA subsidy. Finally, under section 162 of the Act, the rent income generated by an authority was to distributed across different dwellings in an authority's stock through rent relativities reflecting the relativities in the private sector. We now consider the implications of these provisions in turn.

First, the ring-fencing of the HRA ended an arrangement which had existed for 70 years, an arrangement which, as we suggested earlier, had been seen as a reflection both of local taxpayers' legitimate interest in public housing, and of the significance of such housing to the wider community. Henceforth the direct financial involvement of such taxpayers was limited by statute to assistance with a portion of the welfare payments to tenants in receipt of HB. As important, ring-fencing removed a potentially important source of financial choice and flexibility from local decision makers.

Second, the guideline increases, in being based on capital values, represented a return to a market basis for the calculation of rents. The use of capital values rather than the rents actually prevailing in the private sector, however, represented a departure from the precedents set for market-related pricing under the Acts of 1919, 1924 and 1972. Indeed, it can be seen as achieving a more rational basis for rents, in the sense that they would more clearly reflect the value of dwellings than would those rents set in a quantitatively small and distorted private market, an argument which we have considered and developed further elsewhere (Walker and Marsh 1998). By 1995/6 regional variations in average rents reflected much more closely regional variations in capital values than had been the case six years earlier (Walker and Marsh 1995: 4).

Third, the combination of the previously separately calculated HB and exchequer subsidies into one subsidy had two major effects. First, it brought all housing authorities back into the subsidy calculation since all authorities had at least some tenants entitled to HB. Second, it effectively transferred any notional surplus on an authority's HRA back to the exchequer in order to (part) fund that authority's HB subsidy. Tenants receiving HB would still pay the reduced or zero rent to which the HB system entitled them but the authority itself would only receive from the government in return an amount net of the assessed HRA surplus.

The distributional effects of this combined subsidy arrangement in many ways echo those of the 1972 Act in that, as we noted, the 'return' of surpluses to the government gives rise to a series of complex cross-subsidy effects. However, in this case, the cross-subsidy is more explicit than under the 1972 Act. An authority faced with a shortfall in its HB subsidy still has to balance its account. Given ring-fencing, the alternatives with which it is faced are now either to reduce expenditure or to increase income, but the main source for the latter is an increase in rents. Tenants in receipt of HB are protected against such an increase so the increased rents are paid only by those not receiving HB. Consequently, tenants paying full rent can be argued to be part funding, through higher rent payments, the entitlements of those tenants who are in receipt of HB. A further stimulus to higher rents, and thus on tenants' choices, was given by the ability of authorities to spend on capital projects any actual surplus accruing to the HRA, these projects consisting mainly of major repair and improvement programmes. If an authority was unable to invest in such programmes due to the constraints on borrowing imposed by central government, generating extra revenue from rents became an attractive alternative.

The overall impact of the subsidy system depended on the assumptions built into it, particularly in respect of the guideline rent increases that were to be set. In practice, by 1995/6 Metropolitan and Shire districts, and Outer London borough's were each, in aggregate, deemed to be in notional surplus (Walker and Marsh 1997) so that, taken as a whole, central government was no longer providing general, as opposed to tenant-specific support to council housing (Wilcox 1995). The transformation of housing subsidies in the public sector had, in this sense, been achieved. Further, the guideline increases as set not only drew the majority of authorities into assessed surplus but also encouraged a rapid increase in actual average rents from £21.00 per week in 1989/90 to £38.30 per week in 1995/6, the latter being some £4.50 per week above the rent that would have been set had authorities simply followed government guideline increases (Walker and Marsh 1995: 4). Local authorities, thus, felt the need to increase rents at a faster rate than that implied by the guidelines, partly reflecting the use of surplus revenue for major capital and investment projects, as noted above.

The fourth provision of the 1989 Act concerns the requirement for authorities '... to have regard in particular to the principle' (Local Government and Housing Act 1989: s162, (3)) that the rent relativities they set should be set in the light of relativities in the private sector. This is particularly interesting in the context of our discussion here. As we have discussed elsewhere, there are problems with this approach both in principle (Walker and Marsh 1998) and practice (Walker and Marsh 1997). Briefly, there is no reason to believe that the pattern of relativities in the private sector at present, which local authorities are required to 'mirror', reflects an efficient pattern of rents, especially when many landlords in the private sector are not primarily motivated by considerations of profitability (Crook *et al.* 1995: 11 *et seq.*) and many cater for tenants receiving housing benefit. Even if the rents set in the private sector did reflect efficient market outcomes, the legislation itself arguably confuses the issue by defining private sector rents as those '... rents that would be recoverable if they were let ... by *a person other than the authority*' (Local Government and Housing Act 1989: s162 (4), italics added), a definition which thus incorporates not only providers in the private sector *per se* but also NFP providers such as housing associations.

The rationale for restricting local authorities' freedom in rent setting in this manner was to '... encourage a more efficient use of council housing through price signals to tenants ... thereby ensuring that the social rented sector is used as efficiently as possible' (DoE 1996: para. 8.4). This presumably refers to a belief that even if tenants continue to gain access to sector on the basis of some concept of need, they should be encouraged to adjust their choice and consumption of housing within the sector in the light of market-determined relativities. However, even if such households wished to adjust their housing consumption in the light of new relativities set, it is unclear that they would be able to do so. Transfers and, particularly, exchanges within the existing – and shrinking – public sector stock are difficult and time consuming to organize, often relying on a straight swop between households or a large number of empty properties to be successful. Even if the likely effects of HB on blunting rent-based incentives to relocate are ignored, there is still no guarantee that larger households will relocate to larger properties, if that is what is meant by greater efficiency. All the policy would achieve at best is to ensure that those households able to afford the higher relative rents on larger properties would occupy them, whether the households themselves were large or small.

In considering the 1989 Act overall which, it will be recalled, was introduced primarily because central government had lost control over significant aspects of local authorities' housing operations, it can be concluded that it went a long way to restoring the government's power over councils' financial operations in this field. This had been achieved while not, explicitly at least, abandoning the principle that authorities should continue to enjoy a reasonable amount of autonomy in the respect of the manner in which they manage these financial operations.

The return of producer subsidies? Indications of policy change

From the point of view of central government policy more generally this reliance on tenant-specific subsidies posed serious problems. Notwithstanding the increasingly significant contribution to meeting the HB bill that tenants themselves were making, the size of the annual guideline and actual rent increases succeeded in increasing the number of tenants entitled to HB and increasing the size of the entitlements that existing HB recipients could claim. As a result, almost 70 per cent of council tenants were claiming HB in the early 1990s and, nationally, HB became the fastest growing element in the social security budget. Clearly this was likely to create serious tensions between the departments of state at national government level.

On the one hand, the Department of the Environment (DoE) was pursuing a policy of affecting tenants' choices through higher rents and protecting those deemed to be less well off through personal subsidies. On the other hand, the Department of Social Security, and ultimately the Treasury, were faced with paying a large proportion of the costs of those personal subsidies. The way in which these tensions were resolved appears to have been in favour of the latter departments. In November 1994 the DoE announced that council rents had reached 'realistic' levels and that future increases in guideline rents would become progressively smaller. The White Paper published in the following year specified that these increases would be part of a '... move towards rent increases broadly in line with inflation' (DoE 1995: 27). Perhaps more dramatically, the White Paper also put forward a favourable case for general rather than personal subsidies or at least for a better '... balance between helping all tenants through keeping their rents down, and helping individuals through housing benefits' (DoE 1995: 26).

While acknowledging the past benefits of targeting those in need and of possible public expenditure savings that the switch to personal subsidies had achieved, the White Paper identifies two main arguments in favour of a general subsidy to keep down rents: first, a general subsidy can be cheaper over time than paying HB on market rents; second, such a subsidy improves work incentives compared to an HB system which reduces entitlement as income rises. As a result of improved work incentives a general subsidy can reduce benefit dependency more generally (DoE 1995: 26). A recognition of these arguments has meant that issues of pricing social housing have come to be linked closely with debates about citizenship and social exclusion, as discussed in more detail in Chapter 3.

Conclusion

Thus, after 17 years of a housing policy characterized by an increasing reliance on affecting tenants' choices and housing consumption through higher, more market-like pricing, the emphasis may be changing once more. The costs generated by the potential disincentive to work brought about by personal subsidies necessitated by a high rent policy are believed to be outweighing any benefits that those higher rents were intended to achieve. In a situation where over two thirds of tenants are HB claimants and are thus protected from rent increases, a high-rent policy simply draws progressively more tenants into HB, deepens the dependency of existing claimants and correspondingly reduces the numbers of tenants whose choices are likely to be directly affected by those high rents. In a sector where the options in respect of housing consumption which are open to many tenants are increasingly so constrained as to render the idea of freedom of choice virtually meaningless, the government's own options in terms of the form of the appropriate subsidy system are themselves constrained. Certainly, the recent history of local authority housing finance would suggest that higher rents and personal subsidies may help to encourage residualization, but, when residualization has occurred, to continue with such a policy is both costly and inefficient.

References

Bailey, S. (1985) The relationship between cities' housing rents and block grant. *Urban Studies*, 22: 237–48.

Cole, I. and Furbey, R. (1994) *The Eclipse of Council Housing*. London: Routledge.

Crook, A.D.H., Hughes, J. and Kemp, P. (1995) *The Supply of Privately Rented Homes: Today and Tomorrow*. York: Joseph Rowntree Foundation.

Daunton, M.J. (ed.) (1984) *Councillors and Tenants: Local Authority Housing in English Cities, 1919–1939*. Leicester: Leicester University Press.

DoE (1995) *Our Future Homes: Opportunity, Choice, Responsibility*, Cm. 2901. London: HMSO.

DoE (1996) *Housing Revenue Manual*, amendment 3. London: HMSO.

Dresser, M. (1984) Housing policy in Bristol, 1919–30, in M.J. Daunton (ed.) *Councillors and Tenants: Local Authority Housing in English Cities, 1919–1939*. Leicester: Leicester University Press.

Finnigan, R. (1984) Council housing in Leeds, 1919–39: social policy and urban change, in M.J. Daunton (ed.) *Councillors and Tenants: Local Authority Housing in English Cities, 1919–1939*. Leicester: Leicester University Press.

Gibb, K. and Munro, M. (1991) *Housing Finance in the UK*. Basingstoke: Macmillan.

Hansard (1935) vol. 297, col. 376, 30 January.

Hansard (1949) vol. 462, col. 2126, 16 March.

Hansard (1971a) vol. 825, col. 668, 8 November.

Hansard (1971b) vol. 825, col. 671, 8 November.

Hansard (1980a) vol. 979, col. 1459, 21 February.

Hansard (1980b) vol. 979, col. 1475, 21 February.

Harloe, M. (1995) *The People's Home? Social Rented Housing in Europe and America*. Oxford: Basil Blackwell.

Hills, J. (1992) *Unravelling Housing Finance: Subsidies, Benefits and Taxation*. Oxford: Clarendon Paperbacks.

HMSO (1971) *Fair Deal for Housing*, Cmnd. 4728. London: HMSO.

HMSO (1989) *Local Government and Housing Act*, Chapter 24. London: HMSO.

Holmans, A.E. (1987) *Housing Policy in Britain: A History*. London: Croom Helm.

Maclennan, D. (1982) *Housing Economics: An Applied Approach*. London: Longman.

Malpass, P. (1990) *Reshaping Housing Policy: Subsidies, Rents and Residualisation*. London: Routledge.

Malpass, P. and Murie, A. (1994) *Housing Policy and Practice*, 4th edn. Basingstoke: Macmillan.

Merrett, S. (1979) *State Housing in Britain*. London: Routledge and Kegan Paul.

Ryder, R. (1984) Council house building in County Durham, 1900–39: the local implementation of national policy, in M.J. Daunton (ed.) *Councillors and Tenants: Local Authority Housing in English Cities, 1919–1939*. Leicester: Leicester University Press.

Walker, B. and Marsh, A. (1995) *Rent Setting Policies in English Local Authorities*. London: HMSO.

Walker, B. and Marsh, A. (1997) Rent setting in local government. *Local Government Policy Making*, 23: 39–46.

Walker, B. and Marsh, A. (1998) Pricing public housing services in the UK: mirroring the market? *Housing Studies*, 13: 549–66.

Walker, B., Marsh, A. and Dixon, A. (1991) *Housing Finance and Subsidy in Birmingham*. York: Joseph Rowntree Foundation.

Wilcox, S. (1995) *Housing Finance Review, 1995/96*. York: Joseph Rowntree Foundation.

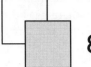

8

A prize of citizenship? Changing access to social housing

David Mullins and Pat Niner

Introduction

This chapter begins by introducing the relationship between citizenship, control and choice and the provision of and access to social housing. It continues by exploring these concepts in relation to two case studies of recent change in policy on access to social housing. The first case study traces the development of homelessness policy over the 20 years since the introduction of the Housing (Homeless Persons) Act in 1977. The second looks at the more recent development of common housing registers as a single access point for housing provided by a number of different social landlords in a locality. A concluding discussion highlights the general dominance of control issues at both central and local levels over access to housing, and this is in turn related to the general scarcity of supply which has emerged as a result of housing's position as the 'wobbly pillar under the welfare state' (Torgerson 1987: 116). The chapter ends by considering the issues arising from the increasingly differentiated nature of the social housing stock, some of which can no longer be considered as a 'prize of citizenship'.

Citizenship and access to social housing

The relationship between citizenship rights and access to social housing has often been a difficult one. There is little disagreement concerning the importance of housing as a basic need (Maslow 1954) and shelter as a human right (United Nations Declaration of Human Rights), or the desirability of avoiding a link between bad housing and poverty. However, there has been less widespread support for state intervention in the production and distribution of housing to achieve the goal of adequate housing for all citizens. In many advanced capitalist societies housing provision has never been fully legitimised as part of the welfare state; see Chapter 6 for a fuller discussion. Torgerson (1987) has argued that, because provision of housing as a commodity and a system of private property rights have usually been a core element of capitalist societies, state intervention in housing is often seen as running against the grain and is therefore open to attack. State assistance with housing can therefore be described as a 'wobbly pillar under the welfare state'. This has led to the 'crowding out' of welfare housing except in times and for groups when market provision proved impossible (Harloe 1995). This residual role has meant that the issue of who should have access to limited state assistance has been a recurrent theme in housing debates.

In Britain, there was a relatively brief universalist period between the Second World War and the 1970s when social housing became a mass tenure which accounted for around a third of all households in 1979. However, this was preceded and succeeded by periods in which access was more socially selective. In the 1920s 'public housing emerged as a tenure serving mainly the rather better off workers and tending to exclude the least well off' (Malpass and Murie 1994: 46). However, in the 1930s the focus switched to slum clearance and more attention was given to affordability issues. After the war there were further periods of general needs provision (1945–53) and slum clearance (1955–64) followed by a period of more dramatic expansion in the late 1960s when public housing was at its most universal. A reminder of the position of social housing in this period is Murie's finding that in 1980 16 per cent of households in the top income decline were local authority tenants (Murie 1996).

The residualization of the social housing sector since 1979 has been well documented (Malpass 1990). Needs-based allocations policies have combined with the expansion of alternative housing options to confine new entrants to the sector to a much narrower range of social groups than in earlier periods (Page 1993; Lee *et al.* 1995). One consequence of this narrower social base has been the tendency of some critics to see social housing as part of a process of exclusion from rather than enjoyment of citizenship rights. For example Bulmer and Rees (1996: 277) refer to 'heavily stigmatised council estates, where only a few of the male inhabitants are in full time work'. They go on to refer to such estates as places where an 'underclass distinguished by its detachment from traditional working class norms may most easily be sought and perhaps found'. However, more considered analyses have revealed a complex relationship between housing tenure and social exclusion, with some of the most disadvantaged areas being of mixed tenure (Lee and Murie 1997); see Chapter 3 for a fuller discussion.

These historical changes in the role of social housing and the profile of tenants indicate the importance of broader public policy changes in shaping the context for access and allocation policies. Smith and Mallinson (1997) have provided further elaboration on this theme by linking macro-level debates about the role of social housing with micro-level issues of discretion and allocation. They argue that most attention has been given in recent years to challenges to the concept of a social housing sector using bureaucratic mechanisms to allocate housing according to need. Extensive research on access to public housing, particularly in relation to race and gender, has indicated a failure to achieve redistributive aims. Meanwhile, challenges from the new right drawing on public choice theories have sought to replace bureaucratic distribution with more market-based mechanisms. Smith and Mallinson contend that more attention should now be given to internal reform of distribution mechanisms within the social housing sector. They return to a long-established theme in studies of access to housing – the role of discretion – using a case study of the assessment of housing and health needs. They conclude that discretion is not so much the problem that rule-based approaches to allocations suggest but rather an operational requirement which may allow bureaucratic insensitivity to be overcome.

Control and access to social housing

This focus on discretion should sensitize us to the power relations involved in access to social housing. Rather than the notion of rights it is the notion of control of access (rationing) which has been in the forefront throughout most of the history of social housing provision in Britain particularly in relation to homelessness (Lidstone 1994). Debates about allocation policies usually appear to be concerned with bureaucratic or professional definitions of need and how these are operationalized (the use of, for example, merit, date order, points schemes, medical assessments). The issue of racial discrimination in access to housing has been well researched, illustrating the impact of these approaches. Formal investigations carried out by the Commission for Racial Equality (CRE) in the early 1980s highlighted the way in which rules and procedures (such as residential qualifications, transfer policies and medical assessment systems) may have a direct or indirect discriminatory effect on housing outcomes (CRE 1984). Henderson and Karn (1984) set these rules and procedures in a wider context illustrating the way in which both formal rules and discretionary decisions were informed by taken for granted moral beliefs. Phillips (1986) demonstrated the importance of organizational constraints operating on housing allocators which mean that as well as meeting housing needs they are faced with the need to reduce the number of empty properties and maximize the chance of offers being accepted. Occasionally these debates have been punctuated by more overt political contests about citizenship rights and responsibilities: for example in the debates around the 1977 Housing (Homeless Persons) Act and parts VI and VII of the 1996 Housing Act which are discussed later in this chapter. Through these episodes we can observe a continuing struggle between competing definitions of citizenship rights and duties, and systems of control or rationing of social housing.

Access to social housing can be seen as a series of control processes. Table 8.1 illustrates how control is exerted at various stages to determine who gets what, where and when. Legislation, regulation, eligibility, prioritization, selection and offer policies all exemplify a rationing approach with control

Table 8.1   Factors controlling access to social housing

Legislation	Basic framework set by central government, e.g. extension of rights through Housing (Homeless Persons) Act 1977, reasonable preference categories for allocations schemes, and exclusion of asylum seekers without 'recourse to public funds' in Asylum and Immigration Appeals Act 1993.
Regulation	Secretary of State, Housing Corporation etc. may set further regulations, e.g. determinations on access to statutory housing registers (under Part VI of Housing Act 1996), performance standards for Registered Social Landlords on access to housing etc., and advice, e.g. *Homelessness Code of Guidance*.
Eligibility	Local policies may further restrict eligibility, e.g. through residence qualifications, age limits, restrictions on housing owner-occupiers etc.
Prioritization	Landlords may use variety of points schemes, group schemes, date order systems etc. to prioritize applications.
Selection	Allocations systems are usually property-led. Discretion important in finding suitable applicant from prioritization systems for given property. Factors other than need e.g. minimizing period property is empty, considering social balance of estate, may play a role at this stage.
Limited offer policies	Applicants' choice may be further restricted by limits to the number of offers they are entitled to in a given period and the way in which offers are made (usually preventing direct choices between alternatives).
Nature of housing stock	Geographical distribution, size, age and type of property play an important part in access processes. Different procedures may be applied to 'difficult to let' properties.
Applicant choices	Differential bargaining power and knowledge used to exploit available choices between areas, landlords, property types etc.

by providers, professionals and the state. The degree of discretion available to local 'gatekeepers' is clearly constrained by the national legislative and regulatory framework. It is also influenced by local factors including the strength of the local economy and housing market and the resulting role played by social housing. Very different considerations apply in gatekeeping access to 'difficult to let housing' than to housing in short supply in relation to need or demand. Considerable variations in local geographies of social housing can result.

Two important dimensions of control are discussed in the examples of access routes into social housing explored in the remainder of this chapter. The first is the interplay between central and local policies in determining outcomes for individuals. The second is the impact of changing power relations at the local level, for example between different providers of social housing and between professional and political stakeholders.

Choice and access to social housing

Having briefly introduced the connections between citizenship and control and access to housing we now consider the role played by choice. Given the dominance of the rationing approaches described above it is perhaps surprising how often the concept of choice is introduced into discussions of access to housing. However, Jeffers and Hoggett (1995) have indicated the role of differential choice and bargaining behaviour by applicants in influencing outcomes. For example, the greater ability of some transfer applicants to wait for an offer they are prepared to accept has long been recognized as a factor affecting the quality of housing received (Maclennan and Kay 1994).

Nevertheless, the way in which choice has been considered in access policies has usually been firmly embedded in a culture of rationing. The most common use of choice is in relation to area choices presented to housing applicants either on initial application to a housing authority or at interview stage. Typically, applicants are invited to select from a list of areas and to prioritize those areas in which they are prepared to accept offers. Housing officers present varying levels of information on the implications of choosing different areas to applicants, but applicants are often encouraged to 'widen their areas of choice' to increase the chances of an early offer. Problems often arise because there is a lack of correspondence between the area codes used by landlords and applicants' own mental maps of the areas that they would choose to live in. Thus while applicants may be asked to express choices at one stage in the process, they usually have little control over how this information is collected or used to influence their rehousing chances. Moreover, factors beyond the immediate control of the landlord such as area characteristics and reputations, and the historical legacy of the housing stock may be even more important than landlord control in mediating the choices expressed by applicants.

Other sorts of choices may sometimes be available to applicants. There may be some choice between different social landlords operating in an area; a choice which has recently widened considerably in theory as a result of quasi-market approaches to funding new social housing. Later in this chapter we examine the extent to which common housing registers have enabled or prevented applicants from making such choices. There may be a choice of occupying dwellings at lower densities than traditional allocation policies would allow (to reduce child densities and allow households to grow). Other examples include the recent involvement of tenants and local managers in local allocation policies (Griffiths *et al.* 1996), and the more long-standing operation of 'sons and daughters policies', both of which seek to avoid the effect of needs-based allocations in breaking up communities. Choice may sometimes play a more significant role in supported and sheltered housing lets, particularly where housing forms part of a 'care package' tailored to an individual's needs (Riseborough *et al.* 1996). However, there are few parallels in the British context to the reported move by Dutch social landlords 'from waiting lists to adverts' (Kullberg 1997) whereby lettings in the non-profit sector are allocated by advertising vacancies in local newspapers and then shortlisting applicants interested in particular properties. The use of more market-based mechanisms of this nature would represent a significant departure from the rationing-based approaches which have continued to dominate in Britain, and produce new trade-offs between fairness and choice.

The purpose of this chapter is to explore the differing perspectives on access to social housing offered by the notions of citizenship, choice and control by taking two examples of policy developments evaluated in research studies carried out by the Centre for Urban and Regional Studies (CURS) at the University of Birmingham. The first example is the development of homelessness policy from the 1977 legislation through to the review of 1996 Act provisions by the incoming Labour government in 1997. Research undertaken over an extended period provides an opportunity to trace the relationship between the implementation of basic citizenship rights and the impact of control mechanisms at central and local levels in the enforcement and abatement of these rights (Niner 1989; Mullins *et al.* 1996; Niner *et al.* 1997). The second example is the more recent development of common housing registers in a number of localities. Such registers act as a single access route to most social landlords with properties in the locality and have often been presented as an enhancement of user choice. An evaluation of some early examples of these schemes provided an opportunity to explore the balance between control and choice in the impact of these partnerships on access to housing (Mullins 1996; Mullins and Niner 1996).

Homelessness case study

Prior to 1977 local authorities, when allocating council houses, had a general duty to give reasonable preference to people who were occupying insanitary or overcrowded housing, had large families or were living under unsatisfactory housing conditions. These general criteria were widely reflected in the definitions of 'need' adopted by authorities for accepting applicants onto their waiting list and/or prioritizing eligible applicants through points schemes or targets. During the 1960s and early 1970s, large numbers of new council tenants entered the sector as a result of slum clearance – between 1965 and 1967 slum clearance rehousing represented 30 per cent or more of total households rehoused in 43 per cent of local authorities in unpublished research commissioned by Central Housing Advisory Committee (Cullingworth Report 1969).

Within this quite loose legislative framework local authorities had enormous amounts of discretion in the way they selected tenants. They had discretion in, for example, who was eligible, how priorities were determined, how a particular applicant was matched to a particular vacancy, the extent of applicant preference allowed, and how the whole system should be administered.

Some of the then current professional concerns about the discretionary operation of allocation processes can be seen from a 1978 report of the Housing Services Advisory Group (HSAG 1978). Having noted the changing context, including generally reducing pressure on the housing stock in many areas, the report spent some time discussing the impact of residential qualifications and other blanket exclusions based for example on age, marital status, tenure or income. These restrictions had been applied in line with notions of rationing scarce resources to meet the greatest needs; however, they had been found to have unintended consequences. These included restrictions on mobility opportunities for the 'adequately housed', the exclusion of certain needs, for example of older owner-occupiers unable to adapt their present homes to meet their needs, and indirectly discriminatory effects on ethnic minorities. Interestingly the report devoted two pages to maximizing consumer choice in allocation policies. Growing quality differences in the stock to be allocated were clearly recognized and a chapter was devoted to 'less desired property'. Part of the solution to the latter problem was seen as removing barriers to eligibility, catering for mobile people and groups such as single people who 'currently have little chance of obtaining council housing' (HSAG 1978: 71). Thus, professional thinking at that time seemed oriented towards offering access to council housing to a wider range of citizens, and offering consumers more choice. A cynical interpretation of the relaxation of control urged by the Advisory Group would refer to the need to avoid vacancies against a background where 'local authorities cannot assume that they can fill whatever they build' (HSAG 1978: 70).

Such issues have loomed even larger for landlords in the late 1990s as demand for social housing has plummeted in some unpopular areas.

Homelessness legislation

The Housing (Homeless Persons) Act 1977 came into effect in England and Wales in December of that year. The Act transferred responsibility for dealing with homeless people from welfare authorities (under the National Assistance Act 1948) to housing authorities. As well as interim temporary accommodation, as required by the 1948 Act, authorities were to secure 'permanent' accommodation for those to whom a full duty was owed. The link with council allocation policies was achieved by adding a further reasonable preference category, namely people to whom the authority owed a homelessness duty, including non-priority homeless people and those found to be intentionally homeless. The legislation was consolidated into Part III of the Housing Act 1985, with slight amendment to counter the effects of a House of Lords decision (the Pulhofer case) in the Housing and Planning Act 1986. Up to the introduction of the 1996 Housing Act, homelessness duties were generally referred to as Part III duties.

The homelessness legislation could be (and was) seen very differently by different parties. On the one hand the Act seemed to represent a significant new citizenship 'right' for those in the greatest housing need of all. At the same time it could be viewed as an unwarranted encroachment on local authority discretion to allocate their housing in line with local priorities, and as a 'queue jumpers' charter' for gaining priority over others on the waiting list. None of these viewpoints actually stand when examined more closely.

The homelessness legislation, while undoubtedly an advance over what went before, was never intended to confer universal rights to assistance. Eligibility for rehousing depended on proven homelessness and priority need, and the homelessness had to be 'unintentional'. In particular the priority need categories – broadly the presence in the household of dependent children, a pregnant woman, or someone vulnerable 'as a result of old age, mental illness or handicap or physical disability or other special reason' – excluded many single people and childless couples. This was directly reflected in the characteristics of homeless people rehoused. For example, in 1991 74 per cent of new tenants who had previously been statutorily homeless comprised families with children compared with 35 per cent of new tenants not previously homeless (Prescott-Clarke *et al.* 1994: 90). The intentionality clause, introduced at the behest of local authorities to reduce the risk of abuse, may have had a deterrent effect. However, its direct impact in terms of rejected applications was relatively modest – only 3.7 per cent of all accepted homeless households in England in 1995 were found to be intentionally homeless (Wilcox 1996, Table 83). The Act also did not confer any right to housing in a local authority of choice. The 'local connection' elements meant that an applicant with no local connection with the authority they applied to but with a connection with another could be referred to that authority for rehousing, unless there was a danger of domestic violence there. Again this was a measure introduced at the behest of local authorities fearing an influx of outsiders with no 'legitimate' call on local resources.

The extent of case law developed on all aspects of the legislation, and especially on intentionality, stands as witness to the challenges to local authorities' interpretations of their duties that have been made by aggrieved applicants. The implementation of homelessness legislation by local housing authorities was found to vary on just about every aspect. For example, in the circumstances in which an applicant would be considered homeless, in definitions of vulnerability, in the extent and form of temporary accommodation used, and in the type of permanent accommodation secured and the number and types of offers considered reasonable to discharge duty. Approaches to intentionality proved especially variable: some authorities looked only for the most blatant instances while others geared lengthy investigations to charting and substantiating all of an applicant's housing actions over several years to identify potential intentional homelessness (Evans and Duncan 1988; Audit Commission 1989; Niner 1989). Political control and pressure of homelessness were found to interact through the exercise of discretion to influence the relative 'liberality' of a particular authority's stance (Niner 1989: 16).

Reducing local service variability and securing fair, consistent and good practice among housing authorities was a prime objective of the third edition of the *Homelessness Code of Guidance* issued by the Department of the Environment (DoE) in 1991. Guidance was more comprehensive than offered by earlier editions of the code, and more stress was placed on service quality reflecting a contemporary public policy agenda emphasizing customer care, quality and performance. While not having the force of law, authorities had to take account of the code as a material consideration when reaching Part III decisions. Research evaluating the impact of the 1991 code (Mullins *et al.* 1996) concluded that homelessness practices were better and fairer in the early and mid-1990s than they had been in the late 1980s. Most authorities had reviewed policies and practices in the light of the code, and the revised code had stimulated changes across all aspects of homelessness practice. Not all observed improvements could, however, be attributed to the code directly. Besides reinforcing trends towards better service quality, the issue of the code and the evaluative research coincided with an increase in housing association completions which had eased the housing supply position in many authorities. Yet despite generally more consistent service, significant variations were still found to exist between authorities in most aspects of homelessness policies and practices. The evaluation noted that because of differences in geography, political control and local housing markets a totally consistent homelessness service might be a chimera.

The extent to which Part III provided a fast track to council housing is also not entirely clear. In some authorities, especially in the south of England, almost all family-sized accommodation was allocated to homeless households rather than to waiting list applicants. Elsewhere, the proportion could be much lower. A number of issues are relevant.

As we have seen, local authorities had a duty to secure accommodation for priority households accepted as unintentionally homeless. This duty was usually discharged by an offer of council housing (Mullins *et al.* 1996). Unintentionally homeless households (and other non-priority homeless and intentionally homeless people) comprised one category to be given reasonable preference in allocating council housing. The extent of preference thought reasonable seems to have related partly to perceptions of homelessness as a legitimate form of extreme housing need to be given priority. It also related to the authority's desire to limit the amount and cost of temporary accommodation to be provided under the homelessness legislation. Depending on housing supply, the latter consideration could in practice mean either the almost total avoidance of any use of temporary accommodation or most homeless people passing through temporary accommodation and staying for significant periods. Mullins *et al.* (1996: 69) found that in just over one authority in ten average stays in temporary accommodation were over a year, while in 14 per cent of authorities the average stay was less than a month. Both perceptions of need and temporary accommodation considerations may underlie the normal absence of explicit priority given to non-priority or intentionally homeless households in allocation schemes.

Authorities differed in the way in which they incorporated homeless people within the total allocations system. Some gave outright priority, either by treating accepted homeless people as a special priority group to be considered for any vacancy before those on the general waiting list, or by awarding them a points score sufficient to bring them to the top of the list. Mullins *et al.* (1996: 97) found that about two thirds of authorities gave outright priority in this way. The remainder used some method of balancing relative needs, perhaps by setting targets or quotas for allocations to different groups. In some cases such targets were designed to ensure that homeless people waited about as long as someone on the waiting list for an offer.

Research has, however, shown that in many authorities if priority was given to the homeless in terms of the speed with which they received an offer then it was at the expense of the extent of applicant choice allowed and the quality of offer. For example, single offer policies were common for homeless people (in 84 per cent of authorities) and fewer offers were made to homeless households than to other applicants in two thirds of authorities (Mullins *et al.* 1996: 94). Homeless people could often express fewer area preferences than other applicants, and this lack of choice could result in the allocation of homeless people to estates where they did not want to live and had no local contacts or support. This has been identified as a factor leading to the development of social segregation and difficult-to-let council estates (e.g. Griffiths *et al.* 1996). Where the homeless include large numbers of ethnic minority households, the same process has been seen to contribute to the concentration of tenants from minority ethnic backgrounds on unpopular estates (CRE 1988).

It is apparent that while homelessness legislation may have provided a partial 'right' to housing, it by no means removed local authority control of allocation processes and it failed to offer much choice to the households affected. At best it changed the rules by which scarce resources (attractive council houses) were rationed.

Legislative change

This section deals primarily with the Housing Act 1996 which significantly changed the law relating to access to council housing and duties owed to homeless people. First, however, we examine three earlier events which affected the rights of homeless people.

A review of homelessness legislation was carried out by the government in the late 1980s (DoE 1989). The premise for the review was that the homelessness net was spread too widely and should perhaps only cover the roofless, and that homeless people were getting unfair priority at the expense of other claimants for council housing. However, the review essentially confirmed the status quo in terms of definitions of homelessness and priority need and left the legislation unchanged. Other recommendations included the development of the revised *Code of Guidance* referred to above, and an enhanced advice service for homeless people (leading to the establishment of the National Homelessness Advisory Service linking regional Shelter Housing Advice Centres with local citizens advice bureaux). Thus, rather than narrowing the service as initially feared in some quarters, the review resulted in a wider service.

The second event reflected developments in immigration rather than housing legislation. The Asylum and Immigration Appeals Act 1993 qualified the homelessness duties of an authority towards asylum seekers and their dependants. This, and developing case law on an authority's responsibilities towards illegal immigrants, overstayers and overseas nationals with no recourse to public funds, was the subject of an addition made to the 1991 *Code of Guidance* in February 1994. Both made clear that assistance under homelessness legislation was to be more closely related in future to 'citizenship' in the form of nationality rights. This theme has been further extended by the Asylum and Immigration Act 1996 and the Housing Act 1996 with its prescription of qualifying persons (for the housing register) and ineligible persons (for homelessness duties). Broadly, persons from abroad and subject to immigration control will only be eligible for housing assistance if they fall into categories specified by the Secretary of State through regulation.

The third event was the 1995 House of Lords decision in the case of Awua (*R. v. London Borough of Brent ex parte Awua*) which had the effect of changing the commonly held interpretations of how an authority could discharge its rehousing duty under Part III. Up to the Awua judgement the general assumption, including that promoted by successive editions of the *Code of Guidance*, was that the accommodation secured for a homeless household should be settled or permanent in order to constitute a discharge of duty. The Awua decision held that such accommodation had to be 'suitable' but that this did not imply any requirement of permanence: an authority's duty could be discharged in as little as 28 days (Arden and Hunter 1996: 52–189). If authorities were so minded, this decision clearly reduced the value of any rights conferred by Part III almost to zero. However, before the impact of the Awua decision had filtered through into housing authority practice, consultation was already taking place which led to Parts VI and VII of the Housing Act 1996, and adjusted rights again.

A consultation paper published in January 1994 (DoE 1994) set out the government's proposals 'for ensuring fairer access to local authority and housing association tenancies' (para. 1.1). Not surprisingly, there were many different strands in the analysis of the existing situation which led to the conclusion that 'fairer access' was required and the subsequent translation to proposed policy change. The main argument was that the scale of rehousing through homelessness had proved to be much greater than ever envisaged when the legislation was introduced in 1977. Priority in allocations given to homeless people had confused the safety-net aspect of the legislation with a fast track to a council tenancy thereby distorting allocations. This was perceived as a problem because of the essential similarities between homeless and waiting list applicants, and the contention that homelessness, while undoubtedly evidence of a short-term crisis, does not necessarily represent evidence of long-term need for social rented housing. Social tenancies should be reserved for people whose 'overall housing needs are substantial and enduring' (DoE 1994: para. 1.1). Other aspects of fairness raised included meeting the needs of 'couples seeking to establish a good home in which to start and raise a family' (para. 3.1) and not penalizing someone who 'takes the initiative in finding alternative accommodation' (para. 2.7) rather than applying to an authority as homeless. The overall intentions of the reforms were to put 'all those with long term housing needs on the same footing, while providing a safety net for emergency and pressing needs' (DoE 1995: 37).

Parts VI and VII of the Housing Act 1996 enacted these proposals and must be seen together. Very broadly, Part VI required that all new lettings to council housing and local authority nominations to housing associations be made through a housing register which all local housing authorities had to maintain. Allocations to secure tenancies could not be made to anyone not on the register. Local authorities had discretion to set their own eligibility criteria for the register, subject to any groups specified by the Secretary of State as being, or not being, eligible. Priority between applicants on the register had to take account of certain 'reasonable preference' categories set out in section 167 of the Act; these did not include being owed a duty under homelessness legislation.

At the same time the 'full' duty towards homeless people was changed by section 193 of Part VII to a duty to provide accommodation for a period of two years (with discretion to continue to provide beyond this if the applicant continued to satisfy the various criteria). Local authority stock (other than hostel or leased accommodation) could not be used to meet this duty, even if let on a non-secure tenancy, for more than two years in any three year period. Housing association assured tenancies could similarly not be used to meet Part VII duties. Even this time-limited duty was avoidable where the local authority was satisfied that there was other suitable accommodation available in their area for an applicant. In these circumstances the duty under section 197 was to give such advice and assistance as was reasonably required to enable the applicant to secure that accommodation for him- or herself. Certain specified groups of persons from abroad and asylum seekers were precluded from any assistance under Part VII (broadly similar groups were also deemed to be disqualified from joining the housing register). Thus the concept of citizenship was here deployed as an exclusionary device to restrict access to rights.

Alongside these changes, two new duties/rights were introduced. Local authorities were to ensure the availability of a free homelessness advisory service aimed at preventing homelessness and providing information about alternatives. Meanwhile, homeless applicants had the right to seek a review of any adverse decision on their case with recourse to the county court on a point of law (previously the only legal redress was through judicial review).

Case study research carried out for Shelter in May/June 1997 on the early impacts of the legislation (Niner *et al.* 1997) allowed us to look again at issues of citizenship rights and local authority discretion in this new context. On the surface at least the rights of the homeless *vis-à-vis* other applicants for social housing were fundamentally changed by the Act in such a way as to remove any structured channel for 'fast track' access. However, the research showed that most authorities had tried with some ingenuity to devise their Part VI priority schemes so as to replicate as far as possible the pre-existing balance between 'homeless' and other applicants in allocations, using the new reasonable preference categories. This was partly driven by the need to keep control of the amount and cost of temporary (two year duty) accommodation needed, but there seems also to have been recognition that homeless people merit priority because of their needs. Despite initial fears of increased secretary of state prescription, the new legislation seemed in the event to have enlarged the scope for local authority discretion. Only one of the six case studies illustrated a major change for applicants – extensive use was being made of section 197 by providing encouragement and assistance (including a rent deposit and damage bond) for applicants to find their own accommodation in the private rented sector. Similar rent deposit schemes were used elsewhere but were thought of as securing two year duty accommodation under section 193.

In 1997 the newly-elected Labour government maintained its opposition to the 1996 Act provisions on homelessness. In November 1997, regulations were introduced to modify homelessness and access policies so that people owed a homelessness duty would again become a reasonable preference category for allocations and any accommodation used under section 197 must be available for at least two years. These provisions restored some of the homelessness rights removed in 1996, and further review was promised. This suggests that while the 1996 Act redefined the legal rights of citizens this had not been accompanied by a redefinition of what can be termed the moral rights of citizens. The legal position was therefore in conflict with the majority view on citizens' rights to housing. As a consequence a change in political control in 1997 resulted in a move back towards the previous interpretation of the legal rights of citizens, thereby reducing the dissonance between their legal and moral rights. In many respects this story is incomplete at the time of writing, and the lessons of the past would suggest that the impact of implementation may be very different to the stated intent of these latest changes.

Common Housing Register case study

The early 1990s saw the development of a number of local schemes to improve coordination of access to social housing. Variously known as common waiting lists (Rea 1993), local housing registers (NFHA 1994) and Common Housing Registers (Binns and Cannon 1996) these schemes adopted a variety of approaches. Nevertheless, all can be seen as responses to the fragmentation of provision of social housing. This had arisen as a result of the quasi-market approach to funding new social housing from the 1980s onwards, and in some areas from stock transfers of local authority housing to housing associations (see Chapter 6).

As a result of these public policy changes a typical local social housing supply may now be extremely fragmented. It may comprise local authority relets, new lettings by regional or national housing associations – some with little previous connection with the area – and relets and new lets of longer-established associations catering for a variety of needs groups (Mullins and Niner 1996). Taking the example of Bristol, Malpass (1997) identified 47 housing associations managing between them 7300 homes in the city, while the city council managed 35,500. The case for better coordination of access to this fragmented local supply is well made by the NFHA based on work in the same city: 'it is unreasonable to expect people in severe housing need to find their way onto the separate waiting lists of all the agencies active in their area when they need housing' (NFHA 1994: 2).

The main question to be addressed in our discussion of common housing registers is their impact of user choice and on patterns of control. We draw on a detailed evaluation undertaken for the Housing Corporation in the mid-1990s (Mullins and Niner 1996). After briefly describing the types of Common Housing Register found in the research we explore the relationship between these schemes and user choice, rationing, central/local control of housing policy and local governance of housing.

Types of Common Housing Register

Mullins and Niner (1996) use the term Common Housing Register (CHR) in a generic sense to refer to various forms of partnership between local authorities and housing associations to receive housing applications and register need using common administrative procedures. These partnerships usually establish a common database to record and process applications for housing, but this need not be computerized and it may be maintained by one agency on behalf of the partnership or by a number of partners using common procedures.

CHRs may develop into common allocations policies where partners also agree to apply common criteria to the assessment and prioritization of need. Housing associations have often favoured participation in common registers but opposed common allocations on the grounds that this reduces their independence. However, even within common allocations arrangements, partners may still apply their own policies to matters such as occupancy standards, bedroom category assessments and estate child densities. Thus, even in common allocations policies the forfeit of control need not be complete. There is therefore a continuum between common registration and common allocations, and it is possible to devise schemes which enable landlords to opt for higher or lower levels of common working. For example a Cornish authority has developed a system allowing the different eligibility policies of local landlords to be applied to a common database of applicants. This allows applicants who do not meet the local authority's requirements regarding residential connections to be considered by housing associations which, in line with Housing Corporation guidance, favour more open access policies.

In practice common registers may vary on a wide range of options. Mullins and Niner (1996) summarize these options in a typology using seven principal dimensions and many possible combinations of options

Table 8.2   Common Housing Registers: dimensions and options

Dimension	Options
Control	Who runs the register? Extent of partnership Governance structure Marketing image Costs and apportionment
Comprehensiveness	Extent of common arrangements Demand groups included Types of property included Inclusion of special needs Inclusion of private sector landlords
Information base	IT system IT access Communication method Monitoring arrangements
Application form	Common form? Standard data items? Single or multiple points of return? Responsibility for data entry?
Home visits	Timing Responsibility
Customer response	Types of information for customers Extent of customer choice Accessibility
Area characteristics	Social housing stock Number of social landlords Lettings Number of applicants registered

Source: Based on Mullins *et al.* 1996.

(see Table 8.2). Meanwhile, Binns and Cannon (1996) have proposed a framework in which potential partnerships can select from these options. Of the seven dimensions, the issue of control was considered to be the most important. In this context key questions of control include who runs and pays for the register, the extent of the partnership, its governance arrangements and its marketing image (Mullins and Niner 1996: 26–7).

Enhancing choice or restoring rationing?

CHRs are frequently discussed as a means of enhancing choice for housing applicants, particularly in publicity material produced by local partnerships. However, the CURS evaluation indicated that they rarely achieve this in practice; indeed they often have the effect of reducing the range of choice available to the determined consumer. The reason for this apparent paradox is that common registers do not change the overall level of housing supply and thus extension of access for some groups has the effect of reducing access for others. Our evaluation concluded that the main advantages of CHRs for customers were not choice but simplicity, convenience and potential access to a wider range of properties. However, these advantages do not flow automatically from establishing a register. For them to be realized there needed to be greater attention to providing information and enabling applicants to make best use of the registers.

Prior to the establishment of the CHR it may have been possible for applicants with quite low levels of housing need to secure accommodation through 'shopping around'. CHRs have reduced the choice of these applicants by opening up lesser-known sources of supply to a wider public. We concluded that the main impact had been to increase fairness by restoring rationing. Even where CHRs did not extend to common allocations arrangements, local authority and housing association interviewees felt that a major advantage of the scheme had been to make best use of the local housing stock to meet housing need. Such advantages apply most strongly in areas of housing shortage, and there may be fewer advantages to landlords in areas of housing surplus. This was confirmed in one of our case studies in an area with significant difficulty in letting social housing. The local authority had decided not to proceed with a CHR mainly because of a lack of demand for social renting in many parts of the city which led the authority to view housing associations as competitors for customers rather than 'partners in meeting housing need'.

Control of Common Housing Registers: central-local relations and local governance

The above evidence leads us to view CHRs more as a mechanism for control of access to social housing than a means of enhancing consumer choice. Two further aspects of control became apparent during the research: first with respect to central/local relations, second with respect to the local governance of housing.

The development of CHRs coincided with a period of policy review by central government. As discussed earlier one of the provisions included in the 1996 Housing Act was to require local authorities to allocate their own lettings and their nominations to housing associations from a single register regulated by the Secretary of State. Progress with local schemes to develop CHRs was undoubtedly slowed in the period between the 1994 Consultation Paper which first proposed creating single registers, and the legislation itself. There were two main reasons for this. First, pragmatically authorities wanted to avoid abortive work on schemes which may have to be recast to comply with any new statutory duties. Second, and more fundamentally, housing associations were reluctant to become involved in schemes which might limit their independence in making their own lets of properties not covered by nominations agreements. Thus attempts by housing associations to preserve their autonomy and control were an important factor in the relatively slow implementation of the concept of CHRs.

Another aspect of the control argument is revealed by examining the governance arrangements for CHRs. CHRs may be seen as an example of the emerging trend towards inter-organizational networks in the provision of local services (Reid 1995). Our research found that the early CHRs tended to be based on rather loose relationships of trust between staff in partner organizations. Governing bodies usually consisted of officers rather than committee members from partner organizations. These bodies became involved in decisions on systems for pointing and prioritization of applications, thus shifting the locus of control over key aspects of access to housing from partner organizations to the partnership. While one authority ran a shadow working party of councillors to ensure that members continued to have an input into access to housing policies, this was exceptional among the evaluation case studies. In our view this raises questions about the accountability and control of social housing resources (Mullins 1996). This may be seen as part of a wider shift from political to professional control, which is taking place across the terrain now occupied by local public spending bodies (Committee on Standards in Public Life 1996) as the new public management (Ferlie et al. 1996) erodes previous concepts of accountability (Greer and Hoggett 1997).

Concluding discussion

Both the examples considered in this chapter indicate the continued importance of control in housing access and allocations. This concluding section explores the underlying paradox of policy developments which are presented as enhancing citizenship and choice while in practice reinforcing control by housing providers and the state.

Taking the homelessness case study first we see that while the 1977 Act appeared to represent a significant augmentation of citizenship rights, this was never universal, was subject to variable local implementation and proved to be vulnerable to political and legal challenge. The interplay between central and local control has been a fascinating element of the emerging story. The various studies undertaken by the authors charting the implementation of the original legislation indicate the influence of complex tactics deployed at both central and local levels in mediating citizenship rights.

At the national level attempts were made to break the link between homelessness and entitlement to permanent housing in 1989 and again in 1994 and vulnerability to legal challenge had already emerged before the latter political changes were implemented in the 1996 Act. The legitimacy of the right to a home in a society where most housing provision has been commodified was always a barrier to making a permanent and positive link between citizenship and housing rights (see Neale 1997 on the importance of an appreciation of the broader social context of homelessness). On the other hand, there was always a possibility (realized in the 1993 Asylum and Immigration Appeals Act) that the concept of citizenship might be deployed as an exclusionary device to restrict the housing rights of those who do not enjoy full citizenship.

At local level the story seems to be much more about rationing practices by local authorities than about allowing or encouraging customer choice. While local political choices have clearly been an important element of this, variations in implementation also reflect substantial variations in the local housing market context and in particular the balance between effective demand and good quality housing which might legitimately be regarded as a 'prize of citizenship'. As Table 8.1 indicated, the nature of the local housing stock will always play a crucial role in the changing pattern of access to social housing. This is primarily because the task of housing allocation is fundamentally about letting properties rather than meeting needs. The really important determinants of the process from the consumers' viewpoint thus occur elsewhere in development and improvement policies for housing and in wider social and economic regeneration programmes for communities.

It is arguable that, as differences in the popularity of the social housing stock increase, choice will become even more difficult to incorporate. There are parallels between the difficulties in applying concepts of consumer choice to homelessness services and in other public services where a degree of insensitivity to consumer demand may be necessary 'in order to protect the interests of those consumers with least resources for either exit or voice – that is, the most vulnerable' (Carter et al. 1992: 175).

There is a considerable gap between rhetoric and reality both in the promise of the 1977 Act to deliver enhanced and consistent citizenship rights and in the gap between the political debate around the 1996 Act and its impact in practice. There is no reason to assume that the gap between the revised regulations issued in November 1997 and the experience of homeless citizens on the ground will be any narrower. It is apparent that the experience since 1977 has been one of shuffling priorities between groups and individuals seeking a limited resource. Throughout most of the period investment priorities bore little relation to the evidence of housing needs and homelessness and thus increasing one set of 'rights' has resulted in a worsening position for others. Each revision of the legislation and guidance since the passage of the Housing (Homeless Persons) Act 1977 has demonstrated the elusiveness of 'fairness' in the context of inadequate resources and competing priorities.

The example of CHRs reinforces our conclusion that even where they are presented as enhancements of user choice, access to housing policies are generally more about rationing and control. Again the context is set by public policy at the national level, but outcomes are determined by local responses to such policy and in particular by local arrangements to control eligibility and priority for rehousing. In this case the national context has been set by policies designed to promote choice for the funders rather than the users of social housing. The development of quasi-market mechanisms encouraging competition between housing associations supplying new homes resulted in fragmentation of provision at the local level. This was particularly the case in the period of expanding new provision between 1989 and 1993 when the Housing Corporation controlled the majority of funding with relatively limited influence from local authorities. The result was a reduced ability of local authorities to impose locally determined priorities on the allocation of housing, and a perceived leakage of supply away from those applicants in greatest need.

In this context the principal attractions of the CHR concept were to simplify access and to re-establish a system of rationing and control to ensure that local housing was allocated fairly to those whom the local authority deemed to be in greatest need. This would build on the mainstream housing provision role of associations, which was already largely delivered through nomination agreements with local authorities. However, some housing associations feared that such arrangements might prevent them from also adopting a complementary housing role whereby they could use their 'own lettings' to meet needs identified in their allocation policies.

However, while reimposing local control was one agenda which produced varying reactions from the suppliers of new housing, it was a second agenda of further centralization of housing allocation policies which had a particular impact on the willingness of housing associations to enter wholeheartedly into CHR partnerships.

In the period between 1994 and 1996 there was considerable uncertainty as to how the government's proposals for a statutory housing register would interact with CHRs. There were fears that participation in CHRs would lead to associations becoming simply 'contractors of the state' with no independent role in access to housing. Thus central policies both produced the need for CHRs and discouraged some potential participation, particularly during a period of uncertainty when it was not clear how much central control of allocations would actually be increased by proposed legislation and direction.

In a number of localities progress in developing CHRs was hampered by conflicts between the strategic interests of local authorities and the desire for greater independence on the part of some associations. However, this should not be overplayed and it has usually been possible to reach compromises between these legitimate interests, particularly where local authorities have not sought to control housing association resources too tightly and where associations have recognized their obligation to use their resources to meet the greatest local needs. Exercises comparing the actual impact of apparently different allocation policies and points schemes have often convinced partners that in practical terms they are usually trying to meet the same or very similar types of need.

The more interesting local control issues to emerge from the evaluation were not so much to do with differences of interest between local authorities and housing associations as with changes in governance arrangements that find parallels in many other aspects of local service delivery. CHRs exemplify the development of new forms of governance of housing (Reid 1995) based on networks and partnerships. One aspect of this development may be a shift in control from formal political and board-level control of access policies to greater autonomy of professionals. Thus, rather than simply an issue of diminishing choice for service users, we may be talking about a diminution of accountability of services to local citizens as a whole (Mullins 1996).

Both of the examples in this chapter demonstrate the difficulty of implementing citizens' rights to housing and consumer choice in a context where supply is limited in relation to needs. They further illustrate the paradox that housing is not generally seen as a central citizenship right and yet there is general agreement that resources should be allocated to those in greatest need. Definitions of need have incorporated a range of wider societal values and may seek to exclude those who do not enjoy full citizenship status. A final difficulty is that this 'prize of citizenship' is highly differentiated. The extent of inequalities which have become embedded within the social housing sector are now huge. Far from seeing social housing as contributing to the achievement of citizenship rights by destroying the link between bad housing and poverty, many writers now regard occupancy of certain parts of the social housing stock as a badge of exclusion preventing participation in wider social benefits (e.g. Bulmer and Rees 1996; Runciman 1996).

It is questionable whether this conjunction of circumstances can continue to be tackled by applying a single set of approaches to control access to different types of social housing in different local contexts. Yet, it seems unlikely that the adoption of more market-based access routes (perhaps based on the Dutch model) to hard-to-let social housing combined with continued strict rationing of the 'real prizes of citizenship' will provide a more satisfactory solution to the problem.

References

Arden, A. and Hunter, C. (1996) *The Housing Act 1996*. London: Sweet & Maxwell.
Audit Commission (1989) *Housing the Homeless: The Local Authority Role*. London: Audit Commission.

Binns, J. and Cannon, L. (1996) *Common Housing Registers: A Good Practice Guide*. Coventry: Chartered Institute of Housing.

Bulmer, M. and Rees, A.M. (eds) (1996) *Citizenship Today: The Contemporary Relevance of T.H. Marshall*. London: UCL Press.

Carter, N., Klein, R. and Day, P. (1992) *How Organisations Measure Success: The Use of Performance Indicators in Government*. London: Routledge.

Committee on Standards in Public Life (1996) *Second Report: Local Public Spending Bodies*. London: HMSO.

CRE (1984) *Hackney Housing Investigated: Report of a Formal Investigation*. London: Commission for Racial Equality.

CRE (1988) *Homelessness and Discrimination: Report of a Formal Investigation into the London Borough of Tower Hamlets*. London: Commission for Racial Equality.

Cullingworth Report (1969) *Council Housing Purposes, Procedures and Priorities*, ninth report of the housing management sub-committee of the Central Housing Advisory Committee. London: HMSO.

DoE (1989) *The Government's Review of the Homelessness Legislation*. London: Department of the Environment.

DoE (1991) *Homelessness Code of Guidance*. London: DoE.

DoE (1994) *Access to Local Authority Housing: A Consultation Paper*. London: Department of the Environment.

DoE (1995) *Our Future Homes*, Cm. 2901. London: HMSO.

Evans, A. and Duncan, S. (1988) *Responding to Homelessness: Local Authority Policy and Practice*. London: HMSO.

Ferlie, E., Ashburner, L., Fitzgerald, L. and Pettigrew, A. (1996) *The New Public Management in Action*. Oxford: Oxford University Press.

Greer, A. and Hoggett, P. (1997) *Patterns of Accountability Within Local Non-elected Bodies: Steering Between Government and the Market*. York: Joseph Rowntree Foundation.

Griffiths, M., Parker, J., Smith, R., Stirling, T. and Trott, T. (1996) *Community Lettings: Local Allocations Policies and Practice*. York: Joseph Rowntree Foundation.

Harloe, M. (1995) *The People's Home? Social Rented Housing in Europe and America*. Oxford: Blackwell.

Henderson, J. and Karn, V. (1984) Race, class and the allocation of public housing in Britain. *Urban Studies*, 21: 115–28.

HSAG (1978) *Allocation of Council Housing*. London: Department of the Environment.

Jeffers, S. and Hoggert, P. (1995) Like counting deckchairs on the Titanic: a study of institutional racism and housing allocations in Haringey and Lambeth. *Housing Studies*, 10: 325–44.

Kullberg, J. (1997) From waiting lists to adverts: the allocation of social rented housing in The Netherlands. *Housing Studies*, 12: 393–403.

Lee, P. and Murie, A. (1997) *Poverty, Housing Tenure and Social Exclusion*. Bristol: Policy Press.

Lee, P., Murie, A., Marsh, A. and Riseborough, M. (1995) *The Price of Social Exclusion*. London: National Federation of Housing Associations.

Lidstone, P. (1994) Rationing housing to the homeless applicant. *Housing Studies*, 9: 459–72.

Maclennan, D. and Kay, H. (1994) *Moving on, Crossing Divides: A Report on Policies and Procedures for Tenants Transferring in Local Authorities and Housing Associations*. London, HMSO.

Malpass, P. (1990) *Reshaping Housing Policy: Subsidies, Rents and Residualisation*. London: Routledge.

Malpass, P. (1997) The local governance of housing, in P. Malpass (ed.) *Ownership, Control and Accountability: The New Governance of Housing*. Coventry: Chartered Institute of Housing.

Malpass, P. and Murie, A. (1994) *Housing Policy and Practice*, 4th edn. Basingstoke: Macmillan.

Maslow, A. (1954) *Motivation and Personality*. New York: Harper & Row.

Mullins, D. (1996) Professional interests rule OK? Wider issues raised by common housing registers. *Agenda*, October: 20–1.

Mullins, D. and Niner, P. (1996) *Common Housing Registers: An Evaluation and Analysis of Current Practice*. London: Housing Corporation.

Mullins, D., Niner, P., Marsh, A. and Walker, B. (1996) *Evaluation of the 1991 Homelessness Code of Guidance*. London: HMSO.

Murie, A. (1996) *Urban and Regional Studies*, Inaugural lecture as chair of Urban and Regional Studies, University of Birmingham. Birmingham: University of Birmingham.

Neale, J. (1997) Homelessness and theory reconsidered. *Housing Studies*, 12: 47–61.

NFHA (1994) *Local Housing Registers*. London: NFHA.

Niner, P. (1989) *Homelessness in Nine Local Authorities: Case Studies of Policy and Practice*. London: HMSO.

Niner, P., White, V. and Levison, D. (1997) *The Early Impacts of the 1996 Housing Act and Housing Benefit Changes*. London: Shelter.

Page, D. (1993) *Building for Communities: A study of New Housing Association Estates*. York: Joseph Rowntree Foundation.

Phillips, D. (1986) *What Price Equality? A Report on the Allocation of GLC Housing in Tower Hamlets*. London: Greater London Council.

Prestcott-Clarke, P., Clemens, S. and Park, A. (1994) *Routes into Local Authority Housing: A Study of Local Authority Waiting Lists and New Tenancies*. London: HMSO.

Rea, S. (1993) *Partnership in Practice: A study of the Common Waiting List Concept*, project for the Institute of Housing Professional Qualification, unpublished but extensively quoted in NFHA (1994) *Local Housing Registers*. London: NFHA.

Reid, B. (1995) Interorganisational networks and the delivery of local housing services. *Housing Studies*, 10: 133–50.

Riseborough, M., Mullins, D. and Marsh, A. (1996) *Creating a Shared Vision: The Housing, Support and Care Needs of Older People in South Warwickshire*, report prepared for JCPT South Warwickshire (subgroup, elderly). Birmingham: Centre for Urban and Regional Studies, University of Birmingham.

Runciman, W.G. (1996) Why social inequalities are generated by social rights, in M. Bulmer and A.M. Rees (eds) *Citizenship Today: The Contemporary Relevance of T.H. Marshall*. London: UCL Press.

Smith, S.J. and Mallinson, S. (1997) The problem with social housing: discretion, accountability and the welfare ideal. *Policy and Politics*, 24: 339–57.

Torgerson, U. (1987) Housing: the wobbly pillar under the welfare state, in B. Turner, J. Kemeny and L. Lundqvist (eds) *Between State and Market: Housing in the Post-Industrial Era*. Stockholm: Almqvist & Wiksell.

Wilcox, S. (1996) *Housing Review 1996/97*. York: Joseph Rowntree Foundation.

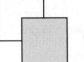

9

Charters in housing: enhancing citizenship, promoting choice or reinforcing control?

Pat Niner

Through the Citizen's Charter the Government is now determined to drive reforms further into the core of the public services, extending the benefits of choice, competition, and commitments to service more widely. The Citizen's Charter is the most comprehensive programme ever to raise quality, increase choice, secure better value, and extend accountability.

(HMSO 1991: 4)

Introduction

The key words 'citizen' and 'choice' in this quotation ensure that some consideration of the *Citizen's Charter* is a must for inclusion in this book. Changes introduced under the *Charter* banner to extend accountability are about defining the information citizens should have access to and the expectations of performance it is reasonable for them to have. They are therefore about giving users some leverage over providers – that is, shifting some control over the service delivered towards service users.

Citizen's Charter proposals include many which are central to major changes that have taken place in social housing in the 1990s, emphasizing the rationale for and cohesiveness of Conservative policy. Proposals affecting tenants include:

- Improved local authority *Tenants' Charter*.
- Opportunities to transfer away from local authority control (the then still extant Tenants' Choice provisions and Large Scale Voluntary Transfer (LSVT) as well as the Right to Buy).
- Stronger tenants' guarantee for housing associations.
- Extending compulsory competitive tendering (CCT) into the field of housing management.

The scope of this chapter is much more modest. It is concerned with the *Citizen's Charter* theme of 'standards', and particularly with initiatives which allow citizens 'to identify the standards of service they can expect, and create pressure for improvement and action where performance is unacceptable' (HMSO 1991: 15). The chapter presents two small case studies of initiatives linked to *Citizen's Charter* philosophy; source material comes from evaluative research carried out for the Department of the Environment (DoE).

The first case study is of the early operation of the 'performance indicator regime', introduced by the Local Government and Housing Act 1989, by which local authorities have to produce annual reports to tenants on their housing management performance (Marsh *et al.* 1993). The second is of the little-known *Park Home Owners' Charter* (British Holiday & Home Parks Association and National Park Home Council 1994) (Niner and Hedges 1996). The context, main provisions and apparent early impact of each are described in the sections which follow. A final section explores the extent to which *Charter* objectives seem to have been met by these initiatives and, in the context of the academic literature, discusses more generally whether they should be seen as enhancing citizenship, promoting choice, shifting the balance of control in favour of service users or, in contrast, reinforcing control by central government.

Reports to tenants: background

Section 167 of the Local Government and Housing Act 1989 required every local housing authority to provide tenants each year with 'such information as may be determined by the Secretary of State relating to the functions of the authority as a local housing authority during that year' (DoE 1990b). A Determination issued in March 1990 (DoE 1990a) spelled out what information had to be provided and further guidance was offered by a Circular issued in September 1990 (DoE 1990b). Local authorities had to provide the first reports for the year 1990–1 within six months of the year end at 31 March 1991.

The background to the new system was set out in a Consultation Paper (HMSO 1989). This started from the premise that 'The Government and local authorities are equally concerned to encourage high standards of housing management and the fullest involvement of Council tenants in this process' (HMSO 1989: 1). Two objectives for the regime were given:

1 To provide useful, up-to-date information for tenants about the performance of their housing authority, to promote their interest and involvement.
2 Through the stimulus of customer demand and interest, and of performance targets and measurement, to enhance standards of housing management.

A number of second-order aims were also quoted in the Consultation Paper.

The Determination required authorities to provide over 150 individual items of information grouped within 28 quantitative indicators in addition to a few non-statistical indicators (for example, information on tenant satisfaction with repairs where available, provisions for tenant consultation and making complaints). While the Circular urged inclusion of targets, comparisons and sub-district level information, these were not statutory requirements. Authorities were free to decide the form of report to be produced, but were reminded that it should be simple and inexpensive.

All local authorities with significant housing stocks produced reports to tenants in the first year, although not all met the deadline. Reports came in all shapes and sizes from the very simple to the elaborate. Leaving aside for the moment apparent outcomes of the regime in terms of its prime objectives, the research suggested that some of the second-order aims were not met. For example, one aim was to permit realistic and relative assessment of performance by neighbouring or comparable authorities. Although the Determination was apparently prescriptive and specific, it left scope for interpretation of the indicator requirements and authorities seem to have used their own definitions to such an extent that any inter-authority comparisons would have been very dubious.

Another aim was to prescribe minimum information requirements while allowing authorities to provide more if they wanted to. While most authorities claimed to have included information over and above that specified, it is possible that no authority actually provided every item of information as specified in the first year. Certainly the DoE's database set up to record and analyse the 28 quantitative indicators showed that for none of the indicators did all authorities provide information in precisely the required form. This suggests, and the research case studies confirmed, that many authorities found producing and disseminating the information a heavy burden (avoiding burdens was another aim) – or would have done had they actually adjusted systems to meet the specification precisely. Paradoxically, authorities with established monitoring and performance indicator systems actually found it most difficult to conform if their own definitions and analyses were different from the statutory requirements. The Determination itself did not help by sometimes specifying indicators in forms slightly different from those already collected for government returns.

The Determination indicators also differed from the housing information required for the *Citizen's Charter* performance indicators across local authority services introduced by Direction in 1992 with the first reports relating to the year 1993/4. These Audit Commission indicators were intended for a general audience and included local authority housing, housing the homeless and processing housing benefit. The housing element has remained broadly similar since it was introduced, but with changes in detail each year. For 1997/8 local authorities must report on ten indicators under the heading 'providing housing accommodation', on three under 'housing the homeless' and five under 'paying housing benefit and council tax benefit' (Audit Commission 1996). Selected indicators are published annually in the form of league tables with change from the previous year also shown. Published tables for the year 1995/6 included the average time taken to relet council homes and the percentage of tenants in rent arrears of more than 13 weeks (Audit Commission 1997).

The publication of performance indicators for housing association tenants took a slightly different course in that, initially, tenants were given the right to demand but not automatically to receive performance information. The range of information was also significantly narrower than that demanded by the 1990 Determination for local authorities. The two systems have come more into line over time as requirements for publication of housing association information have become stricter, and requirements for local authorities have been dramatically simplified by a new Determination issued in 1994 (DoE 1991). This reduced the number of items of information to be produced to about 20, under five broad headings. By this time, however, local authorities had introduced systems for assembling the original information and had tried and tested means of presenting and publishing the indicators; it seems that many authorities continued to provide reports on the same lines as before.

Improvements in the quality of reports produced have been encouraged by the publication of a good practice guide (CURS 1993) and the introduction by the Chartered Institute of Housing of annual competitions for the best reports in various categories (including housing associations). Judging panels have always included tenants, and some authorities have also involved tenants in the development of their individual reports. Tenant reactions to reports in the first year are discussed below.

Reports to tenants: early impacts

The DoE research (Marsh *et al.* 1993) was carried out within a year of the first distribution of reports to tenants. It collected information on local authority and tenant reactions to the new regime. The main conclusions from this very early evaluation were mixed: in some ways the new regime seemed to have been successful, in others it had been much less successful.

Taking the successes first, the fact of producing and distributing reports, many of which reached a high standard of presentation and showed considerable ingenuity in illustrating performance indicators, might be seen as quite an achievement. More particularly, having to produce reports had provided a stimulus for authorities to communicate with tenants; despite duties to consult on management matters, in a few instances this seems to have been for the first time, beyond letters and notifications of rent increases. Most authorities had found the exercise useful either in bringing together performance indicators or in communicating with tenants. Tenants in turn liked the idea of reports in principle and felt that they should have the right to information from their landlord; the great majority thought that their authority should produce a report to tenants the following year. The regime may have induced changes for the better in standards of housing management, especially in authorities not at the time heavily committed to improving service quality, enhancing customer care or regularly involving tenants. Having to produce reports to tenants had:

- changed the organizational culture in some authorities by stimulating a customer-oriented approach to service – sometimes the new regime was seen as a way of selling such a change to elected members;
- introduced or encouraged performance monitoring which could then be developed for internal management purposes, and highlighted areas where performance was poor and thus acted as a spur to service improvement;
- highlighted areas where management information was poor and needed development;
- required authorities to bring together indicators of performance across the service which might previously have been seen in isolation;
- provided a stimulus to thinking about ways of communicating with tenants and a channel for communication which could be built into wider processes;
- acted as a means of communicating with staff in large authorities about what other sections and departments did and what the service as a whole achieved.

These all seem to be positive steps, but all stem from the local authority itself having to collect, assemble, present and disseminate the information in the reports, not from any greater customer demands or interest from tenants as a result of having received the performance information.

It is in this area that the regime was less successful in its first year. There was no evidence that reports had had the effect of stimulating tenant interest and involvement in the housing service. There was no evidence that tenants were becoming more demanding or were pressing for service improvements, or were 'using' the information provided by the reports. Overall, there was very little spontaneous feedback from tenants to authorities on the reports.

There seemed to be three different sorts of factors at work which contributed to this lack of interest and use. First, and most simply, if tenants are to react in any way to information they have to notice, read and understand it. A minority of tenants interviewed in the case study areas had read most or all of the report they had received (assuming that local authorities had succeeded in distributing the reports to all tenants). Overall, two thirds of tenants interviewed actually remembered receiving the report (ranging from 51 per cent to 81 per cent in different areas). Of those who remembered receiving the report only 13 per cent claimed not to have read any of it at all although a further 19 per cent said they had read hardly any of it. Overall, 30 per cent of tenants had read all or most of their report and might be expected to be influenced by it. Again there were differences between local authorities – from 18 per cent to 44 per cent – but even in the most 'successful' area less than half of tenants had read most or all of the report. Readership was higher than average among older tenants, those who were satisfied with their council as landlord, members of residents' associations and those who thought that their landlord kept them well informed. This suggests that any 'message' from the reports was more likely to reach tenants who were already active and well-intentioned towards the authority. Not all tenants who read their reports necessarily understood the contents – just over one in ten of those who read at least part of the report had found it fairly or very difficult to understand.

Qualitative work with groups of tenants suggested that presentation and distribution techniques – for example having a free-standing report with a striking title, not looking like junk mail and including well laid-out text and simple graphics – could increase the probability of reports being noticed, read and understood. However, there undoubtedly remains a fundamental hurdle to stimulating interest and action.

The second sort of factor involved relates to the contents of reports. Not all items of information specified in the Determination were of interest to tenants. Few tenants were interested in stock details, rent arrears bandings (number of tenants owing so many weeks rent, in six bands) or the breakdown of lettings (transfers, homeless and others to new, newly rehabilitated and other dwellings). Some items which attracted great interest did so because of misunderstanding, for example seeing 'debt charges' (interest payments on loans within the housing revenue account) as the cost to the authority of rent arrears, or thinking that all rent arrears would be written off because a figure was included for bad debts written off. Repairs and improvements were topics of interest, although tenants were more concerned with future plans than with past performance. Interest in the future was also apparent more generally – few tenants spontaneously recognized the value of retrospective information on performance. Most were more interested in local policies, procedures, future plans and advice on what to do in case of problems; they were also more interested in information at estate level than for the district as a whole.

This leads directly to the third factor restricting the impact of the reports in stimulating tenant demands for service improvement. How can perform-ance information be used? Is it relevant to know that 98 per cent of housing benefit claims last year were handled within the statutory time limit of 14 days from the point at which all relevant information was provided if your own claim dragged on for two months? Should you complain because your urgent repair took 6 days to complete when the average completion time was 5.5 days? Is it significant that legal costs were 25 pence out of a weekly housing management total of £5.00? Performance information might be viewed as a construct somewhat akin to a map. To make 'use' of it one needs to understand the conventions involved and to see how they relate to everyday life in the same way as one needs to be able to interpret contours, blue and red lines to identify hills and valleys, rivers (or motorways) and roads. In the case of performance information one also, of course, needs some way in which to communicate with the landlord and a landlord able and willing to listen, hear and respond. And the whole exercise must seem to be worthwhile.

While most tenants who had read at least part of their report said that they had found it fairly or very useful, they were much less clear about *how* it might be used. The qualitative work showed that most tenants were not familiar with performance information and were not comfortable with statistical material. There was widespread mistrust of statistics and a con-viction that they could be made to show anything. Where relations were generally poor between tenants and the landlord, anything which seemed to show the local authority in a good light stood the chance of being dismissed as propaganda. In any case, the least satisfied tenants who potentially might have most to complain about were least likely to read the reports. Thus tenant culture and a lack of credibility in some circumstances undermine the potential for reports to fulfil the objectives of the regime in promoting interest and involvement and stimulating customer demands to enhance standards. We will return to these points after introducing the second case study.

The Park Home Owners' Charter: background

Park homes constitute a minority tenure, and very few people will have heard of the *Park Home Owners' Charter*. Yet it provides a good opportunity to examine some of the issues around charters, legal rights, expectations, control and choice. Because of the lack of general knowledge of the tenure, some background information is necessary.

Park homes (residential mobile homes or 'caravans' used for permanent accommodation on home 'parks' or estates of varying size) constitute a very small, very distinct part of the housing market. There were estimated to be about 76,800 mobile homes in England and Wales in 1991 – representing a fraction of 1 per cent of all dwellings (DoE 1991). Their distinctiveness for housing policy purposes lies particularly in their tenure. While a minority of park homes are occupied on tenancies, most residents have a unique form of tenure in which the home is owner-occupied but is located on a 'pitch' which is rented from the park owner. The relationship between the homeowner and the park owner is governed by the Mobile Homes Act 1983. The Act gives the homeowner the right to a written statement of the agreement between himself or herself and the park owner. The 'implied terms' of this agreement (that is, the statutory rights implied by the Act) include security of tenure and rights around selling, giving and bequeathing the home and assigning the agreement. The Act also gives park owners the right to take a commission, currently set at 10 per cent of the sale price, when a park home is sold on site and the agreement is transferred. The agreement between homeowner and park owner also includes 'express terms' which are agreed between the two parties but which are not in themselves rights given by the Mobile Homes Act. The express terms usually include rules about pitch fees, other charges and any rules concerning respective responsibilities and expected behaviour on the park. Pitch fees can be seen as part ground rent, part payment towards park management and maintenance. They are normally reviewed annually and the express terms set out the factors which will be considered – usually inflation as measured by the retail price index (RPI), sums spent by the park owner on improvements for the benefit of the occupiers of the park homes and any other relevant factors.

A survey of park homes and their occupiers in 1990 (Niner and Hedges 1992) found that park homes played two main roles in the housing market: providing convenient, compact homes for single people and couples especially of retirement age, and providing homes for people – sometimes families with children – with few alternatives. In the first role they could be seen as housing of choice, in the second as housing of desperation. Both roles can be traced to their underlying attraction of being cheaper than the nearest bricks and mortar substitute. In the late 1980s the price advantage enabled outright owner-occupiers of conventional properties to sell up, buy a park home in an attractive location and still have a capital sum to help with living expenses. For the more desperate, a park home could provide more space and privacy than a similarly-priced rented room or flat.

Older households were usually highly satisfied with their home, the park and park home life. In the retirement market the chief advantages of park homes are their size, convenience and ease of maintenance relative to many permanent houses. Parks of choice are often located in rural or semi-rural settings. The park owner exercises some control over who comes to live on the park and rules exist to govern behaviour. These factors contribute to creating a sheltered environment, and to the development of a sense of community which some residents felt had disappeared from modern city life. Park homes are less suited to families who often live on the less desirable parks and in older, less well-insulated and equipped homes. Compactness which suits an elderly couple can mean overcrowding and shortage of space for a family with children. For all residents, satisfaction was found to be greatly affected by their views of and relationship with the park owner.

Potential conflicts of interest between homeowner and park owner are inherent in the unique tenure of park homes. The economics of park owner-ship depend on income from three main sources: pitch rents, commission on resale of existing homes, and profit on selling new units. The park owner therefore wants a regular flow of income from pitch rents increasing at least at the rate of inflation. The right to commission on resale of homes is zealously guarded on the grounds that part of the value of the home represents the capitalized value of the right to site the home on the park and park amenity. Replacing older units with new ones is advantageous partly to keep up standards and values and partly to get income from the profit element to be earned by selling a new-sited unit. This profit arises because the selling price of a new unit reflects demand and what people are willing to pay rather than the costs of purchasing and siting the unit, which can be much lower. The desire to replace older units can lead less scrupulous park owners to seek to prevent owners of older homes selling on site and assigning their agreement (which can only be done with the park owner's consent), or even to seek to terminate the agreement on one of the three grounds laid down by the Mobile Homes Act 1983. The first two of these are breaking the tenancy agreement or not living in the park home as the main residence. The third allows an agreement to be terminated, where a court agrees that it is reasonable, if because of its age and condition the home is having a detrimental effect on the amenity of the park or is likely to have such an effect within the next five years. As can be readily appreciated this ground is quite vague and difficult to interpret, and leaves a great deal to the discretion of the courts.

From the homeowners' point of view each of these factors can present difficulties. Regular pitch-fee increases are often resented on the grounds that the park owner does little in the way of management or maintenance to earn an increase; there is little recognition that the park owner needs a return on capital invested. As with service charges in permanent housing, increases can also produce affordability problems for people on low or fixed incomes or pensions. Commission is bitterly resented by many homeowners, again on the grounds that it is totally unearned. Any threat to the homeowner's security of tenure or right to sell his or her home can present problems and disturb a resident's peace of mind.

These potentials for conflict of interest suggest likely difficulties for the Mobile Homes Act in protecting the rights of homeowners satisfactorily. Four factors limit the Act's effective operation. First, many residents (and some park owners) are largely ignorant of the law and its provisions. In these circumstances, it would obviously be unwise to rely on the Act to protect rights many people do not know they have.

Second, there is often a considerable disparity of power, influence and resources between the two 'sides'. While some park owners are as old and poor as their residents, many are large companies with the resources to call upon legal advice in any dispute. As noted, many residents are elderly and have retired to a park home to pursue a 'low input' lifestyle. Residents' associations are not well developed, and some park owners may refuse to negotiate with an association where one exists. The disparity of power, and the fear it can bring, is summed up by a quotation from the 1990 research: 'To a person of 80 years old, the owner walking past and just stopping and peering down each side of her van, that's harassment. That woman's lying awake at nights' (Niner and Hedges 1992: 87).

Third, there is the problem of bringing an issue sufficiently to a head to decide the case. For example, in a dispute about pitch rent increases, the only way to settle the dispute (without the parties agreeing) is for the park owner to take the resident to court for non-payment of the disputed sum. Without decisive court action a dispute can drag on for years, souring relations generally and building up mistrust.

Finally, the fact that the only resort to resolving a dispute is to the courts is off-putting to both parties. Court action is seen to involve bother, costs, delays and uncertainty of outcome. Because cases are rare, many of the more contentious areas of the law are relatively untested and therefore unclear.

Together these factors mean that the 1983 Act does not effectively achieve a balance between the interests of park owners and homeowners. This is not, of course, a unique picture. Precisely the same might be said about landlord/ tenant relations in the private rented sector or leaseholder/freeholder/managing agent relations elsewhere in the permanent dwelling stock. In all those situations there is widespread ignorance of rights, disparity of power, problems in bringing things to a head and reliance on the courts. One important way in which park homes differ is the paucity of legal and other advice available to residents when difficulties arise.

The 1990 survey report giving these insights into the operation of the Mobile Homes Act was published in 1992 and was introduced by a speech by Tim Yeo, then a junior housing minister, to the annual convention of the British Holiday & Home Parks Association (BH&HPA) (one of the two main trade bodies involved in the park home industry). In his speech the minister drew attention to some of the research's main findings and called on the park home industry to draw up a residents' charter, to be produced in consultation with residents, in the belief that 'a demanding Charter ... is the best way to guarantee residents the service they deserve' (Niner and Hedges 1996: 5).

The two main trade associations – the BH&HPA and the National Park Homes Council (NPHC) agreed, seeing it as an opportunity to clarify residents' rights and increase understanding, and no doubt as a way of avoiding the threat of legislative change. The *Charter* was drafted by a joint committee of the two associations with comments from the DoE at various stages. There was limited resident consultation and amendment after which the *Park Home Owners' Charter* was launched in January 1994. Copies of the *Charter* were sent to association members for onward distribution. Publicity was given to the *Charter* in the park homes press, in information leaflets and at exhibitions.

The government's stated aim in encouraging the production of the *Charter* was to tackle problems of ignorance of the law by helping park owners and residents to understand and use the law in a fair and even way. Broadly, the twelve page *Charter* attempts to explain in simple terms the main rights given by the Mobile Homes Act 1983. In this it covers similar ground to DoE Housing Booklet 30 (*Mobile Homes: A Guide for Residents and Site Owners*) but, in intention at least, in a more approachable and user-friendly fashion. Like the *Council Tenants' Charter* (DoE 1992), the *Park Home Owners' Charter* uses typeface distinctions to draw attention to the different status of sections. Thus statutory rights are printed in bold with extensive cross-references to Housing Booklet 30. Italics are used to describe additional rights which 'many park owners also give'. It is not clear whether 'compliance' requires a park owner to provide all the italicised services. Nor is the status clear of sections which are in neither bold nor italic type.

The *Charter* does not set explicit targets for performance, nor does it offer service recipients any form of compensation or redress for non-performance. The BH&HPA and NPHC have made 'compliance' with the *Charter* a condition of membership and have undertaken to use disciplinary procedures against any member who is shown to have breached the *Charter* – although it is not clear what sanctions other than dismissal from membership the associations have. The central role of the trade associations has two important implications. First, it means that the enforcing agency cannot be seen as independent from those likely to be in breach. Second, it means that there is no sanction at all against non-compliance on non-member parks where the *Charter* only applies if the owner chooses. The BH&HPA and NPHC estimate that their membership covers between three fifths and three quarters of all pitches, but does not cover the poorer parks where rights are perhaps most at risk.

The Park Home Owners' Charter: impact

In 1995 the DoE commissioned research to examine the impacts of the *Charter* (Niner and Hedges 1996). The overall conclusions were that the *Charter* was a step in the right direction, but that it made no fundamental difference to relations between park operators and homeowners. The main stumbling blocks to effectiveness were limited familiarity with the *Charter*, the lack of 'bite' to the *Charter* and doubts about its enforcement, its lack of recognition on non-member parks and its perceived lack of independence from the trade bodies representing park operator interests.

Overall, just over three-fifths of park operators interviewed were aware of the *Charter* and just under a quarter had read it all. This average conceals big differences between park owners who were and were not members of the trade associations. Almost all members were aware of the *Charter* and 47 per cent had read it all. In contrast only a third of non-members were aware of the *Charter* and only 5 per cent claimed to have read it all. Among homeowners a third of those interviewed were aware of the *Charter* and 8 per cent had read it all. Homeowners on member parks were better informed than on non-member parks, but the differences were not as great as for the park owners. Just over a third of prospective park home purchasers had heard of the *Charter*.

As noted above, distribution of the *Charter* was from the trade associations mainly through the park operators. Copies did not seem to have been provided to local authorities, Citizens Advice Bureaux or other organizations to whom park home owners might turn for advice. Distribution of copies to existing, new and prospective homeowners was incomplete and patchy. It was almost entirely restricted to member parks. Copies were more likely to be given to prospective purchasers or new residents rather than existing residents, suggesting that park owners saw the *Charter* as a source of initial information rather than a statement of rights of equal relevance to existing homeowners. Distribution even to new residents was partial and seems to have depended to some extent on people asking for a copy (implying that they already knew it existed) and the park operator actually having a stock of booklets available at the time. Awareness at these sorts of levels immediately reduces any potential impact the *Charter* might have.

Most of those who had read at least part of the *Charter* – both park owners and homeowners – thought that it was either very or fairly useful. Most homeowners thought that its usefulness lay in being a point of reference and as a statement of their rights. Park operators referred to helping with problems and disputes, giving insight into mobile-home living and setting standards for the industry. In response to prompted questions, both park operators and home owners thought the *Charter* most valuable as a statement of the rights and obligations of homeowners and as a guide for new homeowners. The *Charter* had actually been used on a tiny minority of parks. Outcomes had not always been successful and depended on the park operator's willingness to negotiate and accept the *Charter*'s guidelines. One case, for example, emerged where a park operator had refused to acknowledge the guidance within the *Charter* despite being a member of one of the trade associations. This raises the question of 'compliance' with and enforcement of the *Charter* provisions.

Neither park operators nor homeowners were entirely clear what 'compliance' with the *Charter* meant. Both parties usually assumed that there was a large element of discretion for park owners and that only the parts grounded in law were binding while the rest was voluntary. It was generally assumed that the *Charter* would not be binding in any way on non-member park owners. The research looked at some of the provisions of the *Charter* over and above those strictly required by the Mobile Homes Act, including provision of information to prospective purchasers, freedom to establish a residents' association, the right of homeowners to receive normal household deliveries directly to their home from companies of their choice and complaints procedures. These extra-legal 'rights' were not given on all parks; they were, however, more likely to be given on member than on non-member parks. Perhaps because of the low levels of awareness of the *Charter* and/or uncertainties as to its status and enforceability, there was little evidence that lack of compliance had been challenged.

The research also concluded that the *Charter* alone could not make up for inadequacies in the law, and that it would be unfair to expect it to do so. Issues around the park owners' right to commission, pitch fee increases, security of tenure and home sales all remain. Indeed one major criticism of the *Charter* might be its unwillingness to address these more difficult 'grey areas' where good practice clarification would be particularly useful. It is perhaps no accident that the *Charter* includes a fairly lengthy explanation (and intended justification) of commission on sales, but is largely silent on the grounds for terminating an agreement, issues around older units, and what a park operator should or should not demand by way of pre-sale surveys, pre-emption clauses or vetting of prospective purchasers when a homeowner wants to sell his or her home. It would presumably be difficult to reach agreement within the trade associations on recommendations in these contentious areas, and even more difficult to consider enforcement.

Discussion

The case study initiatives obviously differ in many ways. For example, simply in terms of scale, there are more council tenants in the City of Birmingham than there are park home residents in England and Wales. One is supposedly a whole 'charter', the other but one element in the wider *Council Tenant's Charter*, being referred to under the heading 'your council must keep you in touch' (DoE 1992). Despite such differences the initiatives share a broad intention: ostensibly each is aimed at improving services by providing information to increase understanding and allow individuals to press for their rights. Neither, of itself, commits service providers to specific service targets nor offers redress for failure.

How then can these case studies be related to the three themes of policy analysis – citizenship, choice and control – with which this book is particularly concerned?

Enhancing citizenship?

Since both initiatives fit explicitly beneath the *Citizen's Charter* banner, one might suppose that they would link directly with enhancing citizenship. In so far as citizenship is defined as being concerned with rights and responsibilities, such a link is not immediately obvious. Neither initiative actually increases rights or defines new obligations (apart from the right of council tenants to receive the performance information itself, which tenants seem to have valued).

However, Symon and Walker (1995: 201) argue that the *Citizen's Charter* actually deals with citizens only as consumers and 'is concerned with enabling individuals to engage in the competitive marketplace, which tends to be the overriding concern with consumerist philosophy'. In line with such a view of citizenship, both initiatives seek to increase awareness of rights or performance in such a way as to enable active citizens to recognize when they are being denied those rights or are receiving below average treatment. In this way citizens (in their role as tenant or park homeowner) are being invited to 'voice' dissatisfaction and press for service improvement. However, the case studies cast serious doubts on the credibility of this chain of reasoning and its effectiveness in practice.

At the very simplest level, the service users must receive and read the information if they are to exercise voice. In neither case had the report or *Charter* actually reached the majority of its target group; the shortfall was particularly marked for the *Park Home Owners' Charter*.

Then, as noted above, there are the questions of topics, style, presentation and credibility which affect whether the information will be absorbed and perceived as relevant. A first step in this might be the involvement of citizens as users in the design and operation of the schemes (Pollitt 1988). The case studies showed that such involvement was largely lacking. This is not, apparently, unusual: Clapham and Satsangi (1992: 72), looking at accountability for housing management through performance assessment, noted that 'no examples are available of performance assessment systems in which consumers have a major influence over the process'. Smith and Walker (1994: 612) examined the impacts of the Welsh equivalent of the report to tenants regime. They argued that the consultative process behind the Determination which involved local authorities and pressure groups resulted in a situation where 'the information in the report is not necessarily that which tenants need to provide them with an understanding of the performance of their landlord'.

Other writers also support our comments above about the language of performance measurement – is it 'actually alien and unintelligible to most citizens, a construct being forced on them by other interests'? (Pollitt 1988: 85). Day and Klein (1987: 243) looked at performance indicators in other service areas and state 'there is ... little evidence that either authority members or the public at large respond to or use such information'. Credibility was also noted as an issue, which again has wider applicability. As Carter *et al.* (1992: 45) comment 'one of the most important attributes of any performance indicator is the credibility of the information on which it is built ... ultimately the credibility ... may reside in the eye of the beholder'. Symon and Walker (1995: 214) noted that 'amongst local authority tenants there was a widespread feeling that it is easy to lie with statistics'. These points are summed up: 'performance indicators have been seen as technical instruments at best and propaganda at worst, and in any case incomprehensible and misleading' (Carter *et al.* 1992: 183).

Interpreting results, and determining what is good or bad performance is also a considerable issue 'when there are no explicit standards' (Carter *et al.* 1992: 46). Symon and Walker (1995: 214) noted that tenants tended to judge 'performance by performance', that is from their own experiences – which may not be a bad strategy in this context. However, even if one can judge whether personal experience is better, the same or worse than an average achieved in the previous year (the information provided in the report) this does not obviously provide guidance on what might/should be done about it. Again, performance information is no substitute for clear service targets and well-publicized rights to redress if those targets are not met (perhaps by a stated margin) for the individual. Reports to tenants may be a step in this direction, but fall well short.

The case studies also suggest that, if citizens are to make an effort to try to press for rights, they must believe that they have some chance of success. Comments made by park homeowners (in unpublished interview notes used for Niner and Hedges 1996) revealed marked cynicism around the whole concept of 'charterism':

'It means nothing to me, the *Citizen's Charter*. I've heard about it on the television. One of Mr Major's ideals.'

'It's usually something that's put out by the government that they don't really want you to have.'

'Looking at it a bit further it's one of these *Citizen's Charter* gimmick type things isn't it? Like one gets in the hospitals. And I don't think it achieves anything.'

If such views are widespread, then few people are likely to be encouraged to be more active by something regarded with such disillusion.

All this is not to say that the provision of information is unwelcome. We are arguing rather that a reliance on enhanced citizenship (within a citizen-consumer perspective), through giving individuals 'voice' by providing that information is unlikely to lead to service improvements *per se.*

However, citizenship can also have connotation beyond the realm of the individual, with an emphasis on collective as well as individual rights (Clapham and Satsangi 1992). 'Citizenship is about people putting aside the personal concerns and considering the wider impacts of decisions on other people and is about citizen participation' (Symon and Walker 1995: 200). The concept of the citizen is also wider than that of the immediate service user, whether in the guise of taxpayer or potential service user (Pollitt 1988).

It should be clear from the case studies that the initiatives explored do not score very well within this wider view of citizenship either. Despite a parallel strand in government policy encouraging tenant participation within public-sector housing management, reports to tenants were directed at the individual, with no specific role for tenant bodies unless a particular landlord chose to involve them. Equally they were directed only towards current, not prospective tenants or other potentially interested audiences. We would argue that, without guidance and support, individual council tenants will have difficulty converting performance information into ammunition to use against their landlord. Birchall (1992: 171) argues that the use of performance information in the reports 'is only going to be as good as the level of effective organisation which tenants have reached'.

The *Park Home Owners' Charter* was intended to be distributed particularly to potential and new homeowners (although in practice distribution was very patchy). Existing homeowners were not identified as a main audience, although the contents would surely have been of great interest to them. Again, there was no recognition of the scope (or need) for any collective dimension. One 'optional' provision of the *Charter* was the 'right' to form or belong to a residents' association, but there was no comparable 'commitment' on the part of the park operator to consult or negotiate with an association.

There is currently some ambiguity over the relative scope for individual and collective action on home parks. This can be illustrated in the history of many disputes about pitch-fee increases. A residents' association takes the lead and seeks to negotiate with the park owner, often about the validity of proposed pitch-fee increases said to be to pay for park improvements but argued by residents to represent arrears of maintenance. The park owner refuses to reduce the increase demanded. One by one, homeowners settle and pay up until only a few committed residents remain in dispute – at which point it is not uncommon for them to be blamed for deteriorating relations between the park operator and residents. In this context, the existence of the

Charter is likely to have little impact, since the information it gives on both residents' associations and pitch-fee increases over and above inflation is extremely non-specific. This would seem to be an opportunity missed.

From this analysis, it should be clear that neither initiative, alone, can be argued to greatly enhance citizenship, whether seen in terms of rights and obligations or citizen-consumer 'voice', or within a wider collective perspective.

Promotion of choice

Neither case study initiative explicitly refers to increasing choice among its objectives. This is, however, an important strand of the *Citizen's Charter* philosophy and each initiative can be examined as it relates to choice.

Choice might be seen within the context of 'supermarket consumerism'. This is a market-based concept which posits the right of consumers to shop around when seeking a new product or if dissatisfied with the existing one. For full applicability it requires free competition, entry and exit – i.e. the consumer can freely switch between services or providers (Clapham and Satsangi 1992). It also implies a well (perfectly?) informed consumer.

Symon and Walker (1995: 211) point out that the reports to tenants regime does not result in published 'league tables' which would be even hypothetically available to interested tenants seeking to shop around. The idea that such performance information could be built into a sort of Which? report of aspects of the housing service is worth considering. One immediate problem is general incompleteness and lack of comparability of the data between authorities noted in the case study above. Comments by Clapham suggest that this is a wider problem: 'difficulties of measurement and interpretation make exercises such as the indicators devised by the Audit Commission to measure local authority performance and to construct league tables of performance potentially misleading. They cannot overcome differences in recording practices and difficulties in the measurement of essentially subjective criteria' (Clapham 1992: 19).

The sheer complexity and variability of the housing management service means that simple, fully comparable indicators are hard to find, less than useful or both. Aldridge, writing in a different context, raises fundamental questions of the worth of a Consumers' Association Which? report approach for such a service. 'The Association's approach is predicated on comparative testing of quality-controlled, standardised, mass-market products. But financial services are not like this. They are abstract and intangible ... They cannot be evaluated by the consumer over an initial trial period ... Any fateful problems usually emerge long after purchase' (Aldridge 1997: 396). Housing management services could very well be substituted for financial services in this quotation, suggesting the inapplicability of a purely rational, objective approach to weighing the performance of different providers.

However, the more fundamental, and widely remarked drawback to seeing housing management services within the concept of supermarket consumerism and choice is the lack of any real exit option for tenants because of alternative 'entry' problems (e.g. Birchall 1992; Clapham and Satsangi 1992; Symon and Walker 1995). A tenant could leave a poorly-performing landlord, but there is then no mechanism whereby that tenant could 'enter' housing in a better-performing authority landlord area. Even within a single authority, transfer systems are not geared to allowing discriminating tenants to identify and move to better-performing estates unless they can also show that they 'need' to move there. Prospective tenants (who are not provided with performance information anyway) have little choice over which local authority to apply to for housing since many councils require applicants to live, work or have some local connection with their area before registering the application. Local connection is similarly enshrined in homelessness legislation. Limited-offer policies, often adopted for households rehoused under the Housing Act 1985 homelessness duties, restrict potential for choice between estates. In so far as better-performing estates are also the most popular (which is likely to be the case) those in most urgent need are least likely to be able to choose to go to such estates. Thus, knowing which local authorities perform the best, or on which estates performance is best, is largely irrelevant to an existing or prospective tenant at the point of move-ment. The alternative to getting an offer on a poorly performing, unpopular estate could be no offer at all, or a very long wait.

Tenants are similarly unable to exercise much choice in the service they receive *without* moving. Tenant consultation, tenant management, housing management CCT and changes in landlord (through Housing Action Trusts, the now-defunct Tenants' Choice or LSVT) all, it could be argued, provide scope for the greater or lesser exercise of choice. The sort of performance information specified in the Determination is tangential to each. Con-sultation is likely to be most useful on specific issues and in specific forums, not on the scatter-gun approach evident in reports to tenants. Poor (or good) performance might provide incentives to tenant management or other change in landlord. However, the experience of poor (or good) performance is likely to be more influential than information about it. While information on prospective managers' performance might well be relevant in considering alternative contractors for a tendered housing management service, this would again need to be much more focused, controlled and guided than that provided by the reports to tenants.

These points suggest that tenants, as informed consumers, might be better placed to make sound decisions about the housing service they receive and from whom they receive it, but that reports to tenants could only be seen as a small step towards this end, perhaps in familiarizing tenants with these sorts of data.

The scope for consumer choice is a little more real when considering the

Park Home Owners' Charter. The trade associations quite explicitly saw the *Charter* as a marketing device which would allow prospective purchasers to decide whether they wanted a park home at all. If they did, the *Charter* should give a marketing advantage to member parks which were offering it over non-member parks which were not. Overall the 'respectability' given by the *Charter* was seen as benefiting the industry as a whole. Very few park owners or homeowners, however, saw the *Charter* as a marketing tool in this way. Low levels of awareness of the *Charter* must in practice reduce any potential it has in this area.

Once on a park as a homeowner, the individual seems to have almost as little choice as the council tenant. Going back to a bricks and mortar home may not be possible for economic or social reasons without a reduction in standards. Moving between parks means selling one home and buying another since, while park homes are 'mobile' to the extent that transport may be physically possible (which in any event is not always true), it is very rare to find a park willing to accept a second-hand home from elsewhere on a pitch. 'Choosing' the standard of service on the park without moving depends on a willing park owner.

This analysis suggests that the case study initiatives are likely in practice to have little real effect in increasing choice.

Reinforcing control?

The final vital link in the chain between information provision and service improvement is the willingness of the landlord or park owner to change in response to voiced pressure from the better-informed consumer. This is where the theme of control comes in. Nothing in either of the case studies suggests that the locus of control or the balance of power has shifted at all due to the initiatives examined. Nothing in these initiatives *makes* a landlord or park owner respond to pressure for service improvement.

The issue of enforcement has been raised particularly in the context of the *Park Home Owners' Charter* – with doubts expressed above about the definition of 'breaches' of the *Charter* as well as the willingness and ability of the trade associations to enforce against members. Essentially, any enhancement of services would stem from positive responses from well-intentioned park owners who share the *Charter* objectives and subscribe to its provisions.

The whole point of 'charters' is that they are not totally grounded on legal rights. They are offering the citizen – whether as tenant, park homeowner, patient, rail traveller and so on – a statement of what he or she can expect, often including something extra (over and above legal rights), or a route to pressing for something extra. The implication must be that charters can only work where both sides, service provider and service user, subscribe to the agreement. A degree of trust between the two parties is necessary if promises are to be credible. Charters may work where there is a commitment to service quality and responsiveness; it is hard to see how they can do much where that commitment is lacking.

A very obvious contrast between the two case study initiatives is relevant here. Reports to tenants are firmly within the public sector, and local authorities can be expected to have a very different outlook from highly commercial park operators in a competitive part of the private sector. *The Park Home Owners' Charter* is essentially a voluntary exercise in self-monitoring (and self-preservation?) by trade associations. Hutton has observed that voluntary codes of practice relying on goodwill and industry self-regulation have proved too frail to ensure quality provision. A particular danger with a voluntary approach is that aggressive predatory firms may gain competitive advantage by opting out, if this is easier or cheaper (Hutton 1995). This seems likely to be true in the home-park industry, and draws attention to the distinction between member and non-member parks and the degree to which this reduces any real value of the *Charter* for homeowners overall. Paradoxically, perhaps as in any attempt at self-regulation, the *Charter* is likely to be most successful for those who need it least.

Looking at the relationship between performance assessment in housing management and landlord accountability to tenants, Clapham and Satsangi (1992: 69) note that 'none of the performance appraisal systems ... seems to offer much in the way of enhancing accountability of the provider to the consumers of housing management services'. Referring specifically to the reports to tenants regime they comment that the introductory circular 'makes only a little progress' in respect of accountability to tenants. This seems to be a widely-shared view (see also Symon and Walker 1995), and is supported by our case study.

Some researchers, however, seem more optimistic about the potential that performance information might have in increasing accountability to consumers – given some change. For example, Clapham (1992: 27) comments that 'performance assessment can be used as a way of empowering users, although this will involve changes in both the way central government regulates service providers, as well as in the service providing agencies themselves'. Again, Pollitt concludes that, in order to bring the consumer into performance measurement, change is needed in the whole context in which performance measurement systems are used. 'The aim is not merely to *please* the recipients of public services (difficult and worthy though that might be) but to *empower* them' (Pollitt 1988: 86, original emphasis). For Carter *et al.* (1992: 183) 'the agenda for the 1990s [is] to rescue the concept of PIs [performance indicators] from the experts and to see whether, and how, it can be integrated into the democratic process'.

There seems to be more support in the literature for the view that performance assessment in the public services is only very secondarily (if at all) about increasing accountability to the service users, and much more about increasing central government's control over services while pursuing a policy of decentralization (to agencies, and downward within organizations). Carter's thesis is that performance indicators offered 'a means of "hands off" control to a Conservative administration committed to the principle of reducing the role of central government, yet confronted by the paradox that decentralisation of services requires tighter central control'. He notes that they are an imperfect instrument of control and 'involve a much resented degree of "back seat driving" on the part of government without, as yet, providing a greater degree of central control over services' (Carter 1989: 136).

How does the report to tenants regime fare in this light? Certainly central government was seen as one of the potential audiences for the reports. If it was ever an intention – which was denied – that comparative performance information would be compiled from the reports or that they would be used in resource decisions, the obvious variability of definitions used by local authorities would soon have made the dangers of this all too clear. Was this one reason behind the decision to greatly simplify the English Determination, perhaps relying on the supposedly more rigorously-audited Audit Commission *Citizen's Charter* indicators for any comparative purposes?

Making use of the resulting information is not, however, the only way in which reports to tenants could be seen as a tool for central control over local authorities. Symon and Walker (1995: 213) argue that it is possible to see the imposition of the regime as 'a "blunt instrument" employed by central government in an attempt to bring about a change in the internal management culture of local authority housing departments'. Our case study suggests that there was limited success here in stimulating consideration of performance measurement, customer care and tenant communication issues, especially in less advanced authorities. However, there is still a very long way to go before this attempt at central influence and control leads to success in our other aspect of control – namely, empowering service users.

References

Aldridge, A. (1997) Engaging with promotional culture. *Sociology*, 31: 389–408.

Audit Commission (1996) *The Publication of Information Direction 1996*. London: Audit Commission.

Audit Commission (1997) *Local Authority Performance Indicators 1995/96*, vol. 2. London: Audit Commission.

Birchall, J. (1992) Council tenants: sovereign consumers or pawns in the game? in J. Birchall (ed.) *Housing Policy in the 1990s*. London: Routledge.

British Holiday & Home Parks Association and National Park Home Council (1994)

Park Home Owners' Charter: Your Guide to Buying, Living in and Selling your Park Home. BH&HPA and NHPC.

Carter, N. (1989) Performance indicators: 'backseat driving' or 'hands off' control? *Policy and Politics*, 17: 131–8.

Carter, N., Klein, R. and Day, P. (1992) *How Organisations Measure Success: The Use of Performance Indicators in Government.* London: Routledge.

Clapham, D. (1992) Evaluation and performance assessment. Unpublished conference paper, 'Exchange of Experience across Welfare Sectors' conference, 19–20 November.

Clapham, D. and Satsangi, M. (1992) Performance assessment and accountability in British housing management. *Policy and Politics*, 20: 63–74.

CURS (Centre for Urban and Regional Studies) (1993) *Producing Reports to Tenants: A Good Practice Guide.* London: HMSO.

Day, P. and Klein, R. (1987) *Accountabilities: Five Public Services.* London: Tavistock.

DoE (1990a) *The Report to Tenants Determination 1990.* London: DoE.

DoE (1990b) *s167(1), Local Government and Housing Act 1989 Housing Management Performance Indicators*, Circular 19/90. London: DoE.

DoE (1991) *Mobile Homes in England and Wales.* London: HMSO.

DoE (1992) *The Council Tenant's Charter: You, Your Home and Your Estate.* London: HMSO.

DoE (1994) *Reports to Tenants – Housing Management Performance Indicators: Revised Determination for 1994/95 and Subsequent Years.* London: DoE.

HMSO (1989) *Published Performance Indicators for Local Authority Tenants (England)*, consultation paper. London: HMSO.

HMSO (1991) *The Citizens' Charter: Raising the Standard*, Cm. 1599. London: HMSO.

Hutton, W. (1995) *The State We're In.* London: Cape.

Marsh, A., Niner, P. and Symon, P. (1993) *An Evaluation of the First Year Experience of the Local Authority Reports to Tenants Regime.* London: HMSO.

Niner, P. and Hedges, A. (1992) *Mobile Homes Report.* London: HMSO.

Niner, P. and Hedges, A. (1996) *Evaluating the Park Home Owners' Charter.* Birmingham: Centre for Urban and Regional Studies, University of Birmingham.

Pollitt, C. (1988) Bringing consumers into performance measurement. *Policy and Politics*, 16: 77–87.

Smith, R. and Walker, R. (1994) The role of performance indicators in housing management: a critique. *Environment and Planning A*, 26: 609–21.

Symon, P. and Walker, R. (1995) A consumer perspective on performance indicators: the local housing authority Reports to Tenants regimes in England and Wales. *Environment and Planning C: Government and Policy*, 13: 195–216.

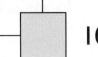

10

More control and choice for users? Involving tenants in social housing management

Moyra Riseborough

Introduction

Tenant involvement in housing has been presented in many different ways and carries a variety of meanings. While it may provide citizens who are the tenants of social landlords with more choice and control over their destiny it may also be little more than an illusion which offers only the semblance of involvement in their landlord's decision-making processes. However, despite these potentially different outcomes, the idea of tenant involvement has an enduring appeal, and there is almost universal agreement that it is a 'good thing'. This chapter examines the slippery notion of tenant involvement, traces its varied origins and forms and, most importantly, seeks to understand its impact on the experience of tenants through an extended case study.

Part of the reason for the ambiguity of tenant involvement lies in the varied origins of current practice. One of these is the involvement of local residents in public service decision making which has been a consistent feature of policy discourse in the UK since the 1960s – see, for example, the Skeffington Report 1968 (Skeffington 1968). Another is the more recent rise of user involvement in social welfare and other public services (Hoyes *et al.* 1994). Yet, as the chapter illustrates these distinct origins have different implications for the meaning and experience of tenant involvement by tenants themselves.

Another important reason why tenant involvement is presented in different ways is that it may be pursued for many different purposes and serves a variety of interests. Hague (1990) refers to the 'elasticity' of the concept which enables it to fit almost any context. Meanwhile, Hoggett and Hambleton (1987) have referred to the interest of both the political left and right in policies to involve the public in decision making, although they are poles apart in their motivation for supporting it. To this extent the prevailing context 'infects' (Somerville and Steele 1995) presentations of tenant involvement and as a result the discourse can subtly turn and change.

To understand the relationship between the discourse, the purpose and the practice of tenant involvement it is helpful to start by considering common definitions and examining the relationship between these definitions and the rise of tenant involvement, including the policy and legislative frameworks which have supported it. This is the task of the first part of this chapter. The second part draws on recent research with older tenants (see Riseborough 1996) as the basis for a critical discussion of whether tenant involvement practices actually lead to more control and choice being exercised by tenants.

What is tenant involvement?

There is general agreement that tenant involvement is essentially concerned with collective rather than individual pursuits (Bengtsson 1994). The phrase is used in this chapter to denote a broad range of processes and practices commonly adopted by social landlords to inform, consult and involve tenants in decision-making activities. These processes include the involvement of tenants as members of management committees and boards (such as estate management boards) and the devolution of some management functions by landlords to organized groups of tenants. However, two types of involvement have largely been excluded from discussion in this chapter – the transfer of total management responsibility or ownership to tenant groups, and cooperative housing. Organized tenant protest is also excluded, except for a brief discussion when considering the provenance of tenant involvement.

There are three main ways in which tenant involvement is located in the literature. The first and most common way of conceiving of tenant involvement in the good practice literature is as a mutual partnership which is assumed to bring benefits for both tenants and landlord. Thus it is depicted as: 'a two-way process involving sharing of information and ideas, where tenants are able to influence decisions and take part in what is happening' (Institute of Housing and Tenant Participation Advisory Service for England (TPAS) 1989: 9).

This view of tenant participation incorporates elements of both information and influence. It carries dangers of ignoring the differential power positions of landlords and tenants, and potentially encompasses a wide range of distinct processes. Some commentators have begun to disaggregate these processes by distinguishing between 'passive' and 'active' processes (Bines *et al.* 1993). Passive characteristics include some of the elements discussed in Chapter 9, such as the provision of information, the setting of performance indicators and asking tenants for their views. Active characteristics refer to tenant co-option onto landlord decision-making committees, devolution of some powers to organized tenant groups and ultimately the devolution of control to such groups.

This leads us on to the second way of understanding tenant involvement which conceives it as a continuum or hierarchy leading to ever greater levels of control (and responsibility) by tenants. Bines *et al.* (1993) employ the notion of a continuum to describe the potential movement from passive to active tenant involvement. This has similarities with concepts found in the planning and community development literature such as Arnstein's (1969) ladder of citizen participation and Broady and Hedley's (1989) community involvement continuum. These writers seek to identify sets of activities most likely to provide tenants/citizens/users with the greatest degree of influence over decision making. Figure 10.1 depicts a series of steps based on the work of these authors showing the expectation of a progression towards higher levels of involvement. The figure embodies the assumption common to much of the literature that progression towards Step 6 is the ultimate aim and that the higher steps are preferable to those below.

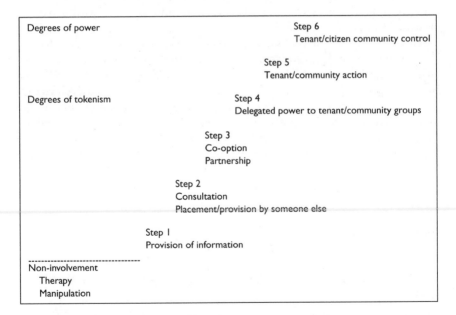

Figure 10.1   Typical model of involvement progression

Source: Derived from Arnstein 1969; Broady and Hedley 1989; Bines *et al.* 1993.

That tenant involvement should aspire to a progression towards tenant control has become a truism of modern social housing management practice. There is no shortage of commentators exhorting social landlords to do this (see, for example, Bartram 1988; Institute of Housing and TPAS 1989; Zipfel 1989; Eversleigh 1994).

While this view is currently dominant, there may be dangers in assuming that all tenants aspire to the highest levels of control and responsibility. A consumerist approach would suggest that provided a good quality of service is available and there are opportunities for redress when things go wrong, most consumers have better things to do with their time than attend committee meetings or manage budgets and staff. It is clearly important that notions of progression through a hierarchy towards control are negotiated with rather than imposed on tenants; the second part of this chapter attempts to demonstrate this through a case study undertaken with older tenants in one large housing association.

A third view of tenant involvement sees it primarily as an accountability mechanism. Here the concern is less with partnership and a hierarchy of participation than with giving tenants and the public some means to find out what decisions social landlords are taking (see, for example, National Housing Federation 1997). Reference to both accountability and tenant control were made in the Housing Corporation's *Tenant Participation Strategy* (1992) which stated: 'The aim ... is to improve accountability to tenants and opportunities for participation and to promote tenant control wherever possible' (p. 23).

This view of tenant participation may be extended to consider the accountability of landlords to groups other than tenants who have an interest in their activities. The Nolan Committee's second report on Local Public Spending Bodies (Committee on Standards in Public Life 1996) develops this notion of accountability by suggesting that housing associations should ensure that their tenant participation strategies are integrated into wider accountability procedures where both tenants and the general public would be the audience. Accountability procedures were also broadened in the report to encompass two dimensions previously identified by Stewart (1993). One was that associations should be capable of giving an account of their actions while the other was that they should be held to account, thus recognizing the range of stakeholders to whom associations have responsibilities, including not only tenants but also the wider public. There are dangers that such approaches may dilute the relationship between landlord and tenant by embracing accountabilities to a wide range of stakeholders, some of whom may have a much less direct interest than tenants. However, the key strengths of the approach lie in enhancing control over the providers of housing, without necessarily overburdening tenants with unwanted responsibilities, and in linking tenant involvement to wider notions of citizenship.

This section has critically reviewed some of the orthodoxies about tenant involvement. Approaches which suggest that there are mutual benefits for landlord and tenant may neglect underlying power and interest differentials. Approaches which suggest the desirability of progression to tenant control may neglect the motivations and interests of tenants and underplay the importance of 'lower levels' of information provision. Approaches based on wider notions of accountability may provide real control and a link with broader citizenship interests, but may dilute the relative importance of the landlord/tenant relationship, as other accountabilities are included. The case study presented in the second part of this chapter explores these issues further. An underlying thesis is that it is important to test ideas about options and processes for tenant involvement with tenants themselves. Such discussion should be sensitive to differences in interests and power between landlord and tenant, and should not make prior assumptions about what are the highest or most desirable forms of involvement. Before introducing the findings of this research, the following section briefly reviews the forces underlying the rise of ideas of tenant involvement in social housing. It is notable that roots relating to self-organization seem to have been over-shadowed in recent years by roots related to the changing social, economic and political context and legislative and regulatory interventions by the state.

The rise of tenant involvement

Any attempt to trace its rise has to acknowledge that tenant involvement falls into two distinct types. One is led by tenants as a form of protest against landlord decisions and the other is led by landlords. Of the two types, organized tenant protest has the longer history although few protests were recorded and published. Some notable exceptions include Moorhouse *et al.* (1972) and Cowley (1979) who examined council tenants' actions to with-hold rent in protest against rent rises, including protest against the introduc-tion of 'fair rents' in 1972, while more recent accounts include Cole and Furbey (1994) and McKenna (1995). There have been many attempts by tenants to take the initiative on tenant involvement, including national organization in relation to specific issues such as rents, tower blocks, and anti-privatization activities, and through ongoing attempts to launch a national tenant body. Arguably these activities have been to some extent 'crowded out' by officially sponsored initiatives. However, the development of the National Tenants Organization in 1977 which joined with the National Tenants and Residents Federation in 1991 to develop a tenant participation charter (Hood and Woods 1994: 64) and the more recent formation of the Housing Association Tenant Organization suggest that the momentum for self-organization will continue to challenge the 'top-down' initiatives of landlords and the state.

As far as social landlords are concerned, limited historical evidence suggests that some were interested in devising tenant involvement strategies in the 1960s and 1970s (Craddock 1975). However, it was not until the 1980s that landlord-led tenant involvement became more widespread and there is little doubt that this was stimulated by central government intervention and legislation (Cole and Furbey 1994). Governmental interventions included the PEP (Priority Estates Project) programme set up in 1979 to deal with 'problem' housing estates, since it was argued that local councils had failed to deal with disrepair and social problems experienced by tenants. Mobilizing tenants could be seen as part of a central government strategy to deal with both physical and social issues. Legislation passed in 1980 and in 1985 provided a stimulus for more landlord-led tenant involvement activities to be initiated. The provisions of the legislation, set out in section 43 of the 1980 and section 105 of the 1985 Housing Acts, were minimal since they placed responsibilities on local authorities and, later in 1985, on housing associations to consult with their tenants on intended housing management changes.

Since 1985 there has been a steady flow of regulatory interventions and financial incentives from central government and the Housing Corporation which have stimulated the growth of tenant involvement activities among a wide range of landlords. The impact of these interventions is indicated in the literature. Work by Cairncross *et al.* (1990a; 1990b) showed that by 1987 80 per cent of local authorities had some formal tenant participation schemes, although this covered all forms of participation including the most basic provision of information to tenants. By 1991/2 more tenant participation activities were being introduced by local authorities and housing associations (Bines *et al.* 1993). For example, it was found that social landlords were commonly providing information for tenants and consulting them, and 78 per cent of local authorities and 75 per cent of housing associations had initiated organized tenants' groups.

For housing associations a major stimulus was provided by the Housing Corporation *Tenant Participation Strategy* (1992) and the Corporation's requirements that registered associations engaged in development should have their own strategies with clear objectives against which to monitor their performance. For all landlords financial incentives included the availability of grants through section 16 of the 1986 Housing and Planning Act. This led many social landlords to appoint tenant participation officers to establish tenant associations and to train tenants (Furbey *et al.* 1996). These grants also stimulated the development of a substantial 'industry' engaged in advising tenants and facilitating participation activities. At the national level bodies such as the TPAS developed as a part of this movement.

For local authorities these developments can be related to a wide range of stimuli. These have included defensive reactions to attacks on local services by Conservative governments in the 1980s and 1990s, the adoption of new programmes which included tenant involvement as an integral element, responses to more general managerial and consumerist strands in public policy, and finally the recognition of the role of tenants as stakeholders in wider political processes.

Local authority landlord reactions to central attacks on services in the 1980s included the development of measures to get closer to tenants and to revitalise local democracy. Decentralization strategies and the development of estate management boards were two examples of this (Cole *et al.* 1988; Burns *et al.* 1994). Later examples of reactions to external threats included activities to organize tenants in the short term to counter the proposals of Tenants' Choice and Housing Action Trusts introduced under the 1988 Housing Act (Woodward 1991; Furbey *et al.* 1996). Most recently the need to involve tenants has arisen from the requirement to consult with tenants before letting contracts under the compulsory competitive tendering (CCT) regime.

New programmes with an integral requirement to involve tenants included stock transfers and other initiatives to regenerate local authority estates. Legislation and guidance on the large scale transfer of ownership of council housing to another landlord insisted that tenants had to be consulted, and the options for and against transfer fairly and impartially presented. This prompted some authorities to involve tenants for the first time, and to engage 'tenants' friends' (consultants) for a brief period before the tenant ballot to decide on stock transfer (Mullins *et al.* 1995). Later, many authorities combined tenant involvement with community development and local economic development activities to take advantage of the Single Regeneration Budget (SRB) and challenge fund opportunities which were introduced in 1994 (Hall *et al.* 1996; Ball 1997). In current urban policy tenant involvement is often cast in a dual role. On the one hand it can provide organized community partners for bids for SRB monies while, on the other, particular resident and tenant groups in certain locations are often identified as people who would benefit from training and employment opportunities through programmes known as 'housing plus'. Housing thus becomes a vehicle to stimulate employment as well as part of the regeneration of the built environment and communities.

More general responses to the new managerialism and consumerism include the adoption of citizens charters and performance indicators which dominated government public policy in the 1990s, and the adoption of user involvement concepts from the wider social welfare field (see Chapter 9).

The 1989 Local Government and Housing Act imposed housing management performance indicators on local authorities and required authorities to publish their performance (including tenant involvement) for tenants on anannual basis. The *Citizen's Charter* introduced in 1991 emphasized consumer interests but was widely criticized for its lack of attention to citizenship (Prior *et al.* 1993; Walsh 1994). The use of managerial tools such as tenant and user satisfaction surveys became commonplace, as did the involvement of tenants and citizens in quality circles or panels on specific aspects of services (Pfeffer and Coote 1991; Skelcher 1993).

The impetus for the re-emergence of user involvement in social welfare services arose from the implementation of care in the community which emphasized choice, empowerment, and normalization to counter insti-tutionalization and dependency (Hoyes *et al.* 1994; Nolan and Caldock 1996). User involvement is most often described as part of the social or health professional assessment and treatment processes (see Walker 1993; Nolan *et al.* 1994). Comparisons between social care user and tenant involvement are most directly drawn in attempts to involve residents in residential care institutions in decisions (Ellis 1993).

A final strand of policy emerged from interest in consumers as stake-holders in the political process (see, for example, Huxham 1996; Barnes 1993). It informed the deliberations of the Nolan Committee and it has become the focus of a critical debate on the role and accountability of quangos and unelected spending bodies – including housing associations – which increasingly provide services to the public (Davis and Spencer 1995; Ewart 1995; Riseborough 1995).

The discussion has so far explained the rise of tenant involvement in the 1980s and 1990s in relation to a variety of stimuli mainly concerning changes in legislation and regulation and the changing role for housing in the broader social, economic and political context. Many of these changes have been contested. Not surprisingly tenant involvement has, therefore, been presented and represented under different guises. Rather less attention has been given to the response of tenants themselves to these initiatives.

Some commentators have suggested that there was a positive response because public services had become bureaucratic and distant from their consumers and tenant involvement provided a way for landlords to recog-nize tenants' legitimate demands. Richardson (1984), for example, asserted that tenant and landlord interests were moving in broadly similar directions. However, Sklair (1975) and Lowe (1986) refer to the effects of the failure of tenants' protest against 'fair rents', during the passage of the 1972 Housing Finance Act, on an emerging national grass roots tenants' association. It depressed tenant-led protest activity and made some concentrate instead on less confrontational relationships with landlords. Saunders (1979) argued that instead of a convergence, social landlords incorporated disaffected tenants into landlord-led tenant involvement activities.

Whether convergence between producer and consumer groups did occur in the evolution of tenant involvement is a contested issue. However, there is little doubt that discourse on tenant involvement since the 1980s primarily focuses on landlord-led efforts to incorporate tenants into structures and processes which will supposedly provide them with some expression of voice Hirschman (1970), a measure of influence and opportunities to participate in decision making. Moreover, tenant involvement commands broad cross-party political support. For example, Burns *et al.* (1994) writing on local authority interest in decentralization and participation, suggest that those on the political left tend to incorporate tenant involvement in strategies to broaden the opportunities available to citizens while those on the right identify tenant involvement as useful consumer activity. Figure 10.2 brings together some of the conflicting representations of tenant involvement which emerge from this chequered history.

So far, the chapter has described tenant involvement, its emergence and the legislative and policy framework which supports it. The discussion has sampled discourse formed by the views of practitioners, policy makers and academics. The second part of the chapter turns to tenants' views and assesses the capacity of tenant involvement to provide tenants with more choice and control. As will be seen the views of tenants challenge some of the representations of tenant involvement that are shown in Figure 10.2.

More choice and control? What tenants say

In 1995 a study involving over 1000 older people living in Anchor Trust properties was undertaken to provide detailed evidence about tenants' views regarding tenant involvement (see Riseborough 1996). At the time the land-lord involved tended to take a paternalistic approach to its provision of housing and services to older people. However, Anchor had been involved in some of the more common tenant involvement activities which were dis-cussed earlier. For example, it provided tenants with information, it carried out regular consultation meetings and had commissioned independent tenant satisfaction surveys which it published to tenants and a wider

---

- A practical activity to engage people-power to deal with run-down housing estates such as the estates action and later the PEP programme introduced by the Department of the Environment from 1979 onwards (Zipfel 1989; Hague 1990).
- An unproblematic partnership between tenants and landlord in pursuit of a mutual interest (Richardson 1984; Institute of Housing and TPAS 1989).
- A process which can empower and constrain tenants (Saunders 1979).
- Part of the response by modern local government and housing associations to (re-)orient themselves to the public and to give an account of their actions (Clarke and Stewart 1987; Housing Corporation 1992).
- An aspect of the public choice brand of consumerism spreading across all public services (Hague 1990).
- Tenants as stakeholders where tenant involvement is a means for social landlords to give an account of their actions and to be held to account for them (Housing Corporation 1992; Committee on Standards in Public Life 1996).

Figure 10.2   Representations of tenant/user involvement

audience (see, for example, Fennel 1986; Riseborough and Niner 1994). In addition, tenants were invited to sit on regional committees and on the board of management. A number of tenant associations existed, although these were primarily social bodies.

The usefulness of these common tenant involvement activities, the appropriateness of common definitions of tenant involvement and their purpose were explored with tenants in qualitative work. The research set out to consider four basic types of involvement: information provision, consultation, tenant representation on committees and devolution of decisions to tenant groups. A less common activity – the use of ballots on important issues – suggested by Anchor tenants was also examined.

Groups of tenants explored the meaning and purpose of tenant involvement and they drew on definitions and representations of tenant involvement which have already been discussed in this chapter (see Figure 10.2). Tenants also examined Arnstein's (1969) ladder, the continuum suggested by Bines *et al.* (1993) and Broady and Hedley's (1989) community involvement continuum (see Figure 10.1).

Anchor tenants for the most part live in sheltered housing which is rarely built as part of an estate plan. The first representation of tenant involvement shown in Figure 10.2 which refers to its usefulness in dealing with run-down housing estates therefore clearly did not apply. Representations that tenant involvement is a purely practical activity which may be pursued by means of an unproblematic partnership between landlords and tenants were heavily contested by tenants. Their responses ran counter to much of the non-academic literature which is purportedly practical and which suggests that tenant involvement is self evidently a good thing. In our research it was impossible to have a meaningful discussion on the usefulness of certain activities without establishing what tenant involvement was for and what it meant. Tenants and researchers grappled with some of the available literature and examples of tenant involvement. Consequently, discussions revealed that the purpose of tenant involvement is far from clear unless tenants know why individual landlords are pursuing it. In the case study, reasons had to be obtained – which involved much discussion with Anchor – and then these reasons had to be explained to the tenants. This part of the research, therefore, indicates that tenants fundamentally questioned the motivation of social landlords 'doing' tenant involvement. One tenant summed this up when he said: 'what's in it for me and what's in it for Anchor?' (Riseborough 1996: 47).

Tenants did not, therefore, take it for granted that their interests and those of landlords would coincide. Comments from tenants on particularly difficult issues, such as their views about changes in Anchor's management practice, provided examples of the kind of subjects where agreement between tenants and the landlord's representatives was unlikely.

In addition, tenants indicated that tenant involvement could be a useful instrument for landlords to exert social control over tenants by, for example, constraining discussion between officers and tenants on contentious issues. These comments echo Saunders' views on the main benefits of tenant action in Croydon during the early 1970s. He contended that the main benefits fell to the state because social control functions are dominant, even where activities are apparently organized to give tenants or users the opportunity to air grievances or to engage in collective struggle (Saunders 1979).

Partnership and power

The Anchor tenants were highly sceptical of the notion that the pursuit of tenant involvement automatically leads to partnerships between tenants and landlords. They pointed out that partnerships develop over time and in that any case there were power differentials between tenants and staff as well as inequalities between individual tenants. For example, while many tenant involvement processes refer to the usefulness of tenant associations and meetings between staff and tenants because they provide opportunities for tenants to voice their views on housing management services and decisions, much depends on the ability and willingness of tenants to do this. Ability to some extent depends on their life experience of attending meetings and their articulateness, both of which raised questions about the usefulness of meetings for less confident, less articulate tenants and for those who were too ill and frail to attend. This suggested that common methods to involve tenants favour particular groups of tenants. It also appeared that these same mechanisms could deepen existing inequalities between tenants.

There appeared to be differences between tenants who were paying full rents and service charges and those who were not. Those who were paying full rents and charges were more likely to feel that they could express a critical view while the others were more reluctant. Not only were the inequalities which people had experienced in their younger lives, such as low income, poor work opportunities and differences in social and economic status persistent in later life, they also formed barriers between tenants. Those tenants who were most willing to attend meetings – including the research discussions – tended to share certain characteristics. Most of them paid some or all of their accommodation costs out of their own pockets and few received even partial housing benefit. In the main they had been owner-occupiers before they came into rented sheltered housing, they were generally very or fairly active with many interests and most were receiving income from occupational or private pensions as well as the state pension. Over three quarters had paid or unpaid experience of management and taking decisions in organizations, including voluntary bodies, and almost all were highly articulate. In contrast those tenants who were less willing to attend discussions and to express a view if they did, tended to be reliant on the state pension as their only source of income and were more likely to be receiving full housing benefit.

Tenants also raised basic questions about the topics and the field of decision making which was created for tenants in tenant involvement strategies. Who, they asked, sets the agenda? Strong views were expressed by tenants on the topics they thought should be part of the agenda for tenant involvement and it was suggested that tenants should be informed about proposed decisions at an early stage so their views could be taken into account before a decision was finally made. Anchor tenants were interested in a broad range of issues and they wanted to influence the content of the agenda. They were interested in matters including appointing staff, service levels, the role of the warden and financial changes. However, as Cairncross *et al.* (1997) confirm, tenant involvement agendas are often extremely narrow. They are usually confined to local management issues which are dictated by professionals who represent the landlord's interests and it is unlikely that professional staff and tenants' interests would necessarily coincide.

Tenants were aware of this divergence in interests and in one discussion group a tenant coined the phrase 'negotiables and non-negotiables' to cover the fact that tenants were keen to know which subjects could be negotiated and which could not. This shrewd comment indicates that older tenants were far from being passive recipients of services. It also indicates they felt that social landlords rather than tenants hold the balance of power. One of the ways this is most palpably demonstrated is through a failure on the part of landlords to involve tenants in the decisions which most affect and concern them. In Anchor's case some of the issues tenants raised, such as being involved in the appointment of staff, are currently being discussed with tenants and efforts are being made to involve tenants in a more equitable way. However, the Anchor study indicates that making changes is a difficult process which may affect the whole of an organization including its culture, staff recruitment and training. Anchor's efforts to recognize these aspects crucially underline the fact that social landlords have to be willing to broaden tenant involvement agendas and to do this in a way that is receptive to tenants' views. Without these movements towards change, tenant involvement has to be seen as, at best, a limited partnership which addresses an agenda which may ignore tenants' concerns.

Yet, through all the twists and turns in the Anchor study tenants repeatedly returned to the theme that tenant involvement was a useful ideal. Saunders (1979) suggested its attractive features include its capacity to disseminate useful information to citizens as well as the hope that it can increase the collective consciousness of groups of people that change is needed. The first of these was frequently referred to by tenants. The second was referred to often at the end of discussions or interviews where tenants commented on the knowledge they had gained or referred to the skills and experience they possessed which would enable them to do tasks better than, or as well as, professional staff and contractors. It is difficult to see how an older tenant consciousness could develop in social rented sheltered housing since the Anchor study underlines the fact that tenants are a heterogeneous group and their differences in status, income, health and education affect relationships between tenants and between tenants and housing staff. As we have seen, tenants distinguished themselves according to age and health/ dependency differences and both dependency and the fear of it appeared to be powerfully divisive. The potential of 'grey' power has not so far been realized in the UK to the extent it has been in the USA (Grayson and Hobson 1995), but there was evidence of a growing awareness of ageism among Anchor tenants and a realization that their consumer and voting power were significant. It is possible that this awareness could begin to overcome the heterogeneity.

Training

Training for tenants to enable them to express their views and to develop tenant groups is often suggested as a way to overcome the difficulties discussed above. In both housing and social care attention to users often denotes a change from traditional paternal provider-user relationships to something which is more equal. Consequently many involvement training programmes are cited which focus on 'empowerment' (Beresford and Croft 1993; Furbey et al. 1996).

However, there are clear differences between the social care model and tenant participation orthodoxy in the treatment of non-involvement by users. Thornton and Trozer (1995), for example, point out that for users of social care services the choice not to take an active part in decisions and meetings is a social right which some of the older and most frail in the population may wish to continue to claim. Walker (1993) and Ellis (1993) writing on the progress of user involvement in community care indicated that power differentials between staff and users are still evident. Moreover they indicate that users are often afraid to speak out because they rely on personal relationships with care professionals and any criticism of these individuals would affect the personal service users receive.

Some Anchor tenants welcomed training provided it would enable tenants and staff to communicate better. Tenants perceived, for example, that officers and tenants sometimes lacked the confidence and the skill to lead meetings. However, it was clear that training would not solve everything and that it would not be welcomed by all tenants and staff. Two key matters that training could not resolve were first ensuring that officers were well informed and briefed so they could answer questions that tenants raised in meetings or in other fora and second, the formation of a common bond. On the second point the heterogeneous nature of the older people in the research sample served to emphasize the lack of common interest between people as tenants. This feature has been remarked on by other researchers, such as Cole and Furbey (1994), in relation to the younger tenant population. Where older tenants are concerned it is often assumed that age provides a common bond, but neither older age nor being tenants provided much of a common bond between the Anchor tenants. Indeed there were indications that tenants' views varied according to their age cohort, gender, income and health or disability. For example, one tenant who was bed-bound (and who was interviewed individually) maintained that, although she had a private income as well as the state pension, she would not say anything that was too critical. She doubted that other tenants would either unless they were paying or they were in pretty good health (Riseborough 1996).

This quote illustrates the sensitive nature of some power differentials which are to some extent peculiar to sheltered and special needs housing provision. They are peculiar in these forms of housing because they stem from non-housing tasks that are performed by resident wardens. Such tasks are rarely codified in tenancy agreements but it is known that warden staff increasingly provide signposting to other care services, advocacy and emergency care and support for short periods of time to tenants (Marsh and Riseborough 1995; Riseborough *et al.* 1996). Since these tasks were not codified, tenants said they were unsure of their rights to expect certain services. Consequently some tenants said they would be unable and/or unwilling to raise these matters in a meeting with staff. One older woman illustrated the point when she observed that 'tenants never know when they might need to call on staff, and so are reluctant to criticize them' (Riseborough 1996).

The issues raised in discussions with tenants also touched on the professional practice of individual members of staff. Issues included a failure to listen or impatience and they provided more evidence that sensitive subjects are difficult for tenants to raise using some of the most common tenant involvement mechanisms like meetings between staff and tenants. On the basis of the research it seems unlikely that training on its own could deal with underlying sensitive issues and matters of fundamental rights. These are aspects which have rarely featured in discussion on tenant involvement, although Saunders (1979) refers to tenant involvement as a process which may empower as well as constrain tenants.

The involvement continuum: tenant priorities

One of the more negative views of tenant involvement is that it is only a consumer or public relations exercise which is not intended to change landlord-tenant relationships. This is partly because some kinds of activities, such as information giving and consultation are dismissed as fairly low-level tenant involvement activities which are consumerist. The Anchor study suggested that tenants do often perceive tenant involvement as a public relations exercise but this may be quite a good rather than a bad aspect of it. From the qualitative and survey work with Anchor's tenants it was clear that tenants attached a high value to information, particularly in plain language. Despite the fact that tenants already received a great deal of information, they wanted more information on financial matters and on the activities and values of Anchor as an organization. Financial matters included the way rents and service charges were worked out and the reasons why charges were increased. Tenants valued information because it enabled them to ask informed questions. Access to information was seen by several interviewees as a prerequisite to any kind of partnership between groups of tenants and the landlord. These findings challenge notions that the provision of information is a low-level or tokenistic tenant involvement activity and suggest instead that having good information is a necessary base for tenant involvement.

In contrast to information-giving, consultation was seen as of limited use by Anchor tenants. In most cases this was because their experience of consultation was not regarded as satisfactory. Their landlord, like other social landlords, is obliged to consult tenants before any major changes, such as rent and service charge increases. However they are not obliged to take tenant views into account. Consequently the Anchor tenants felt they were consulted too late to make a difference and they said the process should either be changed or renamed. If the purpose of consumerism is to smooth over any service delivery problems then consultation exercises at Anchor have backfired and the same may also be true for other social landlords.

Tenants often compared their landlord's efforts at consultation with other consumer experience. They were aware that other services had changed the way they related to customers. Almost all tenants cited examples including complaints procedures and charters of service adopted by former public utilities and many tenants had participated in consumer opinion surveys and generally welcomed these changes. However, tenants commonly made a distinction between something which seemed to be a consumer relations exercise and something which would give them more rights as tenants to challenge things and to make a difference to the outcome. Consultation appeared to do neither.

Tenant representation, or the co-option of tenants onto management committees, was also discussed with the Anchor tenants. This trend has some linkages with the stakeholder notion, which is based on the view that tenants are one of a number of interest groups or constituencies whose interests should be represented in decision making (see National Housing Federation 1997 for further discussion). However, research elsewhere indicates that while the stakeholder idea is attractive, it introduces many practical problems in relation to tenant involvement, for example concerning the formation of constituencies, the process of electing or selecting tenants to represent others and what representation means. Practice is variable, with some associations electing tenant board members from an election of all tenants (see Chapter 6), but most using more limited electorates such as tenant membership which is often low, or co-options from tenant associations which may not be supported by all tenants. Currently, the majority of social landlords select rather than elect tenants and although some advertise these positions and encourage tenants to put themselves forward others do not. The role played by tenants as members of boards of management is also problematic and ambiguous. The requirement for tenant members to pursue the best interests of the association rather than to represent tenants interests is embedded in the constitutions and governing instruments of housing associations. This parallels the conflicts of loyalty faced by local authority nominees on housing association boards (Mullins and McCann 1997). The uncertain role of tenant members was confirmed by a chief executive of a major housing association with a regional committee structure which fed into a board who said that tenant representatives were expected to represent the region's interests on the board, not other tenants (see Mullins and Riseborough 1997 for further discussion).

The Anchor tenants were aware of these problems and were generally not convinced about the usefulness of having tenant representation on boards for two particular reasons. First, because very few of the tenants had received any feedback from existing representatives and second, because representatives were selected and therefore had no mandate to represent other tenants in any case. Thus while the idea of representation and the notion of being stakeholders were regarded as good in principle, there was still a long way to go before they could be regarded as useful or even legitimate in practice.

Returning to the involvement continuum, the last two 'stages' are the devolution of housing management tasks to tenants and tenant control. Some, rather than all, Anchor tenants were interested in taking over particular tasks such as gardening and dealing with contractors in their sheltered scheme or across several local schemes. Tenants were much more interested in having greater influence over the decisions that were made and having some evidence to indicate that their views were listened to by staff. There was little or no interest in having total control over the sheltered scheme or a group of schemes.

With regard to more active forms of participation, such as delegation of power and responsibility to residents' groups, there was a general willingness on the part of many tenants to work towards some sort of partnership with Anchor. However, it was clear that the vast majority of tenants who were interested wanted to participate in specific activities for short periods of time rather than in all activities for prolonged periods. It was also suggested that partnership processes had to be gradually agreed between tenants and between tenants and staff at a local level. Interestingly, tenants suggested three additional processes in partnership building which are often overlooked in standard approaches to tenant involvement. They were:

1 Influence
2 Collaboration
3 Secret ballots

The first process refers to the tenants' wish to influence their landlord's decisions. It was thought that landlords should ask tenants for their views regularly and give their views sufficient weight. The Anchor tenants acknowledged that individual efforts to secure influence could be inequitable since it was likely that the loudest and most articulate tenants would be listened to rather than everyone. However, part of the reason for the inequity was thought to stem from the lack of sufficiently varied opportunities provided by landlords for different tenants to give their views and tenants also had little evidence that their views were taken into account by landlords. A similar point was made by Bines *et al.* (1993) when they indicated that tenant participation was unlikely to give tenants a measure of influence.

The second process suggested by the Anchor tenants was collaboration. Tenants felt that there were particular occasions where joint projects between staff and tenants would be useful to provide a practical way of working together. For example, in scheme design or when major changes were being contemplated in the organization.

The final process proposed by Anchor tenants is rarely discussed in the literature on tenant involvement. Tenants suggested that secret ballots or referendums were the most democratic and independent mechanism which provided all tenants with an opportunity to give an honest opinion on important and sensitive issues such as the role of the warden.

So to some extent tenants confirmed the notion that tenant involvement can be seen as a progression or a series of steps which may eventually result in a partnership between sets of tenants and the landlord's representatives, but they indicated that their interest in tenant control, often seen as the ultimate objective of tenant involvement, was negligible. The reasons for this were partly because older tenants maintained their interests were different to those of younger groups and various kinds of difference were suggested. For example, it was felt that older tenants had shorter time horizons than younger tenants; older tenants wanted to choose the degree of involvement they had; and it was suggested repeatedly that living in sheltered housing was different to living in 'ordinary' housing. But, in addition to these perceived differences the Anchor tenants also referred to their right and preference not to participate in tenant involvement. Reasons for not participating included the fact that tenants were paying professional staff to do management tasks and to take decisions and because tenants had more interesting things to do as part of enjoying retirement. However, rights and preferences not to participate seem to be peculiarly absent from most of the discourse on tenant involvement. This is because the discourse for tenant involvement has taken on a distinctly moral flavour.

The intrusion of morality

Most of the reasons the Anchor tenants gave for not getting involved have received little or no mention in discourse on tenant involvement, although non-involvement in social housing is sometimes portrayed as apathy and evidence of social alienation. The benefits of being involved on the other hand are often depicted in glowing terms. They include building better communities; providing therapeutic communities for older people and those with special needs; overcoming social exclusion; dealing with disrepair; tackling crime and vandalism; and encouraging unemployed social tenants to develop their confidence and skills (see Power 1997; while Cole *et al.* 1997 give a critical discussion). To some extent these benefits can be discerned in other discourses on user involvement in health and social care and in discussion on urban regeneration initiatives which depend on involving local residents, and the overall message in these discourses is that cooperation between ordinary citizens, residents and users together with professionals and politicians will contribute to an improved quality of life for everyone. Opting out is, therefore, not part of the message.

There is little doubt that tenant and user involvement is popular with some groups of tenants. Studies on health and social care show that involvement in decision making has given some of the most disadvantaged and marginalized groups the chance to shape their own lives for the first time (see, for example, Ellis 1993). But, the Anchor study provides the forceful message that it should not be assumed that all tenants need or want tenant involvement. Moreover it suggests that any slavish adoption of tenant involvement practices by social landlords is not to be recommended unreservedly since it may make it even harder for those less articulate and frail tenants to express a view while it also appears to deny tenants the choice – and the right – to become involved on their own terms rather than those of the landlord, or even not at all.

However, the popularization of tenant involvement and the continued pressure on social landlords to ensure that it is introduced and encouraged mitigate against recognizing that there are subtle and sensitive issues which cannot be identified or discussed simply by using standard tenant involvement approaches.

Conclusion

This chapter has pursued the question: does tenant involvement provide tenants with more choice and control? This has also involved considering the value of tenant involvement as an activity to enhance the experience of citizenship. Answers clearly depend on what kind of tenant involvement is being talked about. The chapter has tried to pin this down by identifying the most common kinds of involvement, discussing the most frequent types of practices and procedures, their stated objectives, and the way tenant involvement is represented in discourse. The chapter has drawn on recent detailed empirical research to test out the benefits of tenant involvement from the point of view of older tenants and it has compared their views with those of professional practitioners and academic commentators whose discussions emerge from several different discourses. The evidence presented indicates that answers to the question of whether or not tenant involvement gives tenants more choice and control depend on whose interests are being served by tenant involvement – the tenants', the landlord's or both?

The chapter has illustrated the persistent appeal of tenant involvement despite changes in the social and political context. For example, it has been shown that although some activities are commonly pursued under the guise of tenant involvement it is capable of being represented in various, often contradictory, ways. These representations stem from several rather than one single discourse and each have linkages with other social and political forces. One underlying message is the maxim that tenant involvement is good for you. The moral flavour of this is inescapable, but why have social housing tenants been singled out for special attention?

So far the evidence suggests that social landlords have been directed and pressured to 'do tenant involvement' as a result of central control through regulation and funding. Resident and user involvement has also continued to grow but not on the same scale or with the same degree of central direction and monitoring as for tenant involvement. This suggests that social landlords were not particularly willing in the main to hand over control functions to tenants. It also suggests that social tenants are somehow seen to need to be involved more than those in other tenures. Does this mean that social tenants are perceived as a social problem or are they seen as the victims of structural and pervasive inequality which results in many of them being socially and economically excluded? Either way the implication is that social control is a paramount function of involvement, although the analysis of the issue is different. Consequently, tenants are cast in the role of the oppressed who need to be empowered, are seen as useful unpaid actors who can help solve social problems or are given walk-on parts as consumers. All of these roles were uncovered in the Anchor study but none of them were necessarily of interest to the tenants themselves.

There is evidence that the origins of the recent rise of tenant involvement may be understood as incorporation of tenant activity by the state. However, over time the discourse has become more complex and shifted to accommodate different political arguments. A consistent feature has been the unresolved tension between the notion of tenant involvement as a consumer activity and the notion that it strengthens citizenship. Yet, as Chapter 1 discussed there are also several versions of citizenship and the appropriate balance between rights and obligations. The search for mechanisms to include citizens whose interests are not represented in the parliamentary or local government democratic process dominated discussion in the 1970s under the label of pluralism and re-emerged during the 1990s in the governance debates. This has in many ways brought about a political convergence in favour of tenant involvement. The partnership metaphor which has dominated much practitioner literature on tenant involvement can be seen as a symptom of convergence, although in the Anchor study it was found wanting, not least because of the power differentials already referred to between professional staff and tenants. These have the capacity to be as disabling in the 1990s as power differentials between social care professionals and users were discovered to be in the 1970s (Illich *et al.* 1977). Moreover, the Anchor tenants underlined the fact that partnerships have to be worked out with clear terms of reference that are agreed by both sides – they cannot simply be presumed to exist.

Tenant representation on committees and boards of management was sometimes viewed with outright hostility by the Anchor tenants since the roles of representatives and their duties to other tenants were not clear. This suggests that the popular stakeholder notion is interesting in principle but problematic in practice and further thought needs to be given to the notion to make it work. Likewise, tenant control, which is often seen as the goal of tenant involvement, did not interest tenants at all. The Anchor tenants were suspicious of the motivations that landlords had for pursuing this goal particularly when tenants' rents and service charges remained the same. Taken together these factors suggest that the conceptualization of tenant involvement as a series of progressive steps with tenant control as the goal is not appropriate. It is too simplistic, overlooks time constraints and the other commitments and interests tenants have, denies choice over the degree to which they want to be involved and disregards the interests of tenants who do not want to be involved at all. Moreover these steps may be more effective in increasing citizenship obligations than in enhancing tenants rights as citizens.

This chapter also indicates that tenant involvement cannot solve everything. It cannot tackle fundamental social inequalities and power differentials between tenants and between staff and tenants. The study underlines the fact that the most assertive tenants were 'paying' and felt 'well'. They formed a different relationship with their landlords than those who were dependent on welfare income and who felt in less good health. It is possible that tenant involvement approaches which ignore the existence of inequality between tenants will deepen such inequality.

We used data from a study on older sheltered tenants who are rarely mentioned in published accounts. The discussion has shown that sheltered housing tenants perceive that their experience of housing is distinctive. The study highlighted the need for a codification of the non-housing tasks sheltered staff carry out and the discussion suggests that more care should be taken over the interactions between staff and older people in sheltered housing. Tenant involvement practice makes little or no reference to these aspects at the present time and social care literature is more helpful. In these respects tenant involvement does not offer older sheltered tenants more choice and control. While tenant and staff training may improve communication on less sensitive subjects, the study suggests that where highly personal matters and rights are concerned, tenant involvement practice is unlikely to provide anything extra for tenants of any age.

While some of the misgivings older tenants expressed about tenant involvement may be unique to sheltered tenants the chapter contends that many misgivings over the process, the purpose and the agenda are likely to be shared by younger groups as well. Some of the subtleties revealed in the study are likely to be overlooked because tenant involvement is often based on assumptions about tenants and landlords having common interests and because issues of power and inequality are ignored. These assumptions help to maintain a silence on staff and tenant power differentials as well as on inequalities between tenants. The silence in itself is a powerful manifestation of social control.

Thus, while tenant involvement is an attractive ideal with a persuasive and seductive set of discourses and it serves the interests of some organized groups of tenants, it does not serve the interests of all tenants. Moreover, landlords who usually devise the agenda, process and mechanisms of tenant involvement have vested interests which diverge from those of tenants. This is not to say that tenant involvement is inevitably likely to serve landlord rather than tenants' interests, but it is more likely to unless efforts are explicitly made by landlords to give tenants and staff opportunities to explore the terms of engagement. The 1997 Labour government has indicated its intention to build sustainable communities and overcome social exclusion, so it is likely that tenant involvement will continue to have a prominent role in this new agenda.

Note on the study

The study was a collaborative research exercise with users which involved qualitative and quantitative research instruments. The qualitative work was composed of group interviews and workshops with 90 residents and individual in-depth interviews with 15 other residents. The quantitative work was a postal survey of 1500 other residents. The residents who took part in the study were selected for their representativeness of the Anchor resident population as a whole in terms of their age cohort, gender and the geographical spread of Anchor housing.

References

Arnstein, S. (1969) A ladder of citizen participation. *Journal of American Institute of Planners*, 35(4): 214–24.

Ball, H. (1997) Building on effective partnerships: the paymaster calls the tune?, in M. Riseborough (ed.) *Different Voices. Research and Practice on the Voluntary, Community and Not For Profit Sector: West Midlands Perspectives*. Birmingham: Centre for Urban and Regional Studies, University of Birmingham.

Barnes, M. (1993) Introducing new stakeholders: user and researcher interests in evaluative research. *Policy and Politics*, 21: 47–58.

Bartram, M. (1988) *Council Tenants: Council Initiatives in the Late 1980s*. London: Community Rights Project.

Bengtsson, B. (1994) Tenants dilemma: on collective action in housing. Conference paper, European Network of Housing Research conference, Glasgow, 29 August– 2 September.

Beresford, P. and Croft, S. (1993) *Citizen Involvement: A Practical Guide for Change*. London: British Association of Social Workers/Macmillan.

Bines, W., Kemp, P., Pleace, N. and Radley, C. (1993) *Managing Social Housing*. London: HMSO.

Broady, M. and Hedley, R. (1989) *Working Partnerships: Community Development in Local Authorities*. London: Bedford Square Press for the Coalition of Local Authorities.

Burns, D., Hambleton, R. and Hoggett, P. (1994) *The Politics of Decentralisation: Revitalising Local Democracy*. London: Macmillan.

Cairncross, L., Clapham, D. and Goodlad, R. (1990a) *The Pattern of Tenant Participation in Council Housing Management*, Discussion paper no. 31. Glasgow: Centre for Housing Research, University of Glasgow.

Cairncross, L., Clapham, D. and Goodlad, R. (1990b) *Tenant Participation in Council Housing*. York: Joseph Rowntree Foundation.

Cairncross, L., Clapham, D. and Goodlad, R. (1997) *Housing Management, Consumers and Citizens*. London: Routledge.

Clarke, M. and Stewart, J. (1987) The public service orientation: issues and dilemmas. *Public Administration*, 65(2): 161–77.

Cole, I., Windle, K. and Arnold, P. (1988) *The Impact of Decentralization*, Housing Decentralization Research Project Working Paper 3. Sheffield: Department of Urban and Regional Studies, Sheffield Polytechnic.

Cole, I. and Furbey, R. (1994) *The Eclipse of Council Housing*. London: Routledge.

Cole, I., Gridley, G., Ritchie, C., Simpson, D. and Radley, C. (1997) *Creating Communities or Welfare Housing: A Study of New Housing Association Developments in Yorkshire and Humberside*. York: Joseph Rowntree Foundation.

Committee on Standards in Public Life (1996) *Second Report: Local Public Spending Bodies*. London: HMSO.

Cowley, J. (1979) *Housing for People or for Profit?* London: Stage One Publishing.

Craddock, J. (1975) *Council Tenants' Participation in Housing Management*. London ALHE.

Davis, H. and Spencer, K. (1995) *Housing Associations and the Governance Debate*. Birmingham: School of Public Policy, University of Birmingham.

Ellis, K. (1993) *Squaring the Circle*. York: Joseph Rowntree Foundation.

Eversleigh, J. (1994) *Getting Involved*. London: Association of London Authorities/Association of Metropolitan Authorities.

Ewart, A. (1995) Emerging issues of organisation and strategy in housing associations. Conference paper, Housing Studies Association Conference, University of Edinburgh, September.

Fennel, G. (1986) *Anchor's Older People: What Do They Think? A Survey Amongst Tenants Living in Sheltered Housing*. Oxford: Anchor Housing Association.

Furbey, R., Wishart, B. and Grayson, J. (1996) Training for tenants: 'citizens' and the enterprise culture. *Housing Studies*, 11: 251–70.

Grayson, L. and Hobson, M. (eds) (1995) *INLOGOV Informs On The Third Age*, issue 2, vol. 4. Birmingham: Institute of Local Government Studies, University of Birmingham.

Hague, C. (1990) The development and politics of tenant participation in British council housing. *Housing Studies*, 5: 242–56.

Hall, S., Beazley, M., Burfitt, A. *et al.* (1996) *The Single Regeneration Budget: A Review of Challenge Fund Round II*, Centre for Urban and Regional Studies. Birmingham: University of Birmingham.

Hirschman, A.O. (1970) *Exit, Voice and Loyalty: Responses to Declines in Firms, Organizations and States*. Cambridge, MA: Harvard University Press.

Hoggett, P. and Hambleton, R. (1987) *Decentralisation and Democracy: Localising Public Services*, School for Advanced Urban Studies Occasional Paper. Bristol: University of Bristol.

Hood, M. and Woods, R. (1994) Women and participation, in R. Gilroy and R. Woods (eds) *Housing Women*. London: Routledge.

Housing Corporation (1992) *Tenant Participation Strategy*. London: Housing Corporation.

Hoyes, L., Lart, R., Means, R. and Taylor, M. (1994) *Community Care in Transition*. York: Joseph Rowntree Foundation.

Huxham, C. (ed.) (1996) *Creating Collaborative Advantage*. London: Sage.

Illich I., Zola, I., McKnight, J., Caplan, J. and Shaiken, H. (1977) *Disabling Professions*. London: Boyars.

Institute of Housing and Tenant Participation Advisory Service for England (1989) *Tenant Participation in Housing Management*. Coventry/Salford: IOH/TPAS.

Lowe, S. (1986) *Urban Social Movements*. New York: St Martin's Press.

Marsh, A. and Riseborough, M. (1995) *Making Ends Meet: Older People, Housing Association Costs and the Affordability of Rented Housing*. London: National Federation of Housing Associations.

McKenna, D. (1995) 'Talking gets you nowhere: critical and tenant centred approaches to participation in the management of council housing', unpublished MSc dissertation. Centre for Housing Management and Development, UWCC.

Moorhouse, B., Wilson, M. and Chamberlain, L. (1972). Rent strikes: direct action and the working class, in R. Miliband and J. Saville (eds) *The Socialist Register*. London: Merlin Press.

Mullins, D. and McCann, S. (1997) Stock transfers create conflicts of interest. *Housing Agenda*, July/August: 20–1.

Mullins, D. and Riseborough, M. (1997) *Changing With The Times: Critical Interpretations of the Repositioning of Housing Associations*, School for Public Policy Occasional Paper 12. Birmingham: University of Birmingham.

Mullins, D., Niner, P. and Riseborough, M. (1995) *Evaluating Large Scale Voluntary Transfers of Local Authority Housing: A Final Report*. London: HMSO.

National Housing Federation (1997) *Action for Accountability. A Guide for Independent Landlords*. London: NHF.

Nolan, M. and Caldock, K. (1996) Assessment: identifying the barriers to good practice. *Health and Social Care in the Community*, 4: 77–85.

Pfeffer, N. and Coote, A. (1991) *Is Quality Good For You? A Critical Assurance of Quality in Welfare*. London: Institute for Public Policy Research.

Power, A. (1997) *Estates on the Edge: The Social Consequences of Mass Housing in Northern Europe*. London: Macmillan.

Prior, D., Stewart, J. and Walsh, K. (1993). *Is the Citizen's Charter a Charter for Citizens?* Belgrave papers no. 7. London: Local Government Management Board.

Richardson, A. (1984) *Participation*. London: Routledge and Kegan Paul.

Riseborough, M. (1995) Housing associations: voluntary, charity or non-profit bodies? Conference paper, The National Council for Voluntary Organizations 'Researching the Voluntary Sector' conference, London, 7–8 September.

Riseborough, M. (1996) *Listening to and Involving Older Tenants in Decision Making*. Oxford: Anchor Housing Trust.

Riseborough, M. and Niner, P. (1994) *I Didn't Know You Cared: A Survey of Anchor's Sheltered Housing Tenants*. Oxford: Anchor Trust.

Riseborough, M., Mullins, D. and Marsh, A. (1996) *Creating a Shared Vision: The Housing, Support and Care Needs of Older People in South Warwickshire*, report prepared for JCPT South Warwickshire (subgroup, elderly). Birmingham: Centre for Urban and Regional Studies.

Saunders, P. (1979) *Urban Politics: A Sociological Interpretation*. Harmondsworth: Penguin.

Skeffington, A.M. (1968) *People and Planning*. London: HMSO.

Skelcher, C. (1993) Involvement and empowerment in local public services. *Public Money and Management*, 13: 13–20.

Sklair, L. (1975) The struggle against the Housing Finance Act, in R. Miliband and J. Saville (eds) *The Socialist Register*. London: Merlin Press.

Somerville, P. and Steele, A. (1995) Making sense of tenant participation. *Netherlands Journal of Housing and the Built Environment*, 10: 259–81.

Stewart, J. (1993) Defending public accountability. *DEMOS Quarterly*, Winter.

Thornton, P. and Trozer, R. (1995) *Having a Say in Change: Older People and Community Change*. York: Joseph Rowntree Foundation.

Walker, A. (1993) Increasing the participation of older people in social care: a right and a challenge. Conference paper, the international conference 'Innovation and Participation in Care for the Elderly – Italy meets Europe', Rome, 22–24 May.

Walsh, K. (1994) Citizens, charters and contracts, in R. Keat, N. Whiteley and N. Abercrombie (eds) *The Authority of the Consumer*. London: Routledge.

Woodward, R. (1991) Mobilising opposition: the campaign against housing action trusts in Tower Hamlets. *Housing Studies*, 6: 44–56.

Zipfel, T. (1989) *Estate Management Boards: An Introduction*. London: Priority Estates Project.

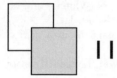

11

Rhetoric and reality in housing policy

David Mullins

Introduction

This book has drawn on the themes of citizenship, choice and control as lenses through which public policy changes can been viewed. The preceding chapters have covered a wide range of issues, and while our main focus has been on housing policy in Britain in the 1980s and 1990s we have also included examples from a longer timespan and a wider range of societies. This has helped us to clarify some of the different ways in which the concepts of citizenship, choice and control have influenced and been drawn on to support specific public policy interventions. It has also provided us with the opportunity to observe the changing definitions of the terms and the new relationships which have emerged as policies underpinned by these ideas have been implemented. In particular it has sharpened our awareness of the range of rhetorical uses of these terms by policy brokers and implementors and of the gaps which frequently begin to appear between rhetoric and reality as these policies are implemented.

This chapter begins by considering some of these rhetorical uses, drawing on examples from the preceding chapters. It then goes on to observe some common conjunctions of citizenship, choice and control. A final section comments on some of the possible reasons for the gap between rhetoric and reality, ending by returning to the question of what drives change in the housing system and the relative importance of policy.

Rhetorical usages: how have the three concepts been employed at political and policy levels?

Choice

A content analysis of a sample of recent housing policy documents in Britain would almost certainly find the incidence of the use of the term 'choice' outnumbering that of the other two members of our conceptual triumvirate many times over. Our case studies include consideration of a government consultation paper *More Choice in the Social Rented Sector* (DoE 1995), while one of the least popular of the third term Conservative housing reforms was inappropriately baptised 'Tenants' Choice'. Advocates of Common Housing Registers often make great play of their potential role in increasing applicants' choice. Similarly, in relation to community care policies, key policy documents such as *Caring for People* (Department of Health 1989a) and *Working for Patients* (Department of Health 1989b) make frequent reference to the importance of increasing user choice (Bartlett and Le Grand 1993). More generally, it has become common to refer to owner occupation as the tenure of choice, and to use this to pursue policies which have promoted the expansion of this sector.

The varied ideological roots of the concept of choice were briefly explored in Chapter 1. For the most part the case studies in the later chapters reflect the dominance of economic thinking in the rationale presented for policies which seek to promote choice in housing policy. These policies draw particularly on behavioural models from economics, which envision individual consumers making rational choices in unfettered markets. There are also strong influences from the public choice critique of public sector bureaucracies, supporting quasi-markets and the fragmentation of social housing provision. In comparison, relatively limited connections are made with either the idea of autonomy embodied in T.H. Marshall's (1950) concept of citizenship or the concepts of 'choice in use' which are closer to Hirschman's (1970) notion of 'voice' than of 'exit'.

Nowhere is the impact of economic thinking about choice more apparent than in policies promoting the extension of owner occupation. There has been a tendency for the concept of choice to be hijacked by advocates of market provision and by supporters of home ownership. Chapter 4 traces the origins and promotion of home ownership in Britain, demonstrating the importance of references to the promotion of individual choice in government publications and political debates on the subject. The failing promises of an increasingly differentiated home ownership sector have been ignored or marginalized in the political discourse. Meanwhile, the putative advantages to the individual and society of home ownership have been expressed in relation to concepts of choice specifically related to tenure.

What this discourse ignores is that choice is not an attribute exclusive to or inherent in any one tenure, and that choice between and within tenures has varied over time and between social groups as a result of a range of contingent factors. Thus, there is a tendency to generalize about the benefits of home ownership, despite the very different experiences of owners in different income groups, household types, geographical locations and property types. The irrelevance of such choices to households dependent on benefits, or on low and unstable incomes is also conveniently ignored. Similarly there is a tendency to emphasize the greater potential choices available to home owners, compared with those in other tenures. Most importantly, the contingent factors associated with the 'golden age' of home ownership, including a rapidly expanding market, continuous rises in property values, tax and fiscal policy advantages, and a social security safety net are frequently underplayed. Thus the strategy of presenting owner occupation as a natural choice has been effective in structuring significant public policy intervention to influence the market. This has ensured the limited relevance to understanding the sector of precisely those free market assumptions on which the ideology is based.

Turning to usages of the concept of choice in relation to social housing, the most striking issues discussed in the earlier chapters are those associated with the demuncipalization and fragmentation of the social housing sector. Chapter 6 discusses the various changes associated with the restructuring of social rented housing in Britain in the 1980s and 1990s. Both the short-lived Tenants' Choice policy and the consultation paper on *More Choice* (DoE 1995) are primarily concerned with reducing the power of monopoly or near-monopoly providers of social housing. Again the underlying reference is to enabling sovereign consumers to make rational choices between a number of alternative potential providers of their housing service. However, in practice these choices have been very constrained. Under both Tenants' Choice and the much more effective Large Scale Voluntary Transfer programme, tenants have only a very limited choice. This occurs at just one point in the process when they are balloted on either changing or retaining their landlord. Nevertheless, the existence of this choice had a substantial impact on their relationship with their new quasi-monopoly landlord after stock transfer. As a result of promises made to secure a positive ballot result, tenants who transferred from the local authority usually enjoyed more favourable tenancy and rent terms than new tenants joining after the transfer.

The recent restructuring of social housing has been much more concerned with extending choices available to the funders of social housing than to the users. This has been achieved through the extension of quasi-market principles to the purchase of new housing developments by the Housing Corporation and, on a smaller scale, by local authorities. The consequences of these arrangements for housing applicants are discussed in Chapter 8. Faced with a wide variety of local social housing providers, it has been argued that applicants' choices can be enhanced by establishing Common Housing

Registers which access lettings from a range of participating landlords. However, the generally limited supply of social housing and dominance of control processes in access arrangements has meant that, in practice, far from consumer choice being extended, it has been reduced – the price paid for the restoration of fair rationing.

Citizenship

Explicit references to citizenship in housing policy discourse have been comparatively rare in the case studies explored in this book. While William Beveridge's *Pillars of Security* (Beveridge 1942) provides a common reference point for discussions about the social rights of citizenship, housing is generally notable by its absence from these debates. The position of housing as a 'wobbly pillar under the welfare state' (Torgerson 1987) is illustrated by the virtual absence of references to housing provision, except as a potential barrier to social inclusion, in a recent volume produced to explore the contemporary relevance of T.H. Marshall (Bulmer and Rees 1996). Attempts by housing providers to resurrect the role of housing in welfare in the late 1990s by picking up on the incoming prime minister's inclusion of housing as one of 'seven pillars of a decent society', has an eerie resonance here (NHF 1997a). However, even where not explicitly presented in terms of the citizenship debate, policies such as the prevention of homelessness, access to housing and indeed the promotion of owner occupation have their rationale in particular conceptions of the social rights of citizenship.

Moreover, an increasing focus of the housing debate on issues of social exclusion and regeneration has arguably rekindled awareness of and reference to citizenship in British housing policy in recent years. Chapter 3 outlined the contours of the debate on housing and social exclusion, and the ambiguous role of housing as a social right of citizenship. It establishes that there has been an increasingly explicit policy focus on programmes to tackle localized social exclusion, for example through the Single Regeneration Budget. A 1997 announcement by the incoming Labour government establishing its Social Exclusion Unit made a direct link between social exclusion and particular housing estates and urban areas. The chapter provides a useful corrective to the view that the relationship between housing and poverty should be viewed in terms of tenure alone.

A cross-national perspective on citizenship and housing is provided in Chapter 2. By comparing differences in the boundaries constructed around citizenship, the social rights of citizenship in Britain, Germany and Australia can be clarified. This introduces the use of citizenship as either an inclusionary or an exclusionary device with formulations such as the Australian 'wage earners' welfare state', and the dominance of patriarchal and racially constructed welfare regimes illustrating the potential social exclusion embedded in popular conceptions of citizenship. Further demonstration of the shifting boundaries of the social rights of citizenship is provided by the case study of homelessness policies in Chapter 8. Over the 20 years since a partial right of citizens to housing was enshrined in legislation by placing duties on local authorities to assist homeless people there has been a continuous contest over the boundaries of these rights. The use of citizenship as an exclusionary device emerges particularly clearly in the interaction between housing and immigration legislation, and specifically in the Asylum and Immigration Appeals Act 1993 which qualified the homelessness duties of local authorities towards asylum seekers and their dependants.

Chapters 9 and 10 review two areas of recent policy development where the concept of citizenship has been used rather more explicitly. However, in both cases its influence has been in the promotion of a rather weak form of political rights rather than social rights. Rather nebulous political rights to be involved and to receive certain specific information from your landlord appear to be increasingly replacing social rights to good quality affordable housing as the focus of concern. This is occurring just as the problem of under-investment in the social housing stock becomes associated with unacceptable levels of disrepair and lack of amenity.

Two examples of the rise of 'charterism' in housing were the requirement for local authorities to publish annual performance reports for their tenants, and the lesser known *Park Home Owners' Charter* for owners of mobile homes. In both cases the language of citizenship disguises a very limited contribution to either the enhancement of the rights and obligations of citizenship or the 'voice' of service users. Like other aspects of the *Citizen's Charter*, these measures are found to have more in common with consumerism, providing information which might theoretically be used by consumers to shop around and 'exit' from unsatisfactory relationships with suppliers (Symon and Walker 1995). In practice, users are often unable to use the information in this way since few of the underlying assumptions of rational consumers negotiating in perfect markets apply to either park homeowners or council tenants.

The rise of tenant involvement was a central feature of policy debates on social housing management in Britain in the 1990s. Again the rhetoric of citizenship has been an important part of a complex policy discourse which led to the adoption of tenant involvement policies by a wide range of social landlords in Britain. One of the myriad of potential benefits claimed for tenant involvement programmes has been their potential contribution to overcoming social exclusion. Yet singling out social housing tenants for this special treatment raises important questions about the citizenship rights of a group who are depicted as oppressed and needing empowerment. Moreover, the lack of account taken of tenants' views in imposing notions such as the desirability of progression towards higher levels of control (and responsibility) for their housing indicates that the practice of tenant involvement has, ironically, been dominated by producer interests and the state.

Control

Not surprisingly, the notion of control has been more rarely used as a rhetorical device in setting the housing policy agenda in the 1980s and 1990s. Arguably the government's main interests in control are twofold: to retain as much as possible for itself, while maintaining the illusion of autonomy and choice for as many other constituencies as possible. If this is the case it is hardly likely that control will feature strongly in the policy rhetoric. Policies openly espousing central control will not attract the support of other constituencies, while policies dispersing control are not likely to be pursued in the first place. Thus our discussion of control issues has been mainly concerned with uncovering the reality behind the rhetoric of policies which espouse choice and citizenship, a subject which we return to later in this chapter. That said there are at least three areas in which there has been a policy rhetoric concerned directly with either control or decontrol.

The first of these areas concerns the finance and regulation of social housing, some aspects of which are discussed in Chapter 7. The ever-present emphasis on achieving value for taxpayers money in housing subsidies, together with the increasing risk involved in privatization programmes have acted as a powerful justification for the need to maintain a strong element of central control. Chapter 7 discusses the impact of these pressures on the financial relationship between central government and local authorities. The chapter describes how throughout the history of council housing, central government has used a mixture of financial incentives and disincentives, and occasionally the force of law, to encourage local authorities to follow central objectives. Periods of crisis in the relationship have occurred when there have been significant differences between central and local objectives and tools of central control have been insufficient to prevail. One example of this was the period prior to the 1989 Local Government and Housing Act when the majority of authorities outside London had zero central subsidy entitlements and were therefore outside central control. A similar crisis for the personal housing subsidy system occurred in the mid-1990s when the full impact of private sector rent decontrol, housing association privatization and reduced capital subsidies saw expenditure on housing benefit rocketing beyond the immediate control of the Department of Social Security. Arguments for central control and regulation are also widely used in relation to the housing association sector, here with additional force to mitigate the risks of increasing levels of private borrowing, and again with variable results in practice (Mullins 1997).

A second context in which arguments for control have been to the fore in recent housing policy is in relation to the accountability of provider organizations. We have already discussed the case of tenant involvement, which is subjected to critical evaluation in Chapter 10. One of the underlying orthodoxies is that tenant involvement should progress towards the highest levels of control by users, apparently regardless of the views or inclinations of tenants themselves. In this respect the tenant involvement orthodoxy is found to differ from that in other social welfare fields where the right to remain a passive consumer is seen as a legitimate aspect of citizenship. The wider question of accountability and control of social housing is discussed in Chapter 6. This has become a central feature of policy rhetoric in recent years as a result of the inclusion of housing in the Local Public Spending Body debate. Fragmentation of new provision, transfers of local authority stock, and a general questioning of the accountability mechanisms of housing associations has led to a significant volume of activity concerning the governance and accountability aspects of control of individual provider organizations. This activity appears to be converging on a stakeholder model, which requires organizations to develop effective accountability arrangements to a wide range of interest groups (NHF 1997b). These developments are in tune with a housing policy climate which is placing an increasing emphasis on meeting objectives rather than the interests of providers. However, the technical problems faced by providers in meeting a range of conflicting accountabilities suggest that new hierarchies of control will emerge.

A third prominent use of the language of control in policy rhetoric is of course in relation to deregulation or decontrol. Nowhere has this rhetoric been more central to housing policy in Britain than in relation to the private rented sector. Chapter 5 reviews the changing policies towards the private rented sector, and the cycle of control and decontrol of private sector rents and tenancy conditions which characterized the approaches of the two main political parties during the post-war years of continuous decline in the sector. The chapter argues that the path of legislative change in this sector provides a vivid illustration of the central themes of this book. While the Conservative Party was espousing the removal of unnecessary controls on landlords and promising an increase in supply and user choice, the Labour Party viewed these controls as an essential element of the social rights of citizenship which should be extended rather than removed (Kemp 1997). The familiar tussle between arguments for regulation and deregulation can be seen in many other areas of public policy, but in few places can the relationship between this rhetoric and the reality of a sector declining for quite unrelated reasons be more apparent. We return to the question of the efficacy of policy in relation to the wider economic forces that have determined the fate of the private rented sector at the end of this chapter.

Relationships between citizenship, choice and control

Concepts of choice used to mask patterns of control

The most frequent interrelationship to emerge from our analysis of the interaction between citizenship, choice and control is the use of a rhetoric of choice to mask a reality of control. Chapter 1 identified the concept of policy stance to highlight the way in which individual policies may be seen as steps in the implementation of a more fundamental programme of change. Perhaps the most significant policy stance identified here has been the adoption by successive Conservative governments of market-based approaches to a wide range of public policy questions. Underlying these approaches has been the dominance of a form of economic thinking which emphasises the role of individual consumer choice, and ostensibly seeks to reduce the role of bureaucratic power. However, many of the policies predicated on this approach have, ironically, relied on the use of bureaucratic controls in their implementation and some have actually had the effect of increasing control.

The most obvious examples of this tendency have involved the use of policies based on a rhetoric of increasing consumer choice to change the balance of power between central and local government. Chapter 7 illustrates the long-term struggle by central government to maintain control over pricing and subsidy decisions in the council housing sector. Chapter 6 identifies the importance of demuncipalization objectives underlying the various privatization programmes from Right to Buy to HATS (Housing Action Trusts) which were promoted in the name of enhancing choice. Despite the rhetoric, the introduction of quasi-markets in social housing has done little to enhance the choices available to individual consumers but has had a significant impact on patterns of control. There has been some debate about whether the resulting fragmentation of social housing services has involved any dispersal of control to the many providers now involved, or simply enabled central government to strengthen its control and weakened the countervailing power of local authorities (Malpass 1997).

The extension of control through policies espousing the promotion of choice has not been confined to central/local relations. Local authority funding and allocation of social housing has also exhibited tendencies towards maximizing control. The concept of the 'enabling authority' has come in for considerable criticism for overemphasizing the levers of power available as local authorities have been 'disabled' by the centralizing processes described above (Malpass 1992). However, some local authorities have secured a short-term ability to perform a genuine strategic role as a result of the capital receipt generated from stock transfers. The different approaches to funding housing association activity adopted by these authorities have ranged from value for money competition to longer-term partnerships with selected partners, particularly the new stock transfer associations (Mullins 1996). Within enabling strategies, many local authorities have been particularly keen to secure control over housing association lets through nominations policies. It is in this context that the presentation of Common Housing Registers (discussed in Chapter 8) as vehicles for applicant choice may be better understood as a means of maximizing control over lettings policies.

Control mechanisms used to enforce social citizenship rights

There is a danger of counterposing the concept of strong central control with that of the enjoyment of social citizenship rights. The area in which strong central control is given most emphasis is in relation to the role of the state in housing subsidy, with an underlying presumption that the purpose of control is to minimize costs to taxpayers and consequently to reduce the chances of assuring the social rights of all citizens. However, there may also be a case for strong central control precisely to ensure that citizenship rights are delivered at the local level.

Again, the homelessness legislation is the clearest example in the book of the impact of strong central controls in securing citizenship rights. While, as we have seen, these rights have been fragile and subject to various challenges, the combination of the legislation and a good-quality Code of Guidance was found to be improving local services to homeless people in the early 1990s. As argued in Chapter 1, the achievement of citizenship rights may involve the transformation of moral rights claimed as part of policy debates into enforceable legal rights. However, as the homelessness argument demonstrates, legal rights may be vulnerable if the legitimacy of their moral basis is questioned, particularly by those able to exert higher levels of control over the political and legislative agenda.

Gaps between rhetoric and policy outcomes

The previous section has already identified the frequent disjunction between the ways in which the concepts of choice, citizenship and control are used to support and promote policy options and the practical outcomes of such policies. Rather than revisiting these arguments, this section briefly identifies some of the underlying factors which have emerged in the chapters that help to explain these gaps.

Unrealistic assumptions

The first set of explanations for the gap between rhetoric and reality lie in the lack of realism in the assumptions upon which the policies are predicated. Economic models based on consumer choice come in for considerable criticism on this count. For example, Chapter 9 draws attention to the failure of charter-based approaches to enable council tenants and owners of mobile homes to use the information provided to exercise 'exit' choices. This highlights the fact that these charters are being applied in situations which bear little resemblance to competitive markets with unfettered opportunities to exercise such choices. Similarly, the requirement introduced by the 1989 Local Government and Housing Act for local authorities to mirror rent relativities in the private sector is justified on the basis of notions of allocative efficiency, however, the policy is based on misplaced assumptions about nature of the private rented sector and a failure to recognize the essential preconditions for such a policy. It is questionable whether relativities in private rents represent an efficient pattern, particularly when the motivations and behaviour of landlords and the distortions generated by the housing benefit system are considered.

Another common factor affecting the realism of policies is the failure to recognize the importance of unequal power relations. This problem can distort both policies based on market choice and those based on broader citizenship ideas. First, the unequal power relations between private landlords and tenants, and the significant impact of housing benefit policy on rental levels at the lower end of the market, provide a lack of incentives for landlords to respond to market signals from dissatisfied tenants. Second, the example of older people living in sheltered housing indicates starkly the inappropriateness of representations of tenant involvement as an equal partnership between landlord and tenant. Not only are there the widely recognized problems of agendas, processes and options being dominated by the landlord, but for some sheltered tenants further inequalities may be introduced by dependence on staff for access to welfare services. Lack of clarity over entitlement to such services and their delivery through relatively informal personal relationships with staff can make it difficult for tenants to play their expected role as critical consumers.

Symbolic policies and the implementation deficit

A second set of explanations for the gap between policy rhetoric and the experience of policy implementation lies in the different purposes and audiences of the two activities. Edelman's (1971) notion of symbolic policies developed to convince particular audiences that 'something is being done' seemed to be particularly apparent in the homelessness case study discussed in Chapter 8. However, in this case the effects of symbolic policies need disentangling from the clear presence of what Pressman and Wildavsky (1973) famously termed the 'implementation deficit'.

Throughout the period of operation of the legislation there were significant differences between the political rhetoric on homelessness and the experience of users of homelessness services. While the 1977 legislation appeared to represent a significant augmentation of citizenship rights, this was always qualified and for many of its proponents represented a symbolic staging post *en route* to more universal rights to housing. Policies developed to diminish rather than enhance these rights also served a symbolic purpose for their proponents. This was particularly apparent in the prolonged review and consultation period prior to the 1996 Act when political proponents of the changes were clearly playing on a different stage to the civil servants charged with the legislative detail. The extent of change in practice was considerably less than the political rhetoric would have led one to expect.

While populist political sentiments such as meeting the needs of 'couples seeking to establish a good home in which to start and raise a family' found their way into consultation papers (DoE 1994: 4), they had limited impact on the form of the resulting legislation.

In both the extension and retrenchment of homelessness rights an implementation deficit was also apparent. The rights established by the 1977 legislation had proved vulnerable to local variations in implementation by local authorities. Local factors such as political control, pressure of housing need, the presence or absence of local advice centres and legal advice were important in producing these variations. The relative autonomy and discretion available to investigatory officers dealing with homelessness enquiries provided a further source of variation. At the national level these rights proved vulnerable to legal challenges, notably in the 1995 House of Lords ruling on the Awua case (*R. v. London Borough of Brent ex parte Awua*) which challenged the previous assumption that homelessness duties had to be met through securing permanent, rather than merely suitable, accommodation. Early research on the implementation of the 1996 Act suggested that a similar implementation deficit applied as local authorities sought to replicate the pre-existing balance between homeless people and other groups in their new allocations policies (Niner *et al.* 1997).

Chapter 2 provides a further contribution to understanding this gap between rhetoric and reality in relation to citizenship rights. Here the importance of pre-existing and underlying aspects of the social structure 'infect' the nature of welfare regimes established to deliver notionally universal citizenship rights. Not only are these rights themselves subject to a continuous contest between interest groups, as in the case of defining statutory homelessness duties for local authorities in Britain, but the very concept of citizenship is itself contested and subject to very different definitions. While the idea of citizenship carries connotations of universalism, in the three societies examined in Chapter 2 this is more rhetorical than real. Boundaries of citizenship are socially constructed and may either exclude some groups completely, as in the case of asylum seekers in relation to social housing in Britain, or offer only an institutionalized second-class status, as in Commonwealth Aboriginal housing programmes in Australia.

A third example of policies presented for different audiences is provided by the deployment of the concept of more choice in social rented housing. The appeal of the rhetoric is quite clearly to the individual consumerist notion of the opportunity to choose between a variety of competing landlords. In practice however the policy is really about introducing quasi-markets to provide greater choice for the funders of social housing. This only becomes apparent when the arrangements for allocation of social housing are considered. The dominance of rationing approaches which restrict consumer choices in the interests of fairness is confirmed in studies of the operation of nominations procedures and common housing registers.

There is also the problem for landlords of how to maximize occupancy of those properties that no one would choose to live in.

What drives change in housing?

In conclusion we return to the question raised in Chapter 1: what drives change in the housing system and how important is the role played by policy? The chapters dealing with the two private tenures in Britain provide fairly powerful evidence to suggest that any explanation of change in housing which addresses itself to housing policy alone is inadequate.

Chapter 4 illustrates that while a favourable set of housing and fiscal policies were the drivers for the rapid expansion of the size of the home ownership sector in Britain in the post-war period, a series of contingent factors have determined the nature of the sector in different periods. Post-war expansion was possible because a cohort of younger households was able to take advantage of a period of full employment and rising earnings. The further development of a mass home ownership sector in the 1980s and 1990s through council house sales and the expansion of ownership down the income scale coincided with less favourable economic conditions. The emergence of arrears and repossessions as serious problems owed at least as much to the macroeconomic climate as to the policy agenda of relentless expansion. In a period of declining fiscal support for further expansion of the sector it is arguable that economic globalization, the liberalization of financial markets, the development of a flexible labour market and further demographic change will in future play a much more significant role in the fate of the sector than anything occurring in the realm of public policy.

Chapter 5 makes an even more convincing case for the limitations of housing policy intervention alone through considering change in the private rented sector. The failure of competing policy stances of regulation and deregulation to make much of a dent in the long-term trajectory of the sector is well established. The limited efficacy of policy interventions is indicated by the high proportion of lettings during the period of rent control which were made outside of the fair rent system. Furthermore, the slight revival of the sector in the 1990s has been widely attributed to the impact of the economic recession and in particular the emergence of 'reluctant landlords' among homeowners who would have otherwise sold or relocated. Factors such as less favourable subsidy treatment in comparison to other housing sectors and uncompetitive rates of return have been seen as central to the long-term decline of the sector. Chapter 5 argues that broader economic and demographic forces have been predominant. However, despite this, housing and related public policies such as slum clearance and housing benefit policy have clearly had a distinct influence during particular periods.

If the private tenures have been subject to a much wider range of influences than housing policy alone, the social housing sector has not been insulated from these forces. The demand for and supply of social housing have been affected by demographic and economic change and by the general treatment of social housing provision as a residual provision for those whose needs cannot be met by the market. The increasing privatization of social housing provision has rendered the sector as vulnerable to market risk as to political risk. For example, housing association rent setting policies are increasingly vulnerable to interest rate movements and to funding decisions by the major financial institutions. The decision by a demutualizing building society to discontinue new lending to the social housing sector and possibly to sell its existing portfolio to another institution provides an indication of such exposure.

While these examples support the need for caution in placing too great an emphasis on housing policy in understanding change in housing, they should not be taken to underplay the role of public policies. The various contributions to this volume have demonstrated the value of careful analysis of both the underlying rhetoric and the implementation process of policies in understanding change in housing. There are signs that new policy agendas may be beginning to be constructed which draw positively on previous experience to develop relevant models for the new millennium.

One message which comes strongly from both the analysis in this book and from contemporary developments in policy thinking is that no one would now expect to achieve significant extensions of universal citizenship rights, individual choices or dispersion of control through housing policy alone. There is widespread recognition that social housing interventions can only be effective when undertaken in conjunction with other policies such as employment, education and health care to tackle patterns of institutionalized discrimination and of the concentration of poverty and deprivation on social housing estates and in the wider community.

Furthermore, there may be less tendency to ignore underlying economic and demographic drivers of change in the policy-making process. In relation to owner occupation there it is now recognized that the virtues of stability, security and sustainability do not accrue naturally to any tenure in a universal way. New approaches are developing which recognize the differentiated nature of the sector and the very different policy interventions required; for example, to meet the repair and security needs of older low income homeowners.

Finally, there is also some evidence of a rediscovery of a broader understanding of citizenship as narrowly-based policies promoting individual self interest are rejected in favour of more collective approaches. Examples may be found in the current preoccupation of housing provider organizations with the (re)discovery of underlying values and purposes, a growing emphasis on the need to establish accountability mechanisms to rebuild trust in both public and third sector institutions, and a growing emphasis on networks rather than contractual or hierarchical relationships.

References

Bartlett,W. and Le Grand, J. (1993) Introduction, in J. Le Grand and W. Bartlett (eds) *Quasi Markets and Social Policy*. Basingstoke: Macmillan.

Beveridge, W. (1942) *Pillars of Security*. London: George Allen & Unwin.

Bulmer, M. and Rees, A.M. (eds) (1996) *Citizenship Today: The Contemporary Relevance of T.H. Marshall*. London: UCL Press.

Department of Health (1989a) *Caring for People: Community Care in the Next Decade and Beyond*, Cm. 849. London: HMSO.

Department of Health (1989b) *Working for Patients*, Cm. 855. London: HMSO.

DoE (1994) *Access to Local Authority Housing: A Consultation Paper*. London: DoE.

DoE (1995) *More Choice in the Social Rented Sector: Consultation Paper*. London: DoE.

Edelman, M. (1971) *Politics as Symbolic Action*. Chicago: Markham.

Hirschman, A.O. (1970) *Exit, Voice and Loyalty*. Cambridge, MA: Harvard University Press.

Kemp, P. (1997) Ideology, public policy and private rental housing since the War, in P. Williams (ed.) *Directions in Housing Policy: Towards Sustainable Housing Policies for the UK*. London: Paul Chapman Publishing.

Malpass, P. (1992) Housing policy and the disabling of local authorities, in J. Birchall (ed.) *Housing Policy in the 1990s*. London: Routledge.

Malpass, P. (1997) *Ownership, Control and Accountability: The New Governance of Housing*. Coventry: Chartered Institute of Housing.

Mullins, D. (1996) *Us and Them: Report of a Survey of Housing Enabling Officers*. Birmingham: Centre for Urban and Regional Studies, University of Birmingham.

Mullins, D. (1997) From regulatory capture to regulated competition: an interest group analysis of the regulation of housing associations in England. *Housing Studies*, 12(3): 301–19.

NHF (1997a) *The Fifth Pillar: Towards New Housing Policies*. London: NHF.

NHF (1997b) *Action for Accountability: A Guide for Independent Social Landlords*. London: NHF.

Niner, P., White, V. and Levison, D. (1997) *The Early Impacts of the 1996 Housing Act and Housing Benefit Changes*. London: Shelter.

Pressman, J. and Wildavsky, A. (1973) *Implementation*. Berkeley, CA: University of California Press.

Symon, P. and Walker, R. (1995) A consumer perspective on performance indicators: the local authority Reports to Tenants regimes in England and Wales, *Environment and Planning C: Government and Policy*, 13: 195–216.

Torgerson, U. (1987) Housing: the wobbly pillar under the welfare state, in B. Turner, J. Kemeny and L. Lundqvist (eds) *Between State and Market: Housing in the Post-Industrial Era*. Stockholm: Almqvist & Wiksell.

Index